FUNCTIONAL NEUROSURGERY

Functional Neurosurgery

Edited by

Theodore Rasmussen, M.D., M.S., F.R.C.S.
Senior Neurosurgical Consultant and Former Director
Montreal Neurological Institute and Hospital
Professor, Department of Neurology and Neurosurgery
McGill University
Montreal, Quebec, Canada

Raul Marino, Jr., M.D.
Professor and Director
Division of Functional Neurosurgery
Hospital das Clinicas
University of São Paulo Medical School
São Paulo, Brazil

Raven Press ▪ New York

Raven Press, 1140 Avenue of the Americas, New York, New York 10036

Made in the United States of America

Library of Congress Cataloging in Publication Data
Main entry under title:

Functional neurosurgery.

   Includes index.
   1. Nervous system--Surgery. I. Rasmussen,
Theodore. II. Marino, Raul. [DNLM: 1. Nervous
system—Surgery. WL368 F979]
RD593.F86   617′.48   77-85871
ISBN 0-89004-228-4

Preface

The primary emphasis of the neurosurgical pioneers during the early years of this century was largely concentrated on the diagnosis and treatment of nervous system *lesions,* neoplastic, traumatic, vascular, and others. Otfrid Foerster, however, concentrated on the study and treatment of disabling epilepsy and pain, *symptoms* of underlying lesions that often did not require treatment for their own sake. Several operative techniques in particular can be considered as the forerunners of what has gradually developed into a subspecialty of neurosurgery, now termed "functional neurosurgery." These include Foerster's introduction of the excision of epileptogenic brain tissue for the treatment of focal epilepsy, anterolateral cordotomy for intractable extremity pain developed independently by Spiller and Frazier and by Foerster, along with the neurosurgical treatment of the pain of tic douleureux, pioneered and developed primarily by Krause, Cushing, Frazier, and Spiller, and by Dandy.

The beginnings of this facet of neurosurgery, however, date back to prehistoric times when trephinations were carried out in many parts of the world, presumably for convulsions, headache, and mental disorders. Trephinations became more widely used by European surgeons in the treatment of epilepsy during the seventeenth and eighteenth centuries as the great variety of potential causes of seizures became more widely known.

At the beginning of the modern era of neurosurgery near the end of the nineteenth century, knowledge of cortical localization arising from the perceptive studies of Hughlings Jackson, Fritsch, Hitzig, and Ferrier, along with the advent of anesthesia, antisepsis, and asepsis, led to the development of more appropriate neurosurgical procedures for epilepsy by Horsley, Krause, Ballance, and other neurosurgical pioneers.

The prodigious and scholarly studies of Harvey Cushing provided the main influence on the subsequent growth of the specialty of neurosurgery during the next few decades, during which time the primary emphasis was on the diagnosis and treatment of *lesions* of the nervous system. In the late 1940s, however, the application of the Horsley-Clarke stereotactic techniques to man led to the effective treatment of a variety of motor disorders, such as parkinsonism, choreoathetosis, torticollis, and hemiballismus for which medical therapy as well as a variety of surgical procedures, central and peripheral, had previously been relatively ineffective. Wilder Penfield's scholarly and progressive refinements of Foerster's cortical resection of epileptogenic cortex gradually led to increasingly widespread acceptance of this surgical approach to certain types of medically refractory focal epilepsy.

Rapid advances in the understanding of neurophysiological mechanisms of the central and the peripheral nervous system have led to further expansion of neurosurgical efforts to alleviate distressing symptoms due to unknown causes or due to lesions or diseases that either require no treatment for their own sake or are untreatable. The development of increasingly refined and sophisticated electronic methods of recording and analyzing the electrical activity of the nervous system and of stimulating it electrically have given further impetus to the development of functional neurosurgery.

The chapters in this volume are intended to give concise overviews of the present state of knowledge and development of the principal, well-established facets of functional neurosurgery. Selected references provided at the end of each chapter will guide the interested reader to more detailed discussions of the individual subjects. The more experimental facets of this field are developing rapidly. The prospects for the future are exciting. We hope that this volume has captured some of this excitement as well as rendered a concise overview of this ever developing field.

Theodore Rasmussen
Raul Marino, Jr.

Contents

CONTENTS

Contributors

H. Thomas Ballantine, Jr., M.D., *Clinical Professor of Surgery (Neurosurgery), Massachusetts General Hospital and Harvard Medical School, Boston, Massachusetts 02114*

Gilles Bertrand, M.D., *Neurosurgeon-in-Chief, Montreal Neurological Institute and Hospital, Professor, Department of Neurology and Neurosurgery, McGill University, Montreal, Quebec, Canada H3A 2B4*

Elizabeth Boone, R.N., *Stereotactic Nurse, Duke University School of Medicine, Durham, North Carolina 27710*

Philip L. Gildenberg, M.D., *Professor and Chief, Division of Neurosurgery, Houston Medical School, The University of Texas, Houston, Texas 77030*

Ida E. Giriunas, R. N., *Massachusetts General Hospital, Boston, Massachusetts 02114*

Jules Hardy, M.D., *Professor of Neurosurgery, Notre Dame Hospital and University of Montreal, Montreal, Quebec, Canada H2L 1M4*

Jeffrey T. Keller, Ph.D., *Director Neuroanatomical Research Laboratory, Research Institute, Christ Hospital, Cincinnati, Ohio, Adjunct Assistant Professor of Anatomy, University of Cincinnati College of Medicine*

Raul Marino, Jr., M.D., *Professor and Director, Division of Functional Neurosurgery, Hospital das Clinicas, University of São Paulo Medical School, São Paulo, Brazil*

Pierre Molina-Negro, M.D., *Associate Professor, Department of Surgery, University of Montreal and Service of Neurosurgery, Hopital Notre-Dame, Montreal*

Walle Nauta, Ph.D., *Professor, Department of Psychology, Massachusetts, Institute of Technology, Cambridge, Massachusetts 02139*

Ayub Ommaya, M.D., F.R.C.S., F.A.C.S., *Head of Applied Research and Acting Chief, Surgical Neurology Branch, N.I.N.C.D.S., National Institute of Health, Bethesda, Maryland, Clinical Professor of Neurosurgery, George Washington University Medical Center, Washington, D.C.*

Hirotaro Narabayashi, M.D., *Professor of Neurology, Juntendo University School of Medicine, Tokyo, Japan*

Blaine Nashold, Jr., M.D., *Professor of Neurosurgery, Duke University School of Medicine, Durham, North Carolina 27710*

Theodore Rasmussen, M.D., M.S., F.R.C.S., *Senior Neurosurgical Consultant and Former Director, Montreal Neurological Institute and Hospital, Professor, Department of Neurology and Neurosurgery, McGill University, Montreal, Quebec, Canada H3A 2B4*

Jean Siegfried, M.D., *Professor of Neurosurgery, University of Zurich, Kantonspital, CH-8091 Zurich, Switzerland*

Gabor Szikla, M.D., *Associate Neurosurgeon in Charge of Research, Department of Functional Neurosurgery, Sainte Anne Hospital Center, Paris, Cedex 14, France*

Jean Talairach, M.D., *Professor of Neurosurgery, René Descarte University, Head of Department of Functional Neurosurgery, Sainte Anne Hospital Center, Paris, Cedex 14, France*

Laughlin Taylor, M.Sc., *Associate Neuropsychologist, Montreal Neurological Institute and Hospital, Lecturer, Neuropsychology, Department of Neurology and Neurosurgery, McGill University, Montreal, Quebec, Canada H3A 2B4*

John Tew, Jr., M.D., *Chairman, Section of Neurosurgery, Good Samaritan Hospital, Cincinnati, an Educational Affiliate of the University of Cincinnati, Director, Neurosurgical Training Program, Good Samaritan and Christ Hospitals, Cincinnati, Ohio*

David S. Williams, B.S., *University of Cincinnati College of Medicine, and Research Institute, Christ Hospital, Cincinnati, Ohio*

William P. Wilson, M.D., *Professor, Department of Psychiatry, Duke University School of Medicine, Durham, North Carolina 27710*

Functional Neurosurgery, edited by T. Rasmussen
and R. Marino. Raven Press, New York © 1979.

Introduction: Functional Neurosurgery as a Specialty

Raul Marino, Jr.

*Division of Functional Neurosurgery, Hospital das Clinicas, University of Sao Paulo
Medical School, Sao Paulo, Brazil*

The drop is a small ocean . . .

—R. W. Emerson

Neurological surgery, as a modern specialty, had its birth as a consequence of important acquisitions of knowledge in the anatomy, physiology, and clinical semeiology of the nervous system. This knowledge was acquired during the nineteenth century. The introduction of neuropathology, the discovery of anesthesia, the control of sepsis, and the development of antisepsis each were important landmarks in the establishment and growth of the specialty. The discovery of X-rays by Röentgen in 1891, followed by the development of other diagnostic procedures, paved the way for the continuing succession of technical advances that gave great impetus to the specialty of neurosurgery, particularly to the modern facets now described as functional neurosurgery.

Major therapeutic progress has sometimes preceded or led to the acquisition of new knowledge on the physiopathologic mechanisms of nervous diseases. The growing field of functional neurosurgery stands out today as one of the more philosophical approaches to medicine. It deals with the awake brain and with the human person who is usually fully conscious on the operating table. Talking to their examiners, the patients themselves guide the hands of the neurosurgeon during his therapeutic maneuvers on the nervous system as he endeavors to alleviate epilepsy, abnormal movements, pain, suffering, and sometimes behavior disorders.

Functional neurosurgery procedures have increased neurological knowledge concerning mechanisms of a variety of cortical functions such as speech, somatomotor, somatosensory, vision, and hearing,—and they have contributed to our knowledge of the function of the deep cerebral structures that modulate abnormal movements, pain, and behavior. Recording, stimulation, and ablation of a variety of areas of the brain in the process of carrying out therapeutic procedures for the relief of functional neurological disorders have enabled neurosurgeons and applied neurophysiologists to study a variety of structures and regions of the human brain. Functional neurosurgery has, then, become not only a productive

1

aspect of classic neurosurgery, but also an important instrument and an indispensable tool for the study of and research on the functioning of the human brain.

This instrument has enabled the neurosurgeon and his team to "listen" to the language of the brain, which is also the language and the music of life itself. Our means of study are still gross and rough, compared to the delicate functions of this organ, but in using them we are learning what epilepsy, pain, abnormal movements, and "emotions" have to tell us regarding certain functions of the brain. It is true that all we know represents only a drop in the ocean, but we also know that sometimes a simple drop of dew may reflect the whole sky.

There is no question in our minds that the study of the brain is the study of man's place in nature. This is the philosophical truth that motivated most of us to study the human brain, the temple and shrine of our thoughts, the most complex, the most perfect, and certainly the most important living structure in our universe.

The brain of man is the map of his destiny, the most beautiful instrument ever created by divine hands. On the dissecting table it is a bare mass of cells and nervous centers perfused with blood, but on the operating table, joined to the body, the awake brain is, in normal life, the only instrument through which man reveals himself and plays the concert of life, conducting the body, and being conducted by the soul. Our nervous cells constitute the link that connects our physical brain with the world in which our consciousness has its roots. Our knowledge of this organ is still meager, but it is already enough for us to understand that the brain may be the seat of our thought, but never its origin. How could a mass of protoplasm compose a sermon?

To date, we are far removed from the mechanistic views of the eighteenth century when LaMettrie (3) concluded that thought was the result of mechanical processes in the brain and in the rest of the nervous system and also from the concepts of Cabanis (1), the so-called father of psychosomatic medicine, who stated that the brain was the organ of thought, "secreting thoughts and ideas as the liver secretes the bile"!

The proper study of the human brain requires that we should first understand its structure before we can ask intelligent questions about its organization and functioning. Only then will we be able to understand the relationship between brain, mind, and life itself.

The findings that to date relate sensation, movements, feelings, and emotions to the brain have not as yet permitted even the most sophisticated neurophysiologist or philosopher to use this knowledge of brain function to resynthesize the phenomenon of everyday life.

The contributions of neurosurgery and its subspecialties to knowledge of the brain and the nervous system are still meager in comparison to the vastness and the complexity of its capabilities; however, we should not forget that more progress has been made in the last few decades than in many previous centuries.

Functional neurosurgery is still a modest branch of the neurosciences, but it has made significant contributions to the discipline and promises to make many more as the discipline advances and is further refined.

Functional neurosurgery has emerged as a result of the need of neurosurgeons, neurologists, neurophysiologists, neuroanatomists, neuropathologists, and psychologists to study the higher functions of the human brain and nervous system in order to provide more effective treatment of a variety of nervous system disorders. More recently a variety of special talents have been recruited to this already complex team. Included in this group are electroencephalographers, biochemists, electronic engineers, and computer experts.

One of the precursors of the term functional neurosurgery was provided by René Lèriche (4,5) when he used the term "functional surgery" to describe some of his interventions on the sympathetic nerves for pain and circulatory disturbances. Lèriche removed the pejorative sense of the term "functional" which was used at that time to designate hysterical or conversion phenomena. He stated that this term should be used to denote function and that where function is present we are "plain pied" on normal and pathological physiology. Since Lèriche's time, there is general agreement that the functional is an important part of pathology and that it may precede or even create the anatomical.

As far as we know, it was one of Lèriche's disciples, P. Wertheimer, who for the first time assembled in a book (6) the present characteristics of functional neurosurgery, granting that name to this division of neurosurgery. In his book, Wertheimer included the physiopathology and treatment of involuntary movements and the surgery for epilepsy, pain, and relief of mental illness. He also included a chapter on the treatment of vascular pathology of the brain and a separate chapter on the treatment of brain edema and alterations of intracranial pressure. He recognized that this separation was, to a certain extent, artificial. He justified this as the need to associate, in his nosological conceptions, the anatomical lesion to the functional changes. According to Wertheimer, functional neurosurgery would be the part of neurosurgery taking advantage of the new neurophysiological acquisitions, and functional procedures would consist of "moderating" and "reformative" interventions, guided by neurophysiological information. Action would be taken toward excitatory and inhibitory phenomena with the aim being the suppression of irritative foci that produce convulsion and the neutralizing of other pathological effects by the interruption of motor paths and sensory paths of nuclei in the surgery for epilepsy, involuntary movements, pain, and mental disorders.

Hughlings Jackson was the first to stress the importance of the correct use of the term functional. He stated: "I have long urged that the term functional should be used as the adjective of the word function. [I remark, parenthetically, that such expressions as that "consciousness is a function of the brain," or any part of it, are illegitimate. Consciousness attends functioning of the brain, or of some parts of it.] "Function is a physiological term; it deals with the 'storing up' of nutritive materials having potential energy, with nervous discharges (or liberation of energy by nerve cells); it has to do with the rates of those liberations, with the resistances encountered, and with different degrees of those resistances." [(2), Vol. 2, p. 472–473]

Jackson continues: "Physiology deals with the dynamics of the organism— that is, with its function. I use the term 'function' with regards to nervous diseases in a strict sense, and never in the way it or its adjective (functional) is used when applied to the symptoms of an hysterical woman, or to minute or transitory changes of structure." [(2), Vol. 1, p. 428]

Jackson emphasizes the correct use of the term *functional* in many other instances in his famous writings: ". . . it is desirable that the term functional should be used with exactness, and that the functional (physiological) changes should be distinguished from the pathological changes producing them." [(2), Vol. 2, p. 472–473]

The aim and objective of functional neurosurgery are to treat, correct, or balance the functions of the brain that are altered toward either hyperfunctional or hypofunctional states. Functional neurosurgical procedures often involve circuits or structures of the nervous system that may frequently be normal except for transient states of altered function. Those circuits are not necessarily the same as those involved in the primary derangement of function. Equilibrium will be reestablished through lesions or stimulation of nervous centers or pathways, as dictated by the origin of the disturbance: biochemical changes, lesions of centers or paths, and so forth, trying to compensate for them through procedures that will reestablish the original balance in the system. The origin of disequilibrium may be vascular, tumoral, degenerative, or infectious, and it may or may not require specific treatment. Main emphasis is given, however, to the correction of the disordered function responsible for convulsions, abnormal movements, pain, mental change, neuroendocrine disturbance, and the like.

Jackson again throws much light on the subject of the normal and abnormal functions of the brain and their pathological bases (2):

. . . . There are two diametrically opposite kinds of functional changes: 1. degrees from slight defect to loss of function; 2. degrees from slight to excessive exaltation of function. The former, negative state of function, exists in cases of paralysis, the latter, positive state of function, in cases of epilepsy, chorea, tetanus, etc. I never use the expression 'disorder of function,' but speak of degrees of negative functional states, and of degrees of states of over-function. The two may coexist. Some elements of the set of motor arrangements, representing a muscular region may have lost function. Whilst other elements of the same set may be in over-function. For example, we find not rarely persisting hemiplegia and occasional convulsion of the muscular region paralyzed.

One advantage of the scheme of investigation by the triple division is that we learn by it where our knowledge is deficient. Indeed, of some cases of nervous diseases it would be commonly said that we know symptoms only. The scheme enables us to separate definitely what we know from what we only suppose. In chorea we know there is the second kind of functional lesion; at any rate, it is an irresistible inference that the movements depend on unduly high instability of nerve cells. But we do not know the site of that lesion, nor the pathological process leading to it. On the anatomy and pathology of chorea all of us have hypotheses only.

We may thus infer that normal function is an interplay between inhibitory and facilitatory functions. The loss of one function may result in a decrease in function of certain other structures and an increase in function in still others.

A *positive symptom* is the result of an exaggerated activity of a certain structure that has been liberated from an inhibitory control that is normally exerted by another structure that has suffered a lesion. Function in this case is exalted, as in the cells of a discharging lesion, hypertonus, tremor, abnormal movements, and central pain. These are, according to Jackson, "hyperphysiological" states. Functional neurosurgery endeavors to correct this abnormal excess of function. It aims primarily to reestablish a broken equilibrium, since the lesion of origin often requires no treatment. For instance, in labyrinthine irritation producing spasmodic torticollis, we will treat structures anatomically intact but functionally out of control (interrupting impulses on nuclcus ventralis intermedius of the thalamus).

In a case with epilepsy of the supplementary motor area, it is implied that neurons in this area are intact and thus able to produce the epileptic seizures. So, the epilepsy is a functional change consequent to the exaggerated function of neuronal mechanisms of this area—the lesion may be in other neurons that act to influence the former. A scar or a calcification is not all epileptogenous zone, but it may result in hyperfunction of neurons and circuits that are adjacent or at a distance.

A *negative symptom* is the result of decrease or loss of function of a certain structure such as hemianopia, hemiplegia, anesthesia, akinesia, or facial palsy. Positive and negative symptoms may exist together, as in the case of a meningioma, causing hemiplegia and epilepsy. When the tumor has been removed, epilepsy may continue, since the surrounding brain tissue is lesioned, or uninhibited, resulting in epilepsy as a functional symptom.

In conclusion, general neurosurgery tends to concentrate on the lesion, rather than on the symptoms, negative or positive. Functional neurosurgery tends to focus on the symptoms, that is, on the abnormal functions which are often positive or hyperfunctional states and which appear at a distance as a consequence of the primary lesion.

Many specialties deal with the human brain, as many insects alight on the prairie flowers. However, only the bees know how to extract the honey. The bees alone are able to do that job and leave the flowers intact without hurting them or making them lose their freshness, allowing the flowers to remain exactly as they were before. This is the hope and aim of functional neurosurgery.

REFERENCES

1. Cabanis, P. J. G. (1802): *Rapports du Physique et du Moral de L'homme.*
2. Jackson, J. H. (1958): In: *Selected Writings of John Hughlings Jackson,* edited by J. Taylor, Vol. 2., p. 376–377. Basic Books, New York.
3. LaMettrie, J. D. de. (1747): *L'homme-Machine.*
4. Leriche, R. (1949): *La Chirurgie de la Douleur.* Masson, Paris.
5. Leriche, R. (1951): *La Philosophie de la Chirurgie.* Flammarion, Paris.
6. Wertheimer, P. (1956): *Neurochirurgie Fonctionelle.* Masson, Paris.

Functional Neurosurgery, edited by T. Rasmussen
and R. Marino. Raven Press, New York © 1979.

Expanding Borders of the Limbic System Concept

Walle J. H. Nauta

*Department of Psychology, Massachusetts Institute of Technology, Cambridge,
Massachusetts 02139, and Mailman Research Center, McLean Hospital,
Belmont, Massachusetts 02178*

In recent years, concepts of the limbic system have undergone a notable amplification, especially as a result of intensive anatomical studies that have drawn the afferent and efferent relationships of the limbic system into sharper focus. Before these more recent developments can be reviewed, it is necessary to deal briefly with the connotation of the term limbic system.

As used here, the term broadly denotes the hippocampal formation and amygdala together with some medial and basal cortical regions connected with these structures either directly or by way of the thalamus (gyrus cinguli, retrosplenial cortex, and parahippocampal gyrus). From these medial regions outward, the border of the limbic system becomes indistinct, and it is particularly difficult to decide whether and to what extent certain parts of the neocortex of the basal frontotemporal region should be considered part of it. Much as the gyrus cinguli is associated especially with the hippocampus by way of direct and indirect fornix projections to the anterior thalamic nucleus, the posterior orbitofrontal cortex is associated with the amygdala by way of a prominent amygdalofugal projection to the medial subdivision of the mediodorsal thalamic nucleus (20,25). The inferior temporal neocortex even receives a direct projection from the amygdala (20,25).

This vagueness presents a fundamental problem in defining the limbic system: unlike the wholly subcortical corpus striatum, much of its expanse forms part of the pallial mantle, and hence gradates into the surrounding neocortex. Despite this difficulty, however, the term, limbic system, has a certain utility, as it denotes an assembly of structures that not only are related by common peculiarities of neural circuitry, but also appear collectively to form part of the neural mechanism determining the organism's internal and overt behavioral responses to its environments. Put in other words, as currently used, the term, limbic system, is based in part at least on a morphophysiological correlation.

It is a matter of preference whether one chooses to extend the term to those diencephalic and mesencephalic structures with which the limbic region of the cerebral hemisphere is known to be associated by largely reciprocal fiber connections. Together, these structures form a subcortical continuum that extends from the septum caudally over the preoptic region, substantia innominata, and hypothalamus and, beyond the latter, throughout a paramedian zone of the midbrain that includes, among other structures, the ventral tegmental area of Tsai and the mesencephalic raphe nuclei. Direct projections leading into this continuum from the cerebral hemisphere originate not only from the hippocampus and amygdala but also from the posterior orbitofrontal cortex.

Anatomical studies of the past 15 years have cleared up at least one long-standing problem: that of the afferent connections of the limbic system with the neocortex. Other studies of recent date have expanded our knowledge of the subcortical ramifications of the limbic circuitry and, more particularly, these studies have brought out previously unknown links with the corpus striatum. The remainder of this chapter will deal with such more recent developments in the anatomical definition of the limbic system.

NEOCORTICAL AFFERENTS OF THE LIMBIC SYSTEM

After the general concept of the limbic system had been explicitly formulated (22,23), it seemed logical to assume that a neural organization of such great behavioral importance would receive substantial projections from the sensory mechanisms of the neocortex. This assumption ultimately proved to be correct, but it is remarkable that the neocortico–limbic connection for a long time remained conjectural. As late as 1958 it was possible to state: "In spite of much speculation, the anatomical substratum for such neocortico–limbic interaction is almost entirely obscure; it would seem to hold a lively challenge for future investigation." (24).

It is true that by that time some fragments of the connection had already been glimpsed. In 1952, Adey and Meyer (1), from a study by the Glees method in the monkey, reported evidence of a projection from the medial frontal cortex through the fasciculus cinguli to the parahippocampal gyrus. Furthermore, a direct projection from the inferior temporal cortex to the amygdala had been reported in 1956 by Whitlock and Nauta (45), likewise in the monkey. Almost 10 years earlier, neurophysiological studies by the method of strychnine neuronography had provided evidence of direct projections from the orbitofrontal cortex to posterior parts of the hypothalamus (34,42), evidence that had soon thereafter been confirmed by anatomical findings (7,41). However, these early observations hardly seemed to satisfy the original expectation of finding substantial projections from all of the sensory areas of the neocortex to the limbic structures at the medial margin of the cerebral mantle. For several years, neuroanatomists, working with fiber-degeneration methods, found themselves frustrated in their attempts to demonstrate such variegated projections to the entorhinal area, the region on the parahippocampal gyrus that since the time of Cajal was known to be the origin of the largest single afferent fiber system of the hippocampus, the temporoammonic bundle. It was not until 1965 that the general pattern of organization of the neocortico–limbic relationship began to be revealed. In that year, Cragg (11) published an important study in the cat, in which he demonstrated a projection from the parietal association cortex (suprasylvian gyrus) to the cingulate cortex, as well as projections from the frontal cortex and temporal cortex to the entorhinal area. This report provided Jones and Powell with a valuable clue (32) when they (14) found that not only the somatic sensory cortex but also the auditory cortex in the cat projects to the suprasylvian gyrus. The question raised by this finding was: could it be that projections from the sensory regions of the cortex converge upon particular association areas that in turn project into the limbic system? Turning to the larger monkey brain, Jones and Powell (18), in a monumental study, were able to show that, indeed, cortico–cortical pathways leading out of all the primary sensory areas of the neocortex, by way of a variable number of intercalated association areas in the parietal, frontal, and temporal lobes, ultimately converge in three places. One of these is the anterior cingulate cortex (areas 24 and 25); a second one is the convexity of the frontal lobe; and the third one is the temporal pole (area TG of v. Bonin and Bailey) and a contiguous strip of medial temporal cortex at the border between the neocortex and the allocortex of the parahippocampal gyrus (area 35). Most recently, Van Hoesen and Pandya (38–40), in a series of important papers, provided a detailed description of the complex pattern of cortico–cortical connections leading from the anteromedial temporal cortex and basal frontal cortex to the entorhinal area, the cortical gateway to the hippocampus.

In hindsight, it does not seem surprising that the neocortico–limbic connection long remained obscure. Quite unlike the neocortical projection to the striatum (caudate nucleus and putamen), which is organized as a system of parallel direct lines originating independently from apparently all cortical areas, the neocortico–limbic connection is characterized by a convergence of concatenated cortico–cortical pathways upon the lower frontotemporal region. The ultimate link to the hippocampus and amygdala thus originates from a limited region of the cortex. It can be inferred from this arrangement that information from the neocortex must reach the limbic system in a highly sequentially processed form. Moreover, the strongly convergent nature of the connection suggests that the information conveyed by it undergoes considerable intermodal integration. It seems likely that the integral contains not only exteroceptive but also visceroceptive elements (27), and thus represents both the organism's external and its internal milieu.

CROSSROADS OF LIMBIC AND STRIATAL CIRCUITRY

Despite their invariable coexistence in the mammalian brain, limbic system (hippocampus and amygdala) and corpus striatum (striatum or caudatoputamen, and pallidum or globus pallidus) have long given the impression of being two mutually isolated neural mechanisms. Until about 25 years ago, these two major components of the forebrain seemed to lack any direct interconnection; for an even longer time, they appeared to have no common sources of afferent supply, and their respective efferent fiber pathways until very recently seemed to have no points of convergence anywhere along their course. To be more specific, until about 20 years ago, known or suspected neocortical afferents to the limbic system were limited to the cingulo–hippocampal connection suggested by Cajal (5) and later by Papez (31), whereas cortical afferents to the corpus striatum were generally believed to originate largely or even entirely from the sensorimotor cortex; neither were any other sources of afferents known to be shared by limbic system and corpus striatum. As to the efferent connections of these two forebrain mechanisms, those of the corpus striatum until only a few years ago were thought to be distributed exclusively to the substantia nigra, subthalamic nucleus, centrum medianum, and VA–VL complex of the thalamus, and to certain mesencephalic regions; see Nauta and Mehler (29) for a review. In none of these distributions did the projections of the corpus striatum seem to overlap the efferents of the limbic system. The latter, instead, have been traced to the anterior and mediodorsal nuclei of the thalamus, as well as to the subcortical continuum formed by the septum, preoptic region, and hypothalamus. They extend caudally beyond the hypothalamus over the ventral tegmental area throughout the paramedian region of the midbrain, partly by way of the medial forebrain bundle and partly also by a more dorsal route composed of the stria medullaris, habenular nuclei, and fasciculus retroflexus. It is important to note that a substantial second component of the medial forebrain bundle deviates laterally from the main bundle and distributes itself largely to more lateral regions of the midbrain tegmentum (see below).

As could have been expected, this initial impression of separateness of the limbic system and the corpus striatum has faded over the past two decades, and at present several forms of association between the limbic system and the corpus striatum can be pointed out. The one detected earliest is a direct connection between these two major forebrain mechanisms: In 1943, Fox (16), from an experimental study by the Marchi method, reported precommissural fornix fibers distributed to the nucleus accumbens septi, a basal forebrain structure which, although in the past regarded by some as part of the septum, nonetheless by cytoarchitectural and histochemical criteria can be interpreted only as a ventromedial subdivision of the striatum. Confirmed in later years by Carman et al. (6) and Raisman et al. (33), this earliest evidence of a direct limbico–striatal connection was amplified more recently by the discovery of additional afferents of the nucleus accumbens originating from the amygdala (13). It is interesting to note that thus far no reciprocating direct striatal projection to the amygdala or hippocampus has been described.

The first evidence of a source of afferents common to the limbic system and corpus striatum appeared in 1956 in the monkey in the form of a projection from the inferior temporal cortex to both the amygdala and ventral regions of the striatum (45). In the two decades since, the cortical afferentation of the limbic system and corpus striatum has been analyzed in considerable detail, and it now seems possible to state that all or nearly all of the neocortex is connected with both mechanisms, either, as in the case of the corpus striatum, by direct corticostriatal fibers originating throughout the expanse of the neocortex (6,19,43,44) and distributed to both caudate nucleus and putamen, or, in the case of the limbic system, by way of variously complex sequences of cortico–cortical connections.

Finally, only very recently has a point of convergence of limbic and striatal efferent systems been demonstrated. The locus in question is the lateral habenular nucleus, a subdivision of the habenular complex long known to receive stria-medullaris fibers originating from the lateral preoptico–hypothalamic region. An autoradiographic study in the cat (17,28) revealed that the nucleus also receives a quite massive projection from the entopeduncular nucleus, the homo-log of the internal segment of the globus pallidus of primate forms. Since the globus pallidus is a major recipient of striatal (caudatoputamenal) efferents, and the lateral habenular nucleus appears to be a principal—if not indeed the principal—source of afferents to the paramedian zone of the midbrain (24; also Herkenham and Nauta, *manuscript in preparation*), this finding suggests the raphe region of the midbrain tegmentum as an ultimate destination of conduction pathways originating in both the limbic system and the striatum. At present, no other loci of confluence of striatal (or pallidal) efferents with limbic conduction pathways are known, but preliminary observations in this laboratory suggest that pallidal fibers may converge with the lateral component of the medial forebrain bundle in the ventrolateral tegmental region containing dopamine cell group A8 of Dahlström and Fuxe (12) (see below).

Outlying Nigral Cell Groups

In the foregoing overview, mention was made of direct projections from the hippocampal formation and amygdala to the nucleus accumbens. In the next section of this chapter, I shall report experimental evidence, obtained in the rat in collaboration with my colleagues Valerie Domesick and Richard Faull, of a second, more indirect but apparently also more widely distributed, conduction route by which the limbic system could be thought to affect the mechanisms of the corpus striatum. Since this route largely leads over the outlying nigral cell groups A10 and A8, a brief review of the anatomical data concerning these cell groups would seem appropriate.

The label, A10, was given by Dahlström and Fuxe (12) to a large, somewhat wedge-shaped group of dopamine cells protruding from the medial half of the pars compacta of the substantia nigra (dopamine cell group A9) in the mediodor-sal direction. Most of the relatively large cells of the A10 group occupy the basomedial midbrain region labeled *ventral tegmental area* by Tsai (36), and their presence appears to have been the main characteristic by which Tsai demar-cated this area from the rostrally adjacent lateral hypothalamic region. Not until 40 years later was the histochemical likeness of these cells to those of the substantia nigra's pars compacta established (12). Shortly thereafter Andén

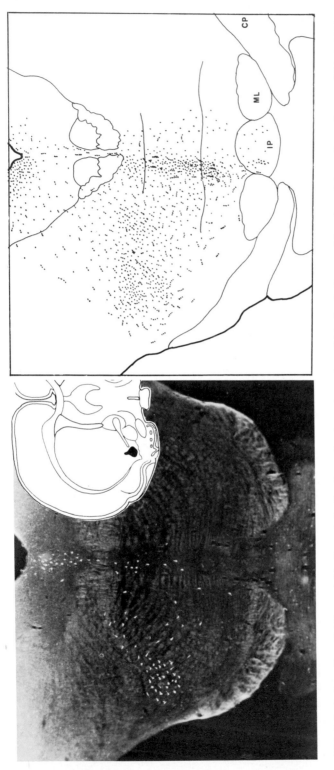

FIG. 1. Left: A section slightly caudal to the substantia nigra, showing retrograde cell labeling in the caudal region of dopamine cell group A8 in a case (RH 27) of HRP injection in the subcommissural striatal pocket *(inset)*. Note trails of sparser labeled cells extending medially from the A8 region. Labeled cells in the tegmental midplane represent caudal part of A10; those in the central gray substance, the dorsal raphe nucleus. (Dark-field photograph, retouched.) **Right:** Charting of radioactive fiber labeling at corresponding level of the midbrain in case RR 89 (inset to Fig. 2, right column). IP, interpeduncular nucleus; ML, medial lemniscus; CP, cerebral peduncle.

et al. (2) reported histochemical and biochemical evidence that cell group A10 projects to the basomedial region of the striatum composed of the nucleus accumbens septi and the olfactory tubercle. In 1971, Ungerstedt (37) added to this the observation that the projection from A10 also involves the central nucleus of the amygdala and the dorsal part of the bed nucleus of the stria terminalis; apparently on the strength of this finding, Ungerstedt introduced the term *mesolimbic system* to distinguish the ascending projection of dopamine cell group A10 from the *nigrostriatal system*— in the narrower sense of that term—consisting of the pars compacta of the substantia nigra (cell group A9) and its projection to the larger remainder of the caudatoputamen. Ungerstedt's view of A10 as a dopamine cell group associated preferentially with the limbic system appears justified by the evidence that A10 projects not only to components of the amygdaloid complex, but also to that part of the striatum that receives its descending (telencephalic) afferents from limbic (hippocampus and amygdala) rather than from neocortical sources. The concept is supported further by the evidence from retrograde cell-labeling experiments that A10 is a major—although not the only—origin of the dopamine fibers innervating that region of the medial cortex upon which the thalamocortical projections of the anterior and mediodorsal thalamic nuclei converge (3). Finally, and perhaps most significant, as a component of the ventral tegmental area, cell group A10 lies embedded in the interstices of the medial forebrain bundle, and hence, among descending fibers originating largely from basal forebrain regions implicated in the subcortical circuitry of the limbic system.

Much less appears to be known about the more caudal outlying nigral cell group A8. This cell group appears to be a dorsal extrusion of the lateral half of the substantia nigra's pars compacta and extends caudally slightly beyond the caudal pole of the substantia nigra. At such caudal levels, it may appear as an independent, somewhat round cell group in the ventrolateral part of the midbrain tegmentum (Fig. 1). It is connected with cell group A10 by irregular cell bridges stretching medially over the medial lemniscus (Fig. 2D); this supralemniscal cell aggregate, sometimes referred to as retrorubral nucleus (4), is considered part of A8 by Palkovits and Jacobowitz (30). That A8, like A9

FIG. 2. (pgs. 14–15) **Left:** An anteroposterior sequence (A–D) of four darkfield photographs (retouched) representing case RH 29 of HRP injection in the nucleus accumbens (injection site shown by *inset*). Note the sparseness of retrogradely labeled cells in the pars compacta of the substantia nigra (dopamine cell group A9). Most of the cell labeling in this case is confined to the ventral tegmental area and corresponds in location to dopamine cell group A10 (A–C); however, the horizontal band of labeled cells dorsal to the medial lemniscus in frame **D** corresponds to the anterior part of dopamine cell group A8. **Right:** Chartings of the autoradiographically demonstrated fiber labeling resulting from a discrete injection of tritiated leucine and proline into the lateral hypothalamus (case RR 89, *inset*). Abbreviations: AON, medial nucleus of the accessory optic tract; CP, cerebral peduncle; FR; fasciculus retroflexus; IP, interpeduncular nucleus; ML, medial lemniscus; MP, mammillary peduncle; ND, nucleus of Darkschewitsch; NI, interstitial nucleus of Cajal; NIII, oculomotor nerve; RN, red nucleus; SNc, substantia nigra, pars compacta; SNr, substantia nigra, pars reticulata; VTA, ventral tegmental area.

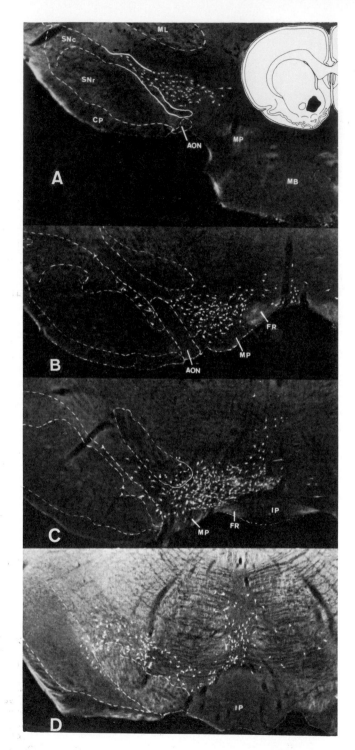

FIG. 2. (See

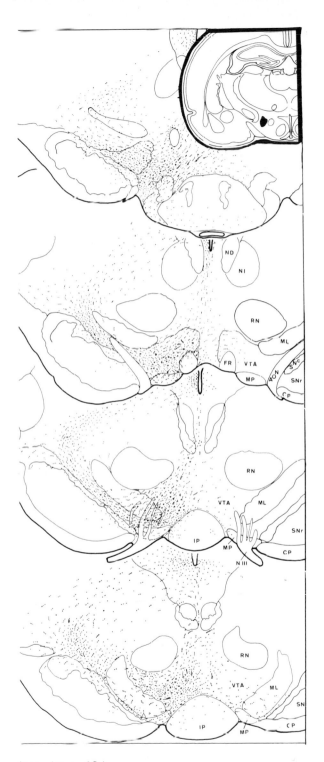

legend page 13.)

and A10, projects to the striatum is documented by Ungerstedt's (37) finding that all three of these cell groups undergo cell loss following massive lesions of the caudatoputamen. Quantitative comparisons of several such cases led Ungerstedt to suggest that dopamine cell group A8, like A9 but unlike A10, projects to the main body of the caudatoputamen rather than to the nucleus accumbens. No further information about the connections of cell group A8 appears to be available at present.

The Present Study

The principal question addressed by the experiments to be described here concerns the relationship of the outlying nigral cell groups (A10 and A8) to the descending conduction pathways directly or indirectly associated with the limbic system. The question arose from the observation that the rostral part at least of cell group A10 is located within the space through which the medial forebrain bundle passes from the hypothalamus into the midbrain. According to findings in earlier studies by fiber-degeneration (24) and autoradiographic (9,35) methods, the descending fibers of the medial forebrain bundle at about this level begin to be rearranged into (a) a medial fiber group that maintains the sagittal orientation of the bundle's hypothalamic trajectory and distributes its fibers to the paramedian zone of the midbrain, and (b) a more lateral subdivision that sweeps laterally and caudally over the dorsal border of the substantia nigra into a ventrolateral tegmental position immediately caudal to the substantia nigra; at this level, it curves in the dorsomedial direction and traverses the cuneiform and parabrachial regions of the tegmentum, with its longest fibers invading the ipsilateral ventral quadrant of the central gray substance. Palkovits and Jacobowitz's (30) illustrations suggest that outlying nigral neurons lie scattered in the path of both the medial and the lateral component of the medial forebrain bundle, but since the scale of these and other chartings does not allow an adequate resolution of topographic relationships, we found it necessary to determine the position of mesencephalo–striatal neurons with respect to descending components of the medial forebrain bundle in more detail by neuroanatomical tracing methods.

Methods

The material on which our report is based was collected in the course of a study of the neural circuitry involving the basal forebrain in the rat. It includes a large number of cases in each of which a small microelectrophoretic injection of tritiated leucine and tritiated proline had been placed in one or the other of a variety of basal structures, in particular the corpus striatum, septal region, substantia innominata, preoptic region, hypothalamus, ventral tegmental area, and substantia nigra; the resultant radioactive labeling of efferent fibers had been recorded autoradiographically by the technique described by Cowan et al. (10). In a concurrent project aimed in particular at the identification of mesencephalo–striatal neurons and the pattern of their projection on the striatum, small deposits of horseradish peroxidase (HRP) were placed by microelectrophoresis in a large variety of loci within the striatum; the resulting retrograde cell labeling was visualized by the Graham-Karnofsky reaction, following, with minor modifications, the protocol described by LaVail et al. (21). More comprehensive reports on these studies will be published elsewhere; for the purpose of the present account, only a few cases need be documented in some detail.

Findings

In this study, retrograde HRP labeling most nearly confined to outlying mesencephalo–striatal neurons (i.e., those neurons of this category that lie outside the limits of the substantia nigra as conventionally drawn) was observed in cases of HRP injection localized to the most ventral region of the striatum. This region includes not only the nucleus accumbens and olfactory tubercle but also the larger, more caudal, remainder of the fundus of the striatum. HRP injected into more dorsal parts of the striatum labeled large numbers of neurons within the substantia nigra proper, but it must be noted that in many such cases additional—and sometimes numerous—labeled neurons appeared in one or the other group of outlying mescencephalo–striatal cells. In general, the findings in these HRP experiments confirmed the results of a concurrent autoradiographic study of the nigrostriatal projection reported in the form of an abstract by Domesick et al. (15).

Figure 2 (left column) photographically illustrates the massive retrograde labeling of outlying nigral cells in a case of HRP injection localized to the nucleus accumbens (case RH 29). The maximal extent of the injection site is shown in jet black in the inset to Fig. 2A. Most cells in this case were labeled vividly enough to be clearly visible in these low-power darkfield photographs, but it was necessary to retouch more sparsely labeled cell bodies. The cell-labeling picture was further enhanced by masking all bright-appearing structures that could be identified in the microscope as nonneuronal cells showing a positive reaction on account of an endogenous peroxidase (erythrocytes, perivascular cells).

Shown alongside these darkfield photographs is a series of chartings of the radioactively labeled fibers (Fig. 2, right column) appearing at the approximately corresponding levels of the midbrain of a rat (RR 89) in which a small injection of tritiated leucine-and-proline had been placed in the lateral hypothalamus. The maximal extent of the injection site is shown in jet black in the inset to the top figure of this column.

These autoradiograms clearly illustrate the trajectory of the hypothalamo–mesencephalic fibers of the medial forebrain bundle. They add several important details to the findings in earlier fiber-degeneration studies. One such additional observation is that some of the fibers deviating laterally, and forming a fiber stratum immediately dorsal to the substantia nigra, actually enter the latter's pars compacta and to some extent even the pars reticulata. This apparent hypothalamo–nigral connection, however, seems only marginal when contrasted with the remarkable topographic correspondence betweeen the descending hypothalamic fibers and the labeled mesencephalo–striatal neurons medial and dorsal to the substantia nigra proper. That this correspondence is not merely a local coincidence is suggested by the strikingly concurrent transposition of both cells and fibers with respect to the medial lemniscus at the level of the caudal one-third of the substantia nigra (Fig. 2D). Rostral to this level, both the labeled mesencephalo–striatal neurons and the laterally deviating hypothalamic efferents are located for the most part ventral and medial to the medial lemniscus (Fig. 2A–C). As the lemniscus, traced caudally, gradually shifts in the ventral and medial direction, the main path of the laterally oriented fibers comes to lead dorsal to the lemniscus. At these same levels, numerous labeled mesencephalo–striatal neurons appear in the same position dorsal to the medial lemniscus (Fig. 2D). It may also be noted that sporadic labeled neurons appear in the contralateral ventral tegmental area in a distribution remarkably similar to that of the relatively few labeled fibers that cross the midline (Fig. 2B–D).

The labeled cells dorsal to the medial lemniscus at the level of Fig. 2D correspond in position to the anterior part of cell group A8 as indicated in Fig. 1 of Palkovits and Jacobowitz (30) (their atlas of catecholamine neurons). At levels immediately caudal to the substantia nigra, Palkovits and Jacobowitz (their Figs. 1d and 2a) indicate the caudal part of dopamine cell group A8. In our case (RH 29, illustrated by Fig. 2), no labeled cells were found in the corresponding ventrolateral tegmental region, but Fig. 1 illustrates a case (RH 27) in which labeled cells did appear in the caudal region in question. In this case, as in several other cases in which the HRP injection was placed in the most ventral striatal zone even farther behind the accumbens level, the cell labeling at more rostral levels of the midbrain was remarkably similar to that shown in Fig. 2, except for labeling of a larger number of cells of the pars compacta. The round aggregate of labeled cells in the ventrolateral tegmentum in Fig. 1 corresponds in location to A8. It will be noted that sparser labeled neurons are loosely scattered over a large triangular region of the tegmentum medial to the more compact ventrolateral cell cluster. Further labeled tegmental cells appearing at this level in and about the median plane probably correspond to the more caudal cells of dopamine cell group A10 as charted by Palkovits and Jacobowitz (30) in their Figs. 1d and 2a. The line of these paramedian cells is continuous dorsally with a likewise paramedian group of labeled cells in the central gray substance that correspond to the dorsal raphe nucleus; it is noteworthy that in all cases of our material HRP, regardless of its injection site within the striatum, was found to have labeled a smaller or larger number of cells in the nucleus raphis dorsalis.

A comparison of the cell-labeling pattern (shown in Fig. 1, left) with the distribution of radioactively labeled hypothalamo–mesencephalic fibers (charted in Fig. 1, right) shows that the location of the more compact ventrolateral cell group corresponds exactly to that of a fairly massive group of hypothalamic efferents that have swept laterally farthest, and from this level caudalward will collectively shift in the mediodorsal direction.

Control Experiments

Since it seemed possible that HRP injected into the striatum could be taken up by dopamine fibers passing through the striatum to the anteromedial cortex, a few control experiments were done to determine whether and to what extent the labeling of nigrocortical neurons possibly resulting from such injections might have affected the interpretation of the present findings. In two rats, eight closely spaced HRP injections were placed in the anteromedial cortex, together spanning the distance from the frontal pole to the anterior border of the granular retrosplenial cortex. The results of this massive injection in both cases confirmed Beckstead's (3) finding that HRP deposited in the anteromedial cortex labels nigrocortical neurons only in the ventral tegmental area and the medial one-quarter of the substantia nigra, pars compacta. Despite the relatively huge size of the intracortical HRP deposits, the number of labeled cells in the ventral tegmental area in both cases was very much smaller than that of the cells labeled in the same area by small intrastriatal HRP injections. It therefore seems safe to conclude that the majority, by far, of the labeled cells shown in Figs. 1 and 2 project to the striatum rather than to the anteromedial cortex. Since any labeled nigrocortical cells would appear scattered in among nigrostriatal neurons, they could not significantly distort the outlines of the nigrostriatal cell groups demonstrated by the present experiments.

Discussion

A fundamental point to be made in discussing the observations reported here is that the HRP method appears to be entirely nonselective with respect to the nature of the neural transmitter synthesized by the neurons it labels. Consequently, the method can give us no clue as to which of the individual mesencephalic neurons labeled in the two cases shown here are actually dopamine neurons; however, even though this fact is acknowledged, it seems fair to assume that at least many of them are. One reason for this assumption is that in many other cases of our large material, HRP injections that were localized to more dorsal parts of the striatum were found to have labeled all or nearly all cells in a corresponding sector of the substantia nigra, pars compacta. There is no reason to suspect that the HRP method is selectively biased against dopamine neurons in other regions of the nigral complex. Furthermore, the topography of the HRP-positive cells shown in Figs. 1 and 2 is compatible, at least, with that of the dopamine neurons indicated in Palkovits and Jacobowitz's (30) atlas. Even though a detailed comparison is made difficult by the difference in resolution of the respective chartings, it seems obvious that most of the neurons labeled in case RH 29 (Fig. 1) correspond to dopamine-cell group A10, for the largest number of these labeled cells are located in the ventral tegmental area of Tsai and along the median plane of the tegmentum. At the level of Fig. 1C, HRP-positive cells appear in the spaces between the more medial bundles of the medial lemniscus; in their charting of a section at this level, Palkovits and Jacobowitz (their Fig. 1b) indicate dopamine cells in exactly the same position. The same charting indicates further dopamine cells lying dorsal to the medial lemniscus, and labeled cells appear in the same position in our Fig. 1C and D. Palkovits and Jacobowitz consider these supralemniscal cells to be part of cell group A8. In several cases not documented here, we could indeed observe that the more laterally situated supralemniscal clusters of HRP-positive cells (Fig. 1D) are directly continuous with the rather compact cell group which appears in the ventrolateral tegmentum at the level of Fig. 2, and whose location corresponds to that of the cell group labeled A8 in Palkovits and Jacobowitz's Fig. 2a.

These comparisons of retrograde-labeling and catecholamine-histofluorescence data seem to justify the conclusion that nondopaminergic tegmento-striatal neurons, if they exist and are labeled by intrastriatal HRP injection, must be confined largely at least to the same tegmental regions that also contain dopamine cells.

The matter has been discussed here at some length for its general interest, even though it is clear that for the purpose of the present study the question as to the chemical characteristics of the tegmental neurons labeled by intrastriatal injection of HRP is of only secondary importance. Of more immediate significance to the general problem outlined in the introduction is the evidence that nearly all these numerous cells lie in the path of descending components of the medial forebrain bundle. The selectiveness of this relationship is remarkable, and thus far no other descending fiber system labeled in our large material has been found to match the distribution of outlying mesencephalo-striatal cells as closely.

Naturally, the question arises as to whether spatial matching implies functional contact between cells and fibers. In this particular instance, such contact is highly probable, for the autoradiographic labeling pattern clearly suggests that the fibers charted in Figs. 1 and 2 do not merely pass through the regions in which labeled cells are distributed. The scatter of grain strongly indicates at least collateral ramification in these regions. Such afferent relationships of the outlying cell groups, all of which lie virtually embedded among descending fibers of the medial forebrain bundle, appear even more likely when it is considered that both the pars compacta and pars reticulata of the substantia nigra, situated along rather than within the fiber path, are invaded by some components of the overlying stratum of hypothalamic fibers (Fig. 1).

In the autoradiographic case RR 89 illustrated here, only that component of the medial forebrain bundle that originates in the lateral hypothalamic region is shown by radioactive labeling. Nearly identical, although less massive, labeling patterns are found in our material in cases of isotope injection in the lateral preoptic region (8,35) or, farther laterally, in certain parts of the substantia innominata. Of particular interest is that such injections, when placed in the nucleus accumbens, label medial forebrain bundle fibers in a pattern that differs from the one shown here only by a much more massive involvement of the substantia nigra, pars compacta. In such cases, laterally directed fibers, instead of following a course dorsal to the substantia nigra, pass through (and very likely terminate in) the medial half at least of the latter's pars compacta. The difference between such cases and the present one suggests that the major source of fibers terminating within the substantia nigra's pars compacta is the nucleus accumbens and adjoining ventral regions of the striatum, whereas the outlying nigral districts receive major inputs from this same ventral striatal region and, in addition, from the lateral preoptico-hypothalamic continuum and substantia innominata. It thus seems that all the regions occupied by dopamine neurons lie in the path of conduction routes associated with the limbic structures of the cerebral hemisphere. Whereas the limbic system could be thought to affect the pars compacta of the substantia nigra mainly by way of ventral parts of the striatum, its conduction lines to the region of dopamine cell groups A10 and A8 would seem to lead over both the ventral striatum and the lateral preoptico-hypothalamic region.

The present study by its limited scope has been able to suggest only one of the probably multiple neural mechanisms that affect the functional state of the nigral complex and, hence, of the striatum. Cell group A8, for example, is shown in both Ungerstedt's (37) and Palkovits and Jacobowitz's (30) atlas also to lie in the path of the ventral fiber bundle ascending from norepinephrine cell groups in the rhombencephalon, and the region of cell group A10 is traversed not only by descending fibers, but also by ascending fibers of the medial forebrain bundle originating in part at least from serotonin cells in the mesencephalic raphe nuclei; however, even in the absence of a more detailed and comprehensive knowledge of the afferent connections of the nigral complex, it seems possible, on the basis of the present findings, to suggest the limbic system as a major source of modulating influence on the interaction between the substantia nigra and the striatum. The functional significance of such modulation must at present remain a matter of conjecture; however, if it is correct to assume that at least one major function of the limbic system expresses itself in the domain of affect and motivation, while the corpus striatum is engaged more in particular in skeletomuscular mechanisms, then it could be postulated that connections such as discussed here may represent the "interface" between motivation and movement.

ACKNOWLEDGMENTS

The studies on which much of this chapter is based were supported by U.S. Public Health Service Grants NB 06542 and MH 25515, and by National Science Foundation Grant BNS 76–81227.

REFERENCES

1. Adey, W. R., and Meyer, M. (1952): An experimental study of hippocampal afferent pathways from prefrontal and cingulate areas in the monkey. *J. Anat. (Lond.),* 86:58–74.
2. Andén, N.-E., Dahlström, A., Fuxe, K., Larsson, K., Olson, L., and Ungerstedt, U. (1966): Ascending monoamine neurons to the telencephalon and diencephalon. *Acta Physiol. Scand.,* 67:313–326.
3. Beckstead, R. M. (1976): Convergent thalamic and mesencephalic projections to the anterior medial cortex in the rat. *J. Comp., Neurol.,* 166:403–416.
4. Berman, A. L. (1968): *The Brain Stem of the Cat: A Cytoarchitectonic Atlas with Stereotaxic Coordinates.* The University of Wisconsin Press, Madison.
5. Cajal, S. R. (1911): *Histologie du Système Nerveux de l'Homme et des Vertébrés.* Maloine, Paris.
6. Carman, J. B., Cowan, W. M., and Powell, T. P. S. (1963): The organization of the corticostriate connections in the rabbit. *Brain,* 86:525–562.
7. Clark, W. E. Le Gros, and Meyer, M. (1950): Anatomical relationships between the cerebral cortex and the hypothalamus. *Br. Med. Bull.,* 6:341–345.
8. Conrad, L. C. A., and Pfaff, D. W. (1976): Efferents from medial basal forebrain and hypothalamus in the rat. I. An autoradiographic study of the medial preoptic area. *J. Comp. Neurol.,* 169:185–220.
9. Conrad, L. C. A., and Pfaff, D. W. (1976): Efferents from medial basal forebrain and hypothalamus in the rat: II. An autoradiographic study of the anterior hypothalamus. *J. Comp. Neurol.,* 169:221–262.
10. Cowan, W. M., Gottlieb, D. I., Hendrickson, A. E., Price, J. L., and Woolsey, T. A. (1972): The autoradiographic demonstration of axonal connections in the central nervous system. *Brain Res.,* 37:21–51.
11. Cragg, B. G. (1965): Afferent connexions of the allocortex. *J. Anat. (Lond.),* 99:339–361.
12. Dahlström, A., and Fuxe, K. (1965): Evidence for the existence of monoamine-containing neurons in the central nervous system. I. Demonstration of monoamines in the cell bodies of brainstem neurons. *Acta Physiol. Scand.,* 232:1–55.
13. De Olmos, J. S., and Ingram, W. R. (1972): The projection field of the stria terminalis in the rat brain: An experimental study. *J. Comp. Neurol.,* 146:303–334.
14. Diamond, I. T., Jones, E. G., and Powell, T. P. S. (1968): The association connections of the auditory cortex of the cat. *Brain Res.,* 11:560–569.
15. Domesick, V. B., Beckstead, R. M., and Nauta, W. J. H. (1976): Some ascending and descending projections of the substantia nigra and ventral tegmental area in the rat. *Neurosci. Abstr.* II, part I, p. 61.
16. Fox, C. A. (1943): The stria terminalis, longitudinal association bundle and precommissural fornix fibers in the cat. *J. Comp. Neurol.,* 79:277–295.
17. Herkenham, M., and Nauta, W. J. H. (1977): Afferent connections of the habenular nuclei in the rat: A horseradish peroxidase study, with a note on the fiber-of-passage problem. *J. Comp. Neurol.,* 173:123–145.
18. Jones, E. G., and Powell, T. P. S. (1970): An anatomical study of converging sensory pathways within the cerebral cortex of the monkey. *Brain,* 93:793–824.
19. Kemp, J. M., and Powell, T. P. S. (1970): The cortico-striate projection in the monkey. *Brain,* 93:525–546.
20. Krettek, J. E., and Price, J. L. (1974): A direct input from the amygdala to the thalamus and cerebral cortex. *Brain Res.,* 67:174–269.
21. LaVail, J. H., Winston, K. R., and Tish, A. (1973): A method based on retrograde intra-axonal transport of protein for identification of cell bodies of origin of axons terminating within the CNS. *Brain Res.,* 58:470–477.
22. MacLean, P. D. (1952): Some psychiatric implications of physiological studies on frontotemporal portion of limbic system. *Electroencephalogr. Clin. Neurophysiol.,* 4:407–418.
23. MacLean, P. D. (1953): The limbic system and its hippocampal formation. *J. Neurosurg.,* 11:29–44.
24. Nauta, W. J. H. (1958): Hippocampal projections and related neural pathways to the midbrain in the cat. *Brain,* 81:319–340.
25. Nauta, W. J. H. (1961): Fibre degeneration following lesions of the amygdaloid complex in the monkey. *J. Anat. (Lond.),* 95:515–534.

26. Nauta, W. J. H. (1962): Neural associations of the amygdaloid complex in the monkey. *Brain*, 85:505–520.
27. Nauta, W. J. H. (1971): The problem of the frontal lobe: A reinterpretation. *J. Psychiatr. Res.*, 8:167–187.
28. Nauta, W. J. H. (1974): Evidence of a pallidohabenular pathway in the cat. *J. Comp. Neurol.*, 156:19–28.
29. Nauta, W. J. H., and Mehler, W. R. (1966): Projections of the lentiform nucleus in the monkey. *Brain Res.*, 1:3–42.
30. Palkovits, M., and Jacobowitz, D. M. (1974): Topographic atlas of catecholamine and acetylcholinesterase-containing neurons in the rat brain: II. Hindbrain (mesencephalon, rhombencephalon). *J. Comp. Neurol.*, 157:29–42.
31. Papez, J. W. (1937): A proposed mechanism of emotion. *Arch. Neurol. Psychiatr.*, 38:725–743.
32. Powell, T. P. S. (1973): Sensory convergence in the cerebral cortex. In *Surgical Approaches in Psychiatry*, edited by L. V. Laitinen and K. E. Livingston, pp. 266–281. Medical and Technical Publishing Co. Ltd., Lancaster.
33. Raisman, G., Cowan, W. M., and Powell, T. P. S. (1966): An experimental analysis of the efferent projections of the hippocampus. *Brain*, 89:83–108.
34. Sachs, E., Brendler, S. J., and Fulton, J. F. (1949): The orbital gyri. *Brain*, 72:227–240.
35. Swanson, L. W. (1976): An autoradiographic study of the efferent connections of the preoptic region in the rat. *J. Comp. Neurol.*, 167:227–256.
36. Tsai, C. (1925): The optic tracts and centers of the opossum, *Didelphys virginiana. J. Comp. Neurol.*, 39:173–202.
37. Ungerstedt, U. (1971): Stereotaxic mapping of the monoamine pathways in the rat brain. *Acta Physiol. Scand.*, 197 (Suppl. 367):1–48.
38. Van Hoesen, G. W., and Pandya, D. N. (1975): Some connections of the entorhinal area (area 28) and perirhinal area (area 35) cortices of the Rhesus monkey. I. Temporal lobe afferents. *Brain Res.*, 95:1–24.
39. Van Hoesen, G. W., and Pandya, D. N. (1975): Some connections of the entorhinal area (area 28) and perirhinal area (area 35) cortices of the Rhesus monkey. II. Frontal afferents. *Brain Res.*, 95:25–38.
40. Van Hoesen, G. W., and Pandya, D. N. (1975): Some connections of the entorhinal area (area 28) and perirhinal area (area 35) cortices of the Rhesus monkey. III. Efferent connections. *Brain Res.*, 95:39–59.
41. Wall, P. D., Glees, P., and Fulton, J. F. (1951): Corticofugal connexions of posterior orbital surface in rhesus monkey. *Brain*, 74:66–71.
42. Ward, A. A., and McCulloch, W. S. (1947): The projection of the frontal lobe on the hypothalamus. *J. Neurophysiol.*, 10:309–314.
43. Webster, K. E. (1961): Cortico-striate interrelations in the albino rat. *J. Anat. (Lond.)*, 95:532–545.
44. Webster, K. E. (1965): The cortico-striatal projection in the cat. *J. Anat. (Lond.)*, 99:329–337.
45. Whitlock, D. G., and Nauta, W. J. H. (1956): Subcortical projections from the temporal neocortex in the *Macaca mulatta. J. Comp. Neurol.*, 106:182–212.

Functional Neurosurgery, edited by T. Rasmussen
and R. Marino. Raven Press, New York © 1979.

Neurology of Brain Functional Disorders

P. Molina-Negro

*Department of Surgery, University of Montreal and Service of Neurosurgery, Hôpital
Notre-Dame, Montreal, Quebec, Canada H2L 1M4*

> If the governing body of this country were destroyed suddenly, we should
> have two causes of lamentation; the loss of services of eminent men; and the
> anarchy of the now uncontrolled people.
>
> —J. H. Jackson, *Evolution and Dissolution of the Nervous System*, 1884

Before entering upon the description of any particular symptom or disease,
it seems convenient to define the meaning of the term "functional." Functional
is often applied to symptoms of a supposedly psychogenic origin. Hysterical
palsy or anesthesia are typical examples. That is a most improper use of the
term. Functional is sometimes used to describe clinical symptoms resulting from
minute or unknown organic changes, or to describe descrete or transitory symptoms of obviously organic lesions.

In 1873, Jackson wrote:

I have for some years used the term functional to describe the morbid alterations of the normal
function of nerve tissue. Therefore, before I speak of these alterations, we must notice what the
normal function of nerve tissue is. Its function is to store up and to expand force . . . There are
but two kinds of alterations of function from disease. Saying nothing of degrees of each, there is
on the one hand *loss of function* and on the other *overfunction* (not better function). In the former,
nerve tissues cease to store up, and therefore to expand force. In the latter, more nerve force is
stored up than in health, and more is therefore expanded; the nerve tissue is highly unstable.
Under the first heading came palsies (akineses), anaesthesiae; under the second, chorea, epilepsies,
tetanus (hyperkineses), neuralgia, etc. . . . (On the anatomical physiological, and pathological investigation of epilepsies, 1873) (11).

In the article entitled "Observations on the Physiology and Pathology of
Hemi-chorea," in 1868, Jackson wrote: "Just as *loss* of function, for instance
palsy, follows *destruction* of nerve tissue . . . so *disorder* of function, for instance
chorea or spasm, results from *instability* of nerve tissue . . ." [(11), Vol. 2, p.
243].

Therefore, according to Jackson, brain functional disorders are *those which
manifest overactivity or overfunction of normal nervous tissue.* Those are symptoms
that Jackson calls positive or plus, as opposed to the negative or minus symptoms
that manifest the loss of function of a destroyed tissue [(11), Vol. 2, p. 7].

GENERAL PHYSIOPATHOLOGY OF BRAIN FUNCTIONAL DISORDERS

It is of paramount importance to keep in mind that all plus or positive symptoms result from overactivity of nervous centers that are, except for overactivity, healthy; in every case, this overfunction is the result of the loss of the control exerted by that part of the nervous system destroyed by the lesion, just as the minus or negative symptoms are the result of the loss of function of the latter.

The normal function of the human nervous system is the result of a competitive equilibrium between its most archaic parts, which it shares with the inferior vertebrates, reptiles, and avians, and the new ones successively acquired with the progression of the evolution. The understanding of human normal and abnormal motor functions is hardly possible without the help of comparative anatomy. All the classic writings are full of references to the theory of evolution. Cajal began his monumental Hystologie du Système Nerveux de l'Homme et des Vertébrés as follows:

> La matière vivante, après d'infinies évolutions, est parvenue à constituer un appareil qui, par son extrême complexité, par les fonctions transcendantes qui lui sont dévolues, semble être l'expression la plus haute de l'organisation animale. Cet appareil est le système nerveux. Nous attarder à la démonstration du rôle capital de ce système serait temps perdu. Dès son apparition chez l'animal multicellulaire, auparavant anarchique et divisé, proie facile de toutes vissitudes du monde ambiant, le système nerveux fait de cet animal, malgré la multiplicité de ses éléments, un être de plus en plus uni, il l'arme de moyens de subsistance et de défense toujours plus nombreux, plus précis, plus puissants, plus synergiques: il lui donne, aux échelons les plus hauts de la série zoologique, ces égides si supérieures de l'intégrité vitale: la sensation, la pensée, la volonté. En un mot, tout esprit synthétique aura conçu que le perfectionnement des éléments nerveux et du système qu'ils composent constitue le perfectionnement même de l'animalité (5).

In the protozoan, there is no nervous system. Irritability is the base for its rudimentary movements. The nervous system appeared first in the Coelenterata and it comprises two neurons: one sensory and one motor. At the same time, purposeful movements of approach, withdrawal, and prehension became possible.

A new element is added in the worms, and "its appearance indicates the enormous progress, the superiority of worms over Coelenterata. This new element is the internuncial or associative neuron" (5). This new element permits the worm to move its entire body and to react immediately to minimal stimuli. As we progress in the scale of invertebrates, we find in the crustacea and arthropoda a greater number of associative neurons making it possible for the animal to perform movements more and more coordinated and defined in relation to the conservation of the individual and species.

In the vertebrates, a new associative neuron is added and it is placed far from the primitive sensory and motor neurons: the psychomotor neuron that constitutes the brain. Fish, thanks to a single striatum that constitutes almost the entire brain, can perform the elegant rhythmic movements of swimming. Reptiles and avians possess a double striatum and a rudiment of brain cortex that make the learning of progressively complex motor and psychomotor tasks possible. Displacement with reptoid, nonrythmic movements, rotation of the head to find the food, a threat, a friend, are now possible; and yet the avian conserves the possibility to perform rhythmic movements with the wings. Birds acquire new possibilities while keeping the old ones. The huge development of the brain and cerebellar cortex in mammals, and particularly the so-called lymbic system or rhinencephalon, provides an anatomical base for complex emotional reactions and social activities and also for bizarre behavior so close to human behavior.

The development of the neocortex in *apes* makes two very important acquisitions possible: language, that is a complex code of communication with sounds and gestures, and purposeful, refined manipulations. Among the superior apes it is probably through improvements of language and manipulation of instruments that primitive man emerges.

It is impossible to decide whether the development of the prefrontal neocortex makes the progress possible or if, more probably, it is the function, the struggle for survival, that conditions the ultimate perfection of the brain. The fact remains that gradually, as new functions and centers developed, the more primitive decreased in importance. But both the old functions and the primitive centers persisted, latent or better dominated by the functions and the centers of higher rank, which appeared more recently.

"One can divide"—says Cajal—"the animal series in neural periods. Unicellular and spongia are the periods of irritability; Coelenterata, the period of two elementary neurons; inferior invertebrates, the period of associative neurons; and the vertebrates, and particularly man, the period of the psychomotor neuron: *each period of course, maintaining and perfectioning the progress of the previous period"* (5).

If the study of phylogenesis helps to grasp the concept of nervous functions in adult humans as the result of superposition and integration of progressively complex functions and structures, ontogeny also throws some light on the subject. In the words of Kuhlenbeck, "the similarities between stages that are merely transitory and embryotic in some forms, but became (although somewhat modified) final, permanent stages in other forms, can be interpreted as strongly suggesting phylogenetic relationships" (12).

The differentiation of the nervous system starts at the beginning of the third week of gestation and around the sixth week, soon after the appearance of the telencephalic vesicle, it is possible to perceive the first movements of the embryo. At the time of birth, the external configuration of the nervous system is almost completed. From the appearance of the Sylvian fissure at 19 weeks, the folding of the cortical mantle increases, and at term more than 50% of the brain cortex is hidden in the depth of sulci that represents more cortical surface than that of any mammal. And yet, the newborn is only able to perform some rudimentary reptoid movements and the rhythmic movements of suction. It is precisely the suction and the strong emotional reactions of pleasure and displeasure of the newborn that certified this appurtenance to the genus of mammals. Gradually, as the folding and myelinization of the cortex increases, new motor and psychic functions appear. The first purposeful manipulation coincides toward the fourth month with the first guttural sound characteristic of primitive speech. Around the sixth month, the hand grasp of the child is firm and he can now remain seated. If carefully carried to a pool, he will naturally swim, even if he is not yet able to walk. Dysmetria and truncal ataxia are normal at this age. Some few months later, both phenomena would be a sure sign of cerebellar disease. Precise manipulation of a finger accompanies at the tenth or eleventh month the first steps and the first meaningful words. Incomplete myelinization of cerebellar hemispheres is manifested by a tendency to fall, while unfinished folding and myelinization of frontal cortex is manifested by startle reactions to all types of stimuli and probably also by myoclonic jerks at the beginning of the sleep. By the end of the second year, myelinization and folding of the brain cortex are practically finished: 75% of the cortex is hidden in the depth of sulci. Simultaneously, the child can do everything: walk, run, swim, throw, and catch, talk, and dance. He will also experience choices, joys, and pains, and he loves and suffers and is afraid or concerned; the harmony of movements and the control of emotions show maturity, achievement of the ontogenic evolution that produces in some few months hundreds of millions of years of phylogenic development. "The ontogeny recapitulates phylogeny" (12).

In the same way that mammal's brain contains a reptilian and a worm primitive brain, the human adult brain includes a proteiform primitive brain, well under control but latent and ready to come to life when the new centers are diseased.

The brain functional disorders appear when the recently acquired centers have lost their function and left the primitive ones uncontrolled. Each brain functional disorder, like uncontrolled behavior, epileptic seizure, or abnormal movements, represents the activity of one normal primitive center left uncontrolled by the loss of function of a new center.

The doctrine of dissolution (or opposed to evolution) of Spencer (19), is at the base of Jackson's doctrine of brain functional disorders. He quotes a sentence of Symond that summarizes very accurately this idea: "Diminished action in one part causes exalted action in another" [(11), Vol. 2, p. 7]. In all brain functional disorders, there is, at a different degree, a subtle blending of negative and positive symptoms, and, it is important to identify each of them correctly in order to locate first the lesion responsible for the negative symptoms and then the centers responsible, through their overfunction, for the positive symptoms. Functional neurosurgery is possible only if we know which structure is responsible for a particular functional brain disorder. Functional neurosurgery does not deal with "negative" symptoms resulting from lesions (that is the aim of general neurosurgery), but with "positive" or "plus" symptoms resulting from the overfunction of otherwise healthy uncontrolled primitive structures.

CLASSIFICATION AND OUTLINE OF BRAIN FUNCTIONAL DISORDERS

The common characteristic of all brain functional disorders is that they result from hyperactivity of a "normal" primitive center, liberated from the inhibitory action of an "abnormal" higher center, seat of the lesion. This definition applies "stricto sensu" to only three conditions: abnormal behavior, epilepsy, and abnormal movements. By analogy, it can also be applied to other conditions, such as central pain, hypertonicity, and some neuroendocrine disorders. Table 1 summarizes the main areas with which functional neurosurgery deals. The inclusion of each one deserves an explanation.

Even the partisan of psychogenesis admits *de facto* that *abnormal behavior* is the expression of overfunction of some brain centers. The routine administration of generous doses of psychotropic drugs is the best argument. Indeed antipsychotics, anxiolytics, and sedatives act by invariably slowing down some presumably hyperactive brain metabolic process. "Human behaviour, violent or peaceful, is always the product of brain environment interaction" (15). It does not matter if one adopts animism or materialism, if one holds dualistic or unitary theories concerning the principle of action of the human being. What matters is the fact that the brain is the vehicle, the final path, the indispensable instrument that makes possible emotions, thoughts, and behavior. Disease, malfunction of those parts of the brain recently acquired in the process of evolution, can result in uncontrolled activity of a portion of the limbic system, substratum of primitive instinctive behavior previously acquired. Obsessive compulsive disorders are but fragmentary hyperfunction of admittedly normal behavior. Therefore, beside environmental investigation, a thorough neurological evaluation must be done in every case of abnormal behavior, and if at the end we cannot perceive any abnormality of brain function, it will probably be focused to be the fault of our methods of investigation. It could be worthwhile to recall that even if environment plays an essential role in the genesis of human behavior "once environment is perceived, it is incorporated into the brain" [(15), p. 140].

Jackson's definition of epilepsy is surely the most commonly accepted. "Epileptic discharges are occasional, abrupt, and excessive discharges or parts of the cerebral hemisphere (paroxysmal discharges)" [(11), Vol. 1, p. 177]. Epilepsy thus defined constitutes a typical, almost the prototype, of brain functional

TABLE 1. *Brain function disorders*

1. Abnormal behavior
2. Epilepsy
3. Abnormal movement
4. Pain
5. Hypertonia
6. Neuroendocrine disorders

disorders. Because the so-called epileptic focus is an overfunctioning normal or partially normal group of neurons. In the investigation of epileptic patients, there is always the temptation when finding a lesion to identify lesion and focus. It is perhaps because of the confusion between the lesion and the focus that restricted surgical excision of the pretended epileptogenic lesion is seldom gratifying. In all Jackson's writing on epilepsy, one can find an almost obsessive concern with this danger. In 1876 he wrote: "A little thought would show two things—first, that local symptoms of necessity imply local disease—and second, that the state of nervous organs or tissues on which a discharge directly depends (the "discharging lesion") is not likely to be easily discovered; for the discharge in convulsion is only an excessive exaggeration of the normal function of the cells and fibers. What we should have to discover is the difference between cells which discharge excessively and those which discharge normally— not a likely thing to be easily discovered. In some cases of epilepsy, we sometimes do not trace even roughly the pathology of the discharging lesion; we may discover no alteration post-mortem of any sort. When we do see a coarse change (tumor, let us suppose), we do not trace the steps by which that coarse change led to the instability of cells of gray matter which the convulsion obliges us to infer to exist. The tumor is not the discharging lesion; it is a foreign body which leads to these changes in gray matter which constitute the discharging lesion" [(11), Vol. 1, p. 219]. The fact that discharging focus lies in the vicinity far away from the destroying lesion depends upon different factors. One of those is probably the more or less primitive origin, both phylogenetically and ontogenetically, of the lesion. Thus in the case of a tumor located in the vicinity of the rolandic fissure, both the destroyed gray matter responsible for the negative symptoms and the overfunctioning gray matter responsible for the bravais-jacksonian seizure would probably lie closely adjacent. Whereas the destruction of a part of the temporal neocortex could result in uncontrolled activity of the most primitive part of the limbic system, far away from the lesion.

It might be pertinent to report the case of a 10-year-old boy who had suffered from childhood from startle epilepsia and such severe behavior disturbances as to require constant surveillance. Abnormal EEG activity in the affected hemisphere led to angiography, which showed a huge cystic lesion in the prefrontal convexity. The corticography during surgery showed some sporadic epileptic activity in the vicinity of the cyst, in an obviously abnormal cortex, and more important epileptic activity close to the middle line in an apparently normal cortex. The decision was made to remove first the cyst and the underlying ulegyric cortex. After surgery, the startle seizures persisted, although they were less violent and less frequent for a while; no obvious change of behavior was detected. A second craniotomy with careful electrocorticographic studies showed a definite epileptic activity in the supplementary motor area, and this was removed. Although the tests for pathology did not show any abnormality, the epileptic seizures stopped after surgery and the behavior of the child became progressively normal. He remains free of epilepsy and is leading a completely normal life 8 years later. The conclusion is that a destroying lesion of the frontal convexity resulted in hyperfunction of a "normal" supplementary motor area responsible for tonic contralateral epileptic convulsion and behavior disorder (10).

Abnormal movements are another good example of a brain functional disorder. Each abnormal movement is but a caricatural exaggeration of a fragment of normal motor activity. Each one represents the uncontrolled activity of a primitive part of the motor system, liberated from control of the newly acquired motor centers. And all progressive neural degenerative disorders which primarily or secondarily involve basal ganglia, will show in the terminal phase a common pattern of flexion dystonia representing the totally uncontrolled activity of the most primitive motor centers, liberated from all striatal and cortical inhibitory influences. According to Denny-Brown, "they represent maintained states of activation of prepontine reflex mechanism" (7).

Pain and particularly "central pain" possesses some characteristics that justify its inclusion, by analogy, in the present chapter. In the past, neurological studies on pain have concentrated on the receptors of pain sensation, spinal tracts, and terminal brain centers. Perception of pain sensation and psycho-affective reaction to pain have been neglected by neurologists and neurophysiologists until recently. Pain is "a perceptual behavioural state of the whole animal" (21). Perceptivity of pain and the reaction to it are the result of a complex integrative process between the different elements of the sensory message of "exteroceptors." Fear arises essentially from past esperiences of pain, and this experience can deeply modify the perception of the pain sensation. The past experience is also responsible for the degree of excitability of the pain path that would control the reaction to pain perception. Surely, pain is the oldest sensation. Reaction to aggression is present even in primitive invertebrates, and the progressive perfection acquired by the nervous system through evolution never abandons the old mechanisms, but simply inhibits them in favor of more complex reaction carried out by new refined associative systems. Unmyelinated, polysynaptic and diffusely distributed pathways represent the old paleo-spino-thalamic system submitted to the inhibitory, modulating control of myelinated fibers of the more systematic neo-spino-thalamic system. Furthermore, the nociceptive sensation, origin of defense or withdrawal reflexes, is submitted to the inhibitory influences of the fibers and center responsible for epicritic sensation. There are many examples to illustrate the disinhibitory character of pain. Causalgia, postherpetic neuralgia, pain of tabes dorsalis, anesthesia dolorosa, and thalamic pain are all conditions in which the lesion predominated in myelinated fibers carrying epicritic and neo-spino-thalamic pain sensations, leaving uncontrolled the diffuse paleo-spino-thalamic pathways responsible for the most primitive sensation of pain. These facts and some further speculation led to the formulation of modern theories of pain, such as the *gate theory* of Melzack and Wall (14), and to the application of neurostimulators in the treatment of pain.

Hypertonia is a condition resulting from numerous lesions located between the spinal cord and the brain cortex having in common this particular trait: they involve pathways or centers that normally exert an inhibitory influence on motor neurons. Antigravity hypertonus, either through direct alpha or reflex gamma influence, is the common underlying status of all hypertonias. Primitive antigravity reactions of labyrinthine origin, present already in primitive vertebrates, are progressively submitted to the influence of neocortex responsible for nonreflex motor activity. In hypertonia, no matter what the localization or nature of the lesion responsible may be, we find overfunction of a "normal" primitive motor system. Again, using the words of Jackson: "The hypothesis starts with the assumption that the spinal centers receive impulses from both the cerebrum and the cerebellum, which impulses in health interfere with one another (inhibit one another). If so, we should not say that the cerebral lesion, or the wasting in certain spinal tracts consecutive upon it, *causes* rigidity; negative lesions can only cause negative conditions in muscles, in this case, paralysis; but on the hypothesis of the cerebral lesion, in other words, loss of cerebral influence on the spinal centers may *permit* the rigidity, for then the cerebellar influence is no longer interfered with and, metaphorically speaking, "flows into the parts deserted by the cerebral influence" [(11), Vol. 2, p. 453].

Neuroendocrine disorders such as pituitary oversecreting diseases are included by analogy among the brain functional disorders, because they result in overfunction of one particular group of pituitary cells, leading to hyperfunctional clinical syndromes; however, the hypothesis of a lack of inhibitory influence from the hypothalamus at the origin of adenoma formation has not yet been demonstrated.

BASIC MECHANISMS AND CLASSIFICATION OF ABNORMAL MOVEMENTS

Abnormal movements represent spontaneous involuntary activity appearing at rest or accompanying voluntary motion. There are but three types of abnormal movements: pure involuntary movement, involuntary movement accompanying voluntary movement, and deformed voluntary movements.

A typical example of the first is the postural tremor characteristic of Parkinson's disease, frequently called resting tremor. Representatives of the second category are attitude tremor and dystonia. A perfect example of the latter is the action myoclonus accompanying some cerebellar lesions. Analysis of the examples given demonstrates that there are but three circumstances in which an abnormal movement can appear: posture, attitude, and movements.

Abnormal Movement During Posture

During posture, there is an absence of voluntary contraction. The limbs are abandoned to the force of gravity. The only detectable activity on the muscles is the reflex antigravity contraction responsible for the permanent tone. Labyrinthine, visual, and proprioceptive impulses are at the origin of reflex antigravity posture.

Elementary antigravity postures are represented in the reticular substance of the midbrain. They are enhanced by cerebellovestibular efferents. There is an increasing evidence that vestibulospinal projections acts predominantly on gamma static motor neurons of extensor muscles. The maneuvers of Jendrassik and Froment selectively increase the vestibulospinal drive, thus leading to increase of antigravity muscle tone. Premotor cortex through fronto-ponto-cerebellar connections probably represent a feedback mechanism that permits the cerebellum to react constantly through the different phases of movements in order to maintain the equilibrium between agonistic and antagonistic muscles. Inhibitory control of posture comes from many sources but fundamentally from the substantia nigra and the neostriatum. Degeneration of nigral cells determines lack of activation of striatal dopaminergic neurons which results in turn in postural plastic hypertonia characteristic of parkinsonian syndrome. In the first stage of Parkinson's disease, there is an exaggeration of postural reflexes with secondary slowness of movements. It is only in the more advanced forms of the disease, when the degeneration involves the neurons of the midbrain tegmentum and the periaqueductal gray matter, that postural reflexes diminish as a manifestation of primary akinesia. Administration of levodopa can dramatically suppress the plastic rigidity if nevertheless there are still nigral and striatal cells capable of using the exogenous dopamine. Surgery produces an analogue effect but through a diametrically opposed mechanism. Instead of reactivating the inhibitory action, like levodopa, surgery diminishes the overactivity of facilitatory structures.

On the other hand, in inferior vertebrates, midbrain reticular formation and paleostriatum are the main motor centers responsible for the primitive rhythmic movements. In superior vertebrates, the activity of this center is subject to the inhibitory influence of the pars compacta of the substantia nigra. Lesions of the latter result in uncontrolled activity of the former, which is manifested clinically by the postural or resting tremor of the parkinsonian syndrome.

Abnormal Movements During Attitude

Attitude can be defined as a posture maintained against the force of gravity with a precise goal. The normal movements represent a continuous change like a kaleidoscope from one attitude to another. Parallel to the relative loss of importance in mammals—and particularly in primates—of the primitive midbrain center, new thalamocortical circuits develop, and these are responsible for nonrhythmic skilled movements of the upper limbs and the face. Simultaneously, new inhibitory structures such as the small cells of putamen and caudate nuclei and the subthalamic corpus Luysii exert an inhibitory control over attitudes or movements of cortical origin. Lesions of the neostriatum will result in a series of abnormal movements that appear precisely during voluntary antigravity postures. The relative importance of the loss of function of parts controlling phasic or tonic mechanisms will condition the different clinical aspects of striatal disease that always predominate in those parts responsible for the most refined and voluntary movements, that of the mouth, the tongue, and the fingers. The subthalamic nucleus exerts its influence over the proximal parts of the limbs, and its lesion results in hemiballismus.

Abnormal Movements During Voluntary Phasic Activity

Execution of voluntary phasic movements, either automatic or conscious, requires an extremely refined control of reciprocal innervation. The first purposeful movements of the child trying to catch one hand with the other shows dramatically the lack of this control. Only after repeated errors and corrections does the child's brain *learn*. And the record of each performance is then carefully kept for future automatic use. The cerebellum is the computer that adjusts carefully, all through the execution of movements, the reciprocal innervation of antagonistic *pairs,* according to the model previously recorded. Cerebellar disease results in disruption of these previous recordings and the loss of adjustment of reciprocal innervation. This control is carried out according to a constant pattern: the cerebellum increases gamma and diminishes alpha motor neuron excitability. Cerebellar dysfunction results in loss of function of the gamma system responsible for the negative symptom and in overfunction of alpha motor neurons responsible for the positive manifestation of cerebellar dyskinesia.

The abnormal movements more frequently encountered have been classified in Table 2 in three groups according to the criteria discussed above. On the other hand, subgroups have been established according to the tonic or phasic, positive or negative character of each symptom.

CLINICAL SYMPTOMATOLOGY OF ABNORMAL MOVEMENT

Since this volume deals only with functional neurosurgery, the discussion that follows will be of "semiology" and not of "nosology." Functional neurosurgery indeed is oriented to symptoms and not to diseases. On the other hand, the discussion will deliberately be devoted to those symptoms that can be successfully suppressed by surgery. In the classification given above, these symptoms belong to the category "positive." (It is obvious that surgery can only correct symptoms resulting in overfunction.) The "negative" manifestations of the loss of function because of a lesion can only be increased by surgery. There are negative consequences of positive symptoms that we can also improve but these seldom contribute to the main goal of the treatment.

We will describe first the tremors that are the main indication for surgery. In second place, the mechanism and the different clinical aspects of torticollis will be discussed. Finally, the different manifestations of cerebellar dyskinesia will be reviewed.

TABLE 2. *Classification of Abnormal Movements*

Characteristics of symptom	Negative	Positive
A. Postural (brain stem)		
Tonic	Akinesia	Parkinsonian rigidity
		Catatonia
Phasic	Akinesia	Postural tremor
B. Attitudinal (Striatum)		
Tonic	Extrapyramidal hypotonia	Dystonia of attitude
		spasms
		dystonia musculorum
		deformans
		torticollis
		Catatonia
Phasic	Extrapyramidal palsy	Chorea
		Athetosis
		Ballism
		Extrapyramidal myoclonus
		Torticollis
		Tremor of attitude
C. Movement (cerebellum)		
Tonic	Cerebellar hypotonia	Decerebration
		"Cerebellar fits" (Jackson)
Phasic	Dysmetria	Cerebellar dyskinesia
		rhythmic myoclonus
		action myoclonus
		movement tremor (or intention)

Semiology of Tremors

In the second century A.D., Galen wrote: "Binas has tremoris species. Primam, quando quescenti homini involuntariis illis et alternis motibus agitantur membra, palpitationem (¶αλμον) dixit, posterionem vero, quae non fit nisi homo conetur partes quasdam movere tremorem (Υρσμ) vocabit" (8) [Two kinds of tremor exist: the first appears while the patient is at rest and consists of involuntary, alternating oscillations of the extremities, and is called "palpitatio"; the second appears only while that individual attempts to move a body part and is called "tremor."] He recognized therefore two types of tremor: the first, the alternating movements that appear in the muscles during rest, and the second, the tremor that appear during voluntary movement of a part of the body. It is only in 1928 that Thomas (20) described the tremor of attitude, which is manifested during the maintenance of a body portion in voluntary contraction against the force of gravity.

If one adopts the restrictive criterion of Dejerine, who defines tremor as "un mouvement involontaire, rythmique et symétrique autour de l'axe d'équilibre du membre" (6) (an involuntary, rhythmic and symmetrical movement about an axis of equilibrium), there are only two types of tremor: the "palpitatio" of Galen and the tremor of attitude of Thomas (20). The first is frequently called "postural" or resting tremor and it corresponds to the tremor most frequently seen in parkinsonian syndromes. The second must be called "attitudinal" tremor and it must be carefully differentiated from Galen's "tremor" which is usually called intention or kinetic tremor, but must be called "movement tremor" according to the definition of Dejerine, however, it is not a true tremor.

The classification of oscillatory movements adopted by the author was originally described in 1971 (17), but the English translation given in Table 3 was published in 1975 (18). The descriptions that follow (a–d) came from this later publication.

(a). *Postural tremor:* Postural tremor appears while the limbs are relaxed with arms alongside the body while reclining, or hanging passively while sitting or walking. In these circumstances, the most important factor from the neurophysiological point of view is the absence of voluntary action. The execution of a voluntary movement, no matter how insignificant, is usually sufficient to stop the tremor. Neglect of this simple observation is the origin of the commonly held notion that tremor persists in repetitive flexion of the arm at the elbow. It is evident that the muscles that flex the elbow are not the same as those that govern movements of the wrist and fingers, which are the immediate effectors of the distal tremor. The latter is, therefore, not affected by movements of the shoulder or the elbow. Even the muscular tension that results from fixing attention on the tremulous limb is usually sufficient in most cases to interrupt, at least momentarily, the tremor. It is also apparent that practically any circumstance favoring relaxation of the affected extremity enhances the tremor.

Postural tremor is one of the symptoms of the parkinsonian syndrome and it is rare to find true postural tremor in other cases of Parkinson's disease. Without involving ourselves in a discussion of the different clinical forms of Parkinson's disease, we can summarize the various aspects of postural tremor by studying it as it appears throughout the evolution of the disease. At the onset, the tremor appears only during fatigue or emotional upset, and it consists of muscular contractions that are more or less rhythmic, rapid, and inconstant. The amplitude remains small and the tremor resembles a physiological tremor or shivering. At this early stage of the disease, it may be difficult to ascertain the diagnosis. Later, the tremor becomes more evident, the contractions assume a greater amplitude, the rhythm becomes slower and more regular, and if the patient maintains a relaxed posture, the tremor will persist. Moreover, electromyography or simple muscle palpation demonstrates the alternating character of the tremor.

TABLE 3. *Classification of oscillatory movements*

A. Tremor
   1. Postural
   2. Attitudinal
   3. Mixed (postural and attitudinal)
B. Movement tremor (intention or kinetic)
C. Vibratory trembling (physiological tremor, normal or exaggerated)

When confronted by an advanced case of Parkinson's disease, one may have the impression that the tremor is mixed, at times postural and at times kinetic. The rigidity may be sufficiently marked that the hand and forearm remain fixed in the original posture during movement at the proximal joints. In these cases, it suffices to ask the patient to move his fingers to abolish the tremor. Similarly, while executing the movement of bringing an index finger close to the nose, the patient's tremor disappears, but once the goal has been attained and maintained, the tremor reappears. The same phenomenon has occurred in this case, and because of the proximal rigidity, the voluntary attitude of the hands becomes, after a few seconds, a relaxed posture. It is only necessary to ask the patient to replace his fingers properly in front of his nose and the tremor disappears.

As the illness progresses to the later stages, one witnesses the gradual disorganization of the tremor. It diminishes in amplitude and regularity and, in many cases, disappears. In short, the patient becomes akinetic and in the process the inverse relationship between tremor and akinesia appears.

Postural tremor is also present in the lower extremities of parkinsonian patients and presents the same characteristics as in the upper extremities, although the rhythm is generally slower (3 to 5 cps). When the tremor of the head is present, it is most often of the affirmative type, characterized by alternating contraction of the neck flexors and extensors. As the illness advances, the tremor diminishes or disappears, possibly because of hypertonia of the flexors maintaining the head in a permanently flexed and rigid posture. Occasionally rhythmical and asymmetrical muscular contractions persist, but these are usually insufficient to displace the head. When the mouth, tongue, and pharynx are affected by the tremor, the speech becomes repetitious, as the patient repeats words or syllables. This phenomenon is referred to as palilalia. Figure 1 shows a cinepho-

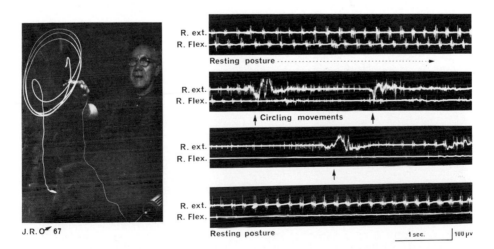

FIG. 1. Cinephotographic and electromyographic recording of postural tremor.

tography and electromyographic recording of an example of postural tremor.

(b) *Attitudinal tremor:* The conditions for the appearance of tremor of attitude are almost diametrically opposed to those of postural tremor. Tremor of attitude is absent when the extremities are being supported or are hanging passively at rest while standing or walking. It manifests itself only while the patient consciously maintains an attitude against the force of gravity and when this attitude is directed toward a precise goal (Fig. 2); it continues as long as the attitude is maintained. Moreover, the more complex the attitude, the greater the intensity of the tremor, as for example in the holding of a glass near the lips or when the patient is impeded from sustaining a definite attitude. The most important neurophysiological consideration is the associated increase in voluntary motor action in carrying out a specific attitudinal objective. The tremor of attitude is distinguished from postural tremor in that the latter appears without voluntary action; however, postural and attitudinal tremor are similar in that neither appears during phasic movement. One may say that both, in a sense, are static tremors.

It is important to differentiate tremor of attitude of the head from postural tremor of the head and also from ataxia of the trunk secondary to cerebellar lesions. The following are criteria used in differentiating the etiology of the tremor.

Tremor of attitude of the head is absent when the head is supported and the muscles of the neck are relaxed. It is apparent that the amplitude of the tremor is directly proportional to the extent of voluntary muscle activity and one can see the progressive increase of the tremor as the patient lifts himself

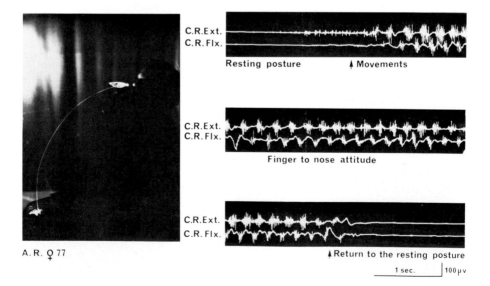

C.R.Ext.
C.R.Flx.
Resting posture   ↟ Movements

C.R.Ext.
C.R.Flx.
Finger to nose attitude

C.R.Ext.
C.R.Flx.
A.R. ♀ 77   ↟ Return to the resting posture

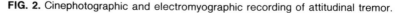

1 sec.   100 μv

FIG. 2. Cinephotographic and electromyographic recording of attitudinal tremor.

from his bed. The tremor may be increased if the examiner, holding the patient's head to impede rotation, asks the subject to turn his head. These characteristics are unlike those seen in postural tremor.

The second characteristic, which in our experience is always present, is that attitude tremor of the head is of the negative type, whereas postural tremor is of the affirmative type. This is because postural tremor is a function of the progravity and antigravity muscles, while tremor of attitude affects the muscles used in turning the head to the side.

The most common type of attitudinal tremor is probably the so-called essential or heredofamilial tremor; however, this is not the only form. Tremor of attitude is also associated with any of the diseases collectively referred to as "pathology of attitude," i.e., it may be present in dystonia of an isolated limb, dystonia musculorum deformans, spasmodic torticollis, athetosis. Tremor of attitude is also seen with cerebral tumors involving the striatum.

A true tremor of attitude is also seen in some patients with multiple sclerosis, but this is infrequent. In most cases, the tremor is referred to as an intention tremor secondary to cerebellar disease. In fact, tremor of attitude is probably caused by a sclerotic plaque in the striatum (unpublished cases).

(c) *Mixed tremor:* A mixed tremor that has both postural and attitudinal characteristics is rarely encountered. With this combination, the tremor manifests itself while the patient is at rest, standing, sitting, or reclining. It is also present whenever the patient assumes an attitude requiring willful maintenance; however, the tremor disappears throughout the execution of purposeful movements.

This type of tremor is encountered in about 1 to 2% of cases of tremors. In half of the cases, there is a relation with Parkinson's disease, but as a rule the disease of patients with mixed tremor has evolved over a period of several years without rigidity, akinesia, dystonia or other symptoms of basal ganglia disease. Figure 3 shows an example of this category.

(d) *Movement tremor:* The distinction made by Galen established an important notion: kinetic tremor was not produced by the so-called "palpitatio" of muscles but was a result of the articular displacements that decompose the movement into irregular shaking excursions. One might argue that every articular displacement has been caused by a muscular contraction and conversely that every muscular contraction engenders the displacement of an articulation. This is not always the case. One may observe the isolated contraction of a muscle or a part of it without articular displacement, and it is the latter that we see with parkinsonian patients. EMG recordings show rhythmic muscular discharges ("palpitatio" of Galen) without the tremor; however, so-called kinetic tremor, while absent without movement, is more apparent whenever the extremity is made to execute bigger movements, because of the coming into play of the greater articulations. This fundamental characteristic is well described by de la Boe, who called it movement tremor ("motu tremulo"). The analysis of EMG recording and cinematography has demonstrated that kinetic tremor is characterized by intermittent, irregular, nonrhythmic contractions and manifests itself

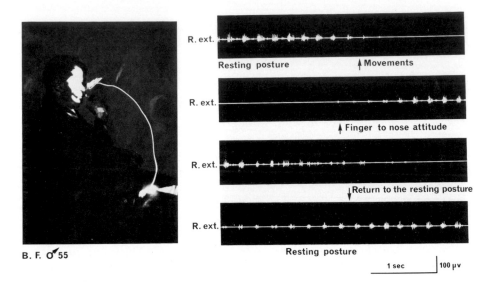

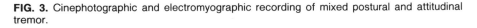

FIG. 3. Cinephotographic and electromyographic recording of mixed postural and attitudinal tremor.

to a greater degree in those muscle groups most directly involved in the voluntary motor control of a movement. It is also apparent that the closer the movement comes to completion, the more violent is the tremor. The tremor ceases once the movement has been completed. On the other hand, if the examiner supports the patient's extremity while he executes the movement, the tremor does not appear and the movement is completed without error. Finally, automatic movements such as swinging the arms while walking are completely without evidence of tremor. Thus, the kinetic tremor is *not* a true tremor since it is neither rhythmic nor symmetrical, and it is not present about a body axis of equilibrium. Figure 4 illustrates this type of tremor in a patient with a posttraumatic Benedikt's syndrome.

It is thought that the cerebellum controls the harmony of voluntary movement by coordinating muscular agonists and antagonists, and by judgment of distance, so that precise movement can be achieved. Disturbance of these mechanisms by a cerebellar lesion produces dysmetria, incoordination and ataxia. The exaggeration of these abnormalities is represented by the kinetic tremor. This tremor is less apparent in diseases of cerebellar afferents. With the spinocerebellar degenerations and tumors of the hemisphere one rarely sees kinetic tremor but merely a moderate degree of ataxia. On the other hand, lesions of the superior mesencephalon which compromise the cerebellar efferents produce involuntary oscillations. These become more violent as the end of the movement is approached and can be easily confused with a true tremor. Photographic and EMG analysis demonstrate that it is no more than a particularly violent, nonrhythmical and asymmetrical ataxia.

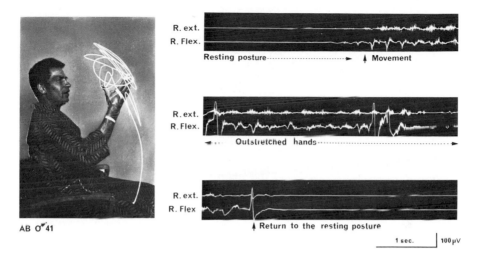

R. ext.
R. Flex.

Resting posture--------------------------► ↑ Movement

R. ext.
R. Flex.

◄··· Outstretched hands--►

R. ext.
R. Flex

AB O⁻41

↑ Return to the resting posture

1 sec.   100 µV

FIG. 4. Cinephotographic and electromyographic recording of movement tremor.

Torticollis

Spasmodic torticollis can be defined as an involuntary rotation of the head because of the loss of function of a structure which normally inhibits this movement. The great number of muscles participating in the lateral orientation of the head and the variable participation of each one from case to case explain the almost infinite variety of clinical forms. We can indeed find rotation alone or combined with different degrees of tilting, flexion, or extension of the head. Definition of the degree of participation of muscles is of paramount importance for the choice of the surgical technique and it must be done with the help of electromyography and blocking techniques (2,16). Before that, there is, nevertheless, one important question to answer: namely to establish for each case if it is a pure torticollis or if it is only a symptom of the torsion dystonia syndrome. Although I am personally convinced that both forms share a common physiopathology, there is a profound difference of character. Pure torticollis represents a self-limited disease frequently nonprogressive. Like the tremor of attitude which is frequently associated in the patient himself or in the family, it represents a striatal dysfunction transmitted by heredity according to a dominant autosomal mode. Torsion dystonia is the clinical manifestation of a remarkable progressive degenerative disease, frequently inherited also as a dominant autosomal trait, known with the denomination of dystonia musculorum deformans. Torticollis represents in this case only one of the many clinical symptoms of the disease. Usually, but not always, phasic torticollis (abnormal movements of rotation) belongs to the first category, while tonic torticollis (abnormal immobile attitude of the head) is, as a rule, a manifestation of the dystonia musculorum deformans.

Since the main source of stimuli for the rotary motion of the head is the

TABLE 4.
Classification of
spasmodic torticollis

A. Peripheral
   1. Vestibular
   2. Spinal
B. Central or striatal
   1. Tonic
   2. Phasic
C. Psychogenic

vestibular system, irritative lesions of this system, located either in the peripheral or central pathways, can provoke a torticollis. Careful investigation of vestibular function must be done in each case of pure torticollis (1).

Finally, since the sternocleidomastoid is one of the most powerful muscles involved in rotation of the head, an irritative lesion of the spinal nerve could result in a torticollis, just as irritation of facial nerve provokes hemifacial spasms, irritation of trigeminal nerve provokes trigeminal neuralgia, and as irritation of vestibular and cochlear never provokes vertigo and tinnitus.

Psychogenia has progressively lost importance as the cause of torticollis. The denomination of "torticollis mentallis" given by Brissaud in 1895 has been long since forgotten (4).

Psychogenia is in torticollis the equivalent of dental caries in trigeminal neuralgia: a diagnosis and treatment applied to the patient before the correct diagnosis is made. For the sake of completeness, however, it will be retained in the following classification of the disease torticollis (Table 4).

Cerebellar Dyskinesia

Movement or intention tremor has already been described as the last form of tremor. It represents the most common form of uncontrolled cerebellar lesion.

The second form of cerebellar dyskinesia that can be treated by surgery is the cerebellar myoclonus. According to Bonduelle (3), the more general and uncommitting definition of myoclonus will be "that of a sudden sharp involuntary muscular jerk." There are many forms of abnormal movements that can be included in this definition. According to the localization of the lesion responsible and to the underlying physiopathology, all myoclonus belongs to one of these four categories: epileptic myoclonus, extrapyramidal disease, cerebellar lesions, and spinal cord lesions. All types of myoclonus have in common the fact that they represent an overfunction release phenomenon, but only extrapyramidal and cerebellar myoclonus are "stricto sensu" abnormal movements, according to the definition that we adopted.

Extrapyramidal myoclonus is the most elementary form of basal ganglia disease. It seldom appears isolated. Usually it is one of the symptoms, often unnoticed, accompanying striatal diseases. The association of myoclonus with attitudinal tremor, particularly of the head, and with torsion dystonia, is well known. In these cases, myoclonus is precisely the symptom that responds better to surgery.

In cerebellar disease, myoclonus is a major manifestation. The common characteristic to all types of cerebellar myoclonus is its relation with voluntary movement. They are all action myoclonus. When the limbs are abandoned to the force of gravity or sustained in static attitude and even in action ("manoeuvre du geste accompagné"), the myoclonus, as the other manifestation of cerebellar dyskinesia, diminishes or disappears. That is the case of the myoclonus of the "dyssynergia cerebellaris myoclonica" of Ramsay Hunt and of the "action myoclonus" described by Lance and Adams (13) in hypoxic encephalopathy.

All types of cerebellar lesions—degenerative, tumoral, and traumatic—can be accompanied by myoclonus. But myoclonus is never an acute manifestation of those diseases. It takes months after the appearance of the negative symptoms. A patient of mine with severe head injuries that led to a Benedikt's syndrome with bilateral movement tremor, in which a stereotactic lesion of the ventro-oralis posterior successfully suppressed the tremor on one side, a palatal rhythmic myoclonus in association with an action myoclonus of the upper extremity ipsilateral to the thalamic lesion appeared 4 months after surgery and 10 months after injury. The pathologic results showed a bilateral olivary pseudohypertrophia. Two small traumatic lesions of one dentate nucleus and the contralateral brachium conjunctivum explain the secondary degeneration of the olives in this remarkable case. Guillain and Mollaret described in 1931 (9) the triangle formed by the red nucleus and the olive of one side with the dentate nucleus of the opposite side, the involvement of which is the common pathological feature of palatal myoclonus.

SUMMARY

The description of an apparent heterogeneous group of pathologic conditions under the heading brain functional disorders seems justified by the existence of a common underlying physiopathology. Indeed, all of them appear as the result of hyperfunction of some "normal" primitive center deprived of the inhibitory control of a superior center, "abnormal" as a result of some lesion. Brain functional disorders must be treated by functional neurosurgery, the goal being to reestablish normal function through action in the normal, yet overfunctioning center. Therefore, in the presence of a brain functional disorder, the critical point is not, as in general neurosurgery, to find a lesion, but to understand a mechanism. Functional neurosurgery can only be applied once that is achieved. That probably justifies the length and the rather philosophical approach of this chapter.

REFERENCES

1. Bertrand, R. A., Molina, P., and Hardy, J. (1977): Vestibular syndrome and vascular anomaly in the cerebello-pontine angle. *Acta Otolaryngol.,* 83:187–194.
2. Bertrand, C., Molina, P., and Martinez, S. N. (1978): Unilateral combined stereotactic and peripheral surgery in spasmodic torticollis. *Appl. Neurophysiol. (in press).*
3. Bonduelle, M. (1975): The myoclonia. In: *Handbook of Clinical Neurology,* Vol. 6, edited by P. J. Vinken and G. W. Broyn, p. 761. Elsevier, New York.
4. Brissaud, E. (1895): *Leçons sur les Maladies Nerveuses.* Recueilliés et publiées par H. Meige. Masson, Paris.
5. Cajal, S. R. (1952): *Histologie du Système Nerveux de l'Homme et des Vertébrés.* CSIC., Madrid.
6. Dejerine, J. (1902): *Sémiologie du Système Nerveux,* pp. 667–681. Masson, Paris.
7. Denny-Brown, D. (1975): Clinical Symptomatology of Basal Ganglia Diseases. In: *Handbook of Clinical Neurology,* Vol. 6, edited by P. J. Vinken and G. W. Bruyn, p. 153. Elsevier, New York.
8. Galenus: De Tremore. Chart. Tome VII, pp. 200–201 (quoted by J. Parkinson: "Essay on the Shaking Palsy," Sherwood, Neely, and Jones, London (1917).
9. Guillain, G., and Mollaret, P. (1931): Deux Cas de Myoclonies Synchrones et Rythmées Vélo-Pharyngo-Laryngo-Diaphragmatiques. Le problème anatomique et physiopathologique de ce syndrome. *Rev. Neurol.,* 2:545–566.
10. Hardy, J., Marino, R., and Molina, P. (1974): Epilepsie Sursault et Foyers Corticaux Multiples. Guérison d'un cas. Société de Neurochirurgie de Langue Française.
11. Jackson, J. H. (1958): In: *Selected Writings of John Hughlings Jackson,* edited by J. Taylor, Vol. 1, p. 93. Basic Books, New York.
12. Kuhlenbeck, H. (1967): *The Cerebral Nervous System of Vertebrates,* p. 154. Academic Press, New York.
13. Lance, J. W., and Adams, R. D. (1963): The syndrome of intention or action myoclonus as a sequel to hypoxic encephalopathy. *Brain,* 86:111–136.
14. Melzack, R., and Wall, P. D. (1965): Pain mechanisms . . . a new theory. *Science,* 150:971–979.
15. Mark, V. H., and Ervin, R. F. (1970): *Violence and the Brain.* Harper and Row, New York.
16. Molina, P., Bertrand, C., Martinez, S. N., and Hardy, J. (1974): Controlled Lesions of VOI and Adjoining Structures in Stereotactic Surgery of Spasmodic Torticollis. Presented at the Harvey Cushing Society, St. Louis.
17. Molina-Negro, P., and Hardy, J. (1971): Etude Sémiologique des Tremblements. *Union Med. Can.* 100:879–895.
18. Molina-Negro, P., and Hardy, J. (1975): Semiology of Tremors. *Can. J. Neurol. Sci.,* pp. 23–29.
19. Spencer, H. (1901): The principles of psychology. Appleton & Co., London.
20. Thomas, A., and Long-Landry, E. (1928): Deux Cas de Tremblement d'Attitude du Membre Supérieur. *Rev. Neurol.,* 1:585–587.
21. Wall, P. D. (1976): Modulation of pain by non-painful events. In: *Advances in Pain Research and Therapy,* Vol. 1, p. 14. Raven Press, New York.

Functional Neurosurgery, edited by T. Rasmussen
and R. Marino. Raven Press, New York © 1979.

Frontiers of Functional Neurosurgery in Biomedical Research

Ayub K. Ommaya

*Surgical Neurology Branch, Section on Applied Research, National Institute of Neurological
and Communicative Disorders and Stroke, National Institutes of Health,
Bethesda, Maryland 20014*

There is little doubt that functional neurosurgery is rapidly becoming the
field in which neurosurgeons can make major contributions to medical research
in the neurosciences. Based primarily on our own experience with functional
neurosurgery at the National Institutes of Health (NIH), I would like to offer
a classification of what I consider to be the existing and potential scope of
techniques available to the neurosurgeon and then discuss how such methods
can be used in research as well as in practice. Three general classes of technique
are involved, i.e., *physical, chemical,* and *biological.* To date, the contribution
of the physical techniques of stimulation and lesion making have provided the
major part of our contribution to medicine and biological research, particularly
in the fields of epilepsy, pain, and certain psychiatric conditions. It should be
noted, moreover, that neurology itself has always been based on the use of
the classical technique of lesion analysis. The use of chemical techniques has
been only tentatively approached, and truly biological methods remain at the
conceptual stage. I will discuss each set of existing and potential techniques,
not in an attempt to review exhaustively all the possibilities, but to consider
with a few examples what I think are unique opportunities offered by each
method and approach, and how each method may help not only to uncover
facts by itself but also serve to generate ideas suitable for testing with the other
modalities. This aspect will be illustrated by a brief description of our hypothesis
for consciousness and cognitive functions based on our observations in functional
neurosurgery. In conclusion, I will touch upon an important issue which is
particularly relevant to functional neurosurgery and which we always have to
bear in mind, namely, the boundary, real or imaginary, between medical research
and medical practice.

PHYSICAL METHODS

The classical techniques of functional neurosurgery include the utilization
of controlled ablation or stimulation of specific areas with subsequent behavior
analysis compared to preoperative observations. The power of such methods

was first clearly demonstrated by Fritsch and Hitzig in the nineteenth century and pioneered by the father of both structural and functional neurosurgery, Sir Victor Horsley. Our work at the NIH over the past 15 years has centered primarily on the study of the mechanisms for memory, language, and other cognitive functions in man, primarily based on our experience in treating patients suffering from epilepsy, intractable pain, and involuntary movements. Two sets of studies will be briefly summarized: the first consists of observations aimed at uncovering the contribution of the cingulum and medial temporal structures to memory mechanisms in man, and the second consists of a double-blind evaluation of the effect of cerebellar stimulation in the treatment of epilepsy. The first study was carried out by Dr. Fedio and myself and the second by Dr. Van Buren with Drs. Wood, Oakley, and Hambrecht.

Contributions of Limbic System Structures to Memory Mechanisms in Man

Three groups of neurosurgical patients formed the basis for this study, each group having either depth stimulation or therapeutic resection of specific limbic structures. The first series consisted of patients with intractable pain undergoing stereotactic bilateral cingulotomy using chronic indwelling stimulating or lesion-making electrodes. The second series consisted of patients with intractable epilepsy with suspected bitemporal foci undergoing bitemporal stereotactic implantation of chronic electrodes in the temporal lobe and hippocampus for further diagnostic evaluation. The third group of patients consisted of subjects who had undergone a unilateral left or right subtotal temporal lobectomy for the relief of intractable psychomotor epilepsy.

Surgical removal in all the cases measured 5 to 6 cm along the lateral temporal cortex from the tip of the temporal pole, the resection invariably involving the temporal gyri and varying portions of both hippocampus and hippocampal gyri. The cognitive tests that were used were also administered to a group of normal volunteer subjects for comparison with the lobectomy patients. The test procedures used are given in detail in a forthcoming article of mine (8); these procedures consisted of a set of separately administered verbal and nonverbal tasks. The verbal tests consisted of familiar objects which had to be named and recalled in a serial order, and the nonverbal objects were 20 sets of random complex forms of structures which did not lend themselves easily to verbal description.

Results of Stimulation and Lesion Formation in the Cingulum Bilaterally

The data clearly showed that left cingulum stimulation disrupted short-term verbal memory quite markedly as compared to the minimal effects associated with stimulation of the right cingulum or of the frontal white matter on either side. The results of the nonverbal tests showed a reversal of this effect with the right cingulum stimulation disrupting nonverbal short-term memory much more than equivalent stimulation of the left cingulum; however, it was found that stimulation of the frontal white matter from either the right or left side appeared to disrupt short-term nonverbal memory equally. This white matter effect was not significantly less than that produced by right cingulum stimulation. This observation was of key significance in the development of our unitary hypothesis for the mechanism of consciousness and of higher cerebral functions, which is presented in a subsequent section of this chapter. In striking contrast to these effects of stimulation on the cingulum, postoperative analysis of the cingulumotomy patient's performance on Memory and I.Q. tests, after lesions had been completed, failed to reveal any significant deficit whatsoever. Thus, memory scores as well as verbal and perceptual organization factors for intelligence were unaffected by bilateral cingulumotomy. The lesions were made with radio-frequency heating bilaterally and were large enough to be recognized easily at subsequent CT scanning.

Effects of Stimulation of the Temporal White Matter, Amygdala, and Hippocampus on Memory

Stimulation in either the right or left anterior temporal white matter could not disrupt short-term memory as tested by the verbal and nonverbal tests described above. Neither did such stimulation disrupt the performance of the patients on three separate tests of perception and learning. Electrical stimulation of the amygdala at sites plotted to be within this structure on both the right and left sides also were without effect on the perception or recall of the verbal and nonverbal material described above. Of particular interest was the observation that temporal lobe stimulation in the hippocampus with identical parameters produced negligible effects on memory performance. In contrast to a base line of prestimulation performance at an error rate of 5 to 10% on both verbal and nonverbal tasks, bilateral hippocampus stimulation was associated with only a very slight increase in errors (between 12 and 16%) both on the verbal and nonverbal memory task. The effect in any event was markedly less than that seen with cingulum stimulation. At no time did we observe aphasia or perceptual disturbances during stimulation of the left or right hippocampus.

The Effects of Right or Left Temporal Lobectomy on Learning and Memory Processes

Our results with the verbal and nonverbal tests were almost identical to those found by Milner in the much larger material from the Montreal Neurological Institute. Patients with a right temporal lobectomy required many more trials to learn nonverbal material as compared to normal patients or patients after left temporal lobectomy. Conversely, left temporal lobectomy patients had greater difficulty in learning verbal material compared to the remaining groups. Our investigations thus confirmed and extended the evidence for lateralization of verbal and nonverbal functions, but brought out a new factor which had not been sufficiently recognized in the earlier investigations. This was the identification of a greater disruptive effect only on nonverbal material by stimulation of the white matter bilaterally as compared to the more strictly localized effect on verbal material with stimulation from the left side. In addition, our findings distinguished an immediate or short-term memory mechanism which can, for example, be defined by the digit span of the individual from an apparently separate mechanism responsible for developing a "supra-span" or learning of more complex memoranda, as previously described by us (3,4). Whether the supra-span secondary mechanism is defective after temporal lobe lesions by virtue of inability to store or consolidate new memoranda or simply by an inability to retrieve items from normally continuing storage has not yet been decided. However, we were able to bring out clearly the dissociation between the short-term memory span for both verbal and nonverbal material, which always remained intact after temporal lobectomy, and the longer-term inability to learn complex (or supra-span) memoranda, which is always disrupted after temporal lobectomy.

These findings tend to support the idea of a dual mechanism for memory. The contrasting effects of cingulum stimulation and cingulum lesions on short-term memory are probably best explained by postulating a downstream effect on limbic structures in the temporal lobe. Because of the anatomical projection of the cingulum to the hippocampal gyrus and the lack of interference with memory by direct hippocampal stimulation, we believe that the mesocortex of the hippocampal gyrus is the critical zone for memory coding.

Our hypothesis is that there is a dual role for the limbic system in memory. The more ancient inner limbic ring, which includes fornix, amygdala, and hippocampus, is primarily concerned with providing the emotive or affective "tagging" of new memoranda probably via hypothalamic mechanisms. More specific coding for memory is the function of the outer limbic ring, which includes the cingulum, hippocampal gyrus, and uncinate bundle. The cingulum is postulated as functioning primarily as a connecting system between the affective coding of the inner limbic ring, primarily by the hippocampus, and the retrieval coding of the outer limbic ring, primarily by the hippocampal gyrus. This would explain why stimulation in the cingulum would interfere with memory. The crucial function of the hippocampal gyrus in memory fits with all the published data on patients with amnesia and lesions of the hippocampal complex. Such anatomical data have previously been interpreted rather loosely as indicating that it is the hippocampus which is significant for the memory defect seen in patients with lesions of this zone. On close examination of the data, however, it is clear that none of these patients had lesions, which spared the hippocampal gyrus.

The only publication we have been able to find which clearly described lesions made selectively in the hippocampus only, in 7 patients, with sparing of the hippocampal gyrus is that by Gol and Fabish (5), who failed to observe the type of severe memory defect seen by Scoville and Milner after bitemporal lobectomy. We have not found any data on the effect of lesions confined to the hippocampal gyrus alone. It is proposed, therefore, that coding of memoranda for retrieval from storage is carried out by the hippocampal gyrus via the associative neocortex. This associative neocortex functions as a necessary part of the retrieval system for memory in the temporal lobe by storing clues to the reconstruction of experience from a separate storage system. This postulate fits with the established fact that the associative neocortex cannot be the site for storage of the elements of memory itself because temporal lobectomy does not produce significant and permanent retrograde amnesia, such a deficit being clearly seen only in conditions where diffuse neocortical injury is produced, e.g., in cerebral concussion and electroshock therapy (9).

Neuronal storage of memory itself may well be located within the primary sensory cortices from which stimulation can never elicit the memory itself but only modality specific elements of the original trace. Access to such a cortical storage system is available via the associative neocortex of the temporal lobe, where stimulation can produce either a recreation or distortion of experiences, as first observed by Penfield. The demonstration of visual experiential responses and déjà vu phenomena obtained primarily from the nondominant hemisphere fits well with the demonstrated localization of nonverbal mechanisms for memory in the minor hemisphere. We can thus suggest that the cortical area for language is essentially a highly developed part of the retrieval system for word memory, while memories not describable by words are coded for retrieval in a much wider area bilaterally but predominantly on the side opposite to the hemisphere mediating speech and language.

Evaluation of Cerebellar Stimulation in the Treatment for Epilepsy by Double-Blind Stimulation and Biological Criteria (12)

This study, conducted by Van Buren and his associates in our branch, was carried out on 5 patients who were selected as having intractable and medically refractory seizures that had persisted for a period of between 8 to 23 years without remissions. Severe socioeconomic handicaps with an average of over one seizure per day while under hospital observation characterized these patients. All patients had combinations of partial and general seizures with focal and/or bilaterally synchronized epileptic activity consistently found on multiple electroencephalograms. The technique for implantation of the stimulating electrodes and the mode of stimulation were those described by Cooper (2). An attempt was made to evaluate the effect of the stimulation on seizures using a double-blind method as well as assessments of the patient's overall behavior as obtained from the patient's immediate family. In addition, levels of two neural transmitters, GABA and norepinephrine were estimated in the spinal fluid.

Results

No patients were rendered free of seizures. An analysis of these data, comparing seizure frequency before and after cerebellar stimulation, showed no significant alterations that could be attributed to the stimulation or to any of the conditions during the period treatment. Indeed, there was an increase in seizure frequency when the stimulation was on in the late postoperative period, suggesting progression of the patient's disease with time. There was thus clear evidence, at least in this group, that cerebellar stimulation does not have any significant effect on the frequency or severity of seizures. The results of electroencephalographic examination in these patients also confirmed the clinical data. Examination of intelligence and memory functions in these patients showed no change after the implantation and subsequent stimulation.

A totally different outcome was found when the patients' families were asked to give their opinion. Although none of the patients' seizures improved, the families felt that their functional status *was* improved in a way that they could not clearly define. They described such things as increased alertness, more interest in surroundings, and decreased intrafamily strife. They also felt the seizures were less severe, were of shorter duration, and seemed to be upsetting the patients less. In complete contrast to the monitored observations on the ward, they felt that the frequency had reduced while the patients were at home. The general family evaluation, therefore, over the approximately 2-year period of cerebellar stimulation, was positively enthusiastic. Evaluation of the spinal central excitatory state by measurement of H reflexes and the tendon-vibrating responses showed no significant effects.

Extremely interesting data were obtained from evaluation of the cerebrospinal fluid (CSF) neural transmitter levels. The norepinephrine levels in the spinal fluid were found to rise and the GABA (gamma-aminobutyric acid) levels were found to fall with the cerebellar stimulation. In 3 patients, cerebellar biopsy showed atrophy of Purkinje's cells and there was a suggestion that the degree of cerebellar atrophy might be related to the neural transmitter responses in that the greatest rise in norepinephrine was seen in the patient whose biopsy showed the greatest amount of Purkinje's cell retention (75% as compared with normal subjects and relative to the other patients who retained less than 25%). The increased levels of norepinephrine in the CSF noted in these patients receiving cerebellar stimulation could have produced a general mood enhancement and behavior improvement which is opposite to the decline in CSF levels of a norepinephrine metabolite which has been recorded in cases with depression. This work suggests, therefore, that the overall improvement which impressed the family may be related to the relief of the depression associated with the chronic seizure state in these patients. This study also emphasizes the importance of the placebo effect and may indeed suggest one avenue to a study of the mechanisms of such effects.

CHEMICAL APPROACHES IN FUNCTIONAL NEUROSURGERY

The studies with stimulation and lesion techniques described above are good examples of how valuable data may be gathered in the course of treatment and diagnosis. The suggestion of a nonspecific but potentially useful effect on the neural transmitter levels by cerebellar stimulation is also important because it serves to show that behavior can be very precisely modulated by the more diffuse effects of endogenous or exogenous chemical substances; e.g., analogs of brain peptides or neurotransmitters are available and waiting to be tested. One of the difficulties in evaluating the effects of such intraventricular and intrathecal neurosurgical pharmacotherapy has been the lack of a good model that can be directly compared to man. We have recently published our method for the long-term study of intraventricularly or intrathecally administered drugs and intracranial pressure in the rhesus monkey (13). We would suggest that this model is uniquely suited to those pharmacological investigations that are required in order to provide avenues of application of this type of functional neurosurgery in man. By cannulating the fourth ventricle and spinal subarachnoid space without a direct puncture of the nervous tissue, we have been able to obviate the artifacts produced by such hitherto unavoidable brain injury in previous models. Sterile and chronic access to the ventricular CSF or to the CSF without tissue damage is thus allowed and we have confirmed that mixing of injected drugs with lateral ventricular cerebral fluid is complete and predictable. The model is shown in Figs. 1 and 2 and the results of the initial application of our primate model to the pharmacokinetics of methotrexate injected into the spinal fluid are presented in Fig. 3. The disappearance curves for intraventricularly injected methotrexate in our animals were compared with those determined in 93 patients with subcutaneous reservoirs who were receiving methotrexate for meningeal leukemia. The curves for our monkey model are almost identical to those for man, and the absolute concentrations are a proportion of the dosage as compared to the human data. These encouraging data provide us with a tool that can be used to study a number of other systems.

In collaboration with Dr. Floyd Bloom of the Salk Institute, we are currently

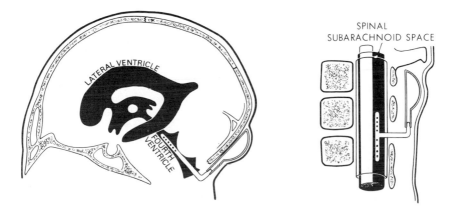

FIG. 1. Placement of catheters in subarachnoid and ventricular spaces and mode of connection to chronically indwelling subcutaneous CSF reservoirs. (From ref. 13, with permission.)

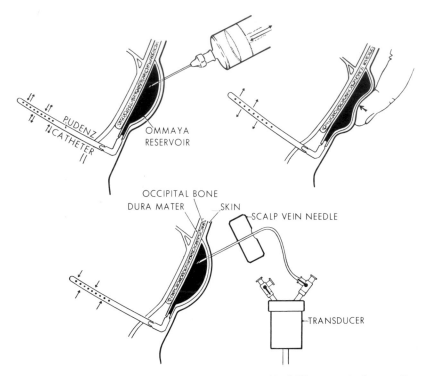

FIG. 2. Techniques of fluid sampling and/or injection with CSF reservoir *(upper diagrams)* and of CSF pressure monitoring *(lower diagram).* (From ref. 13, with permission.)

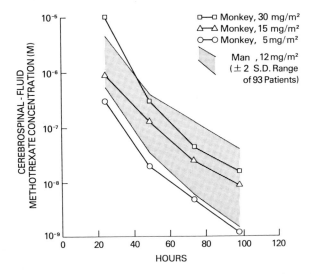

FIG. 3. Plot of methotrexate concentration versus time in human and monkey CSF. Note close correspondence of drug levels from time of injection to time of disappearance. (From ref. 13, with permission.)

investigating the effects of endorphins in this model. The possible application of such techniques to the problems of chronic pain and addiction are obvious. It is not unreasonable to speculate that the development of neurosurgically controlled pharmacotherapy will most probably enable the development of a type of functional neurosurgery that is much less invasive and more specific in the control of a number of disease conditions such as epilepsy, pain, and possibly even behavioral and psychiatric disorders than has hitherto been possible with physical methods.

BIOLOGICAL TECHNIQUES AND FUNCTIONAL NEUROSURGERY

This is probably the most exciting avenue for functional neurosurgery that remains to be developed at this time. By the term *biological* I mean primarily the use of *transplantation* techniques, which are aimed not at altering brain functions by surgical removal or stimulation of a particular site, but by direct addition of exogenous functioning tissues that can provide factors deficient in that brain and that may fulfill very specific purposes. Two areas in which observations have been recently made are particularly pertinent. The first is the use of grafts from the peripheral nervous system introduced into the central nervous system. A fundamental contribution in this area has recently been published by Blakemore, who has demonstrated that Schwann's cells transplanted from sciatic nerve into the CNS (central nervous system) can remyelinate CNS axons (1). Blakemore prepared small localized areas of primary demyelination in experimental areas that do not normally demyelinate as a model for the persistently demyelinating plaques of multiple sclerosis. Using a portion of the animal's own sciatic nerve as a source of viable Schwann's cells, he was able to show that these nerve transplants provided the source for remyelination of the naked axons. The most marked effects occurred with axons close to the transplanted cells, with distant axons remaining unmyelinated. The implications of these observations for human neurology, and particularly for the treatment of multiple sclerosis by functional neurosurgery, are clearly evident. We are currently conducting experiments in our laboratory to replicate these experiments in a model for traumatic demyelination in the rhesus monkey.

A second set of observations utilizing the technique of peripheral nerve transplants into the CNS has been published by Kao in a series of pioneering observations made over the last 5 years. Using dogs, he has shown that it is occasionally possible to obtain regeneration of a neurologically useful type across a completely crushed spinal cord in the dog, provided a peripheral nerve graft is used 1 week after the initial crushing lesion (6). This key step of delaying the nerve graft for 1 week after initial injury allows the grafted nerve to function as a source of Schwann's cells which can myelinate the axons emerging from the transected cord. The axons can now do so because of removal of the postinjury cavitation debris and an apparently weaker neuroglial scarring reaction. Because of the difficulties of interpreting neurological recovery in dogs, since dogs have significant reflex mechanisms for walking and standing at the spinal cord level, we have decided to replicate the nerve-grafting study in the subhuman primate, in which paraplegia was induced. Currently, 12 rhesus monkeys have undergone spinal cord crushing and nerve grafting using a modification of this technique which is evaluating the relative merits of a variety of Schwann's cell source transplants in conjunction with a study of the effect of pulsed high-energy radio-frequency waves on cord healing.

Finally, Teuber has drawn our attention to recent unpublished observations that certain brain structures, e.g., the hippocampus in mammals, can accept permanent implants of nerve cells secreting various neurotransmitters (11). The implications of such a combination of biological and pharmacotherapeutic approaches should also be of interest to the functional neurosurgeon.

It is obvious, from this brief review of some of the ways in which functional neurosurgery may grow, that the young neurosurgeon entering this field will have to develop his skills not only in the classical techniques of lesion making and neural stimulation, but he will also have to learn methods in the fields of pharmacology and neurobiology. Only in this way can neurosurgeons remain in the forefront of biomedical research.

A HYPOTHESIS FOR THE MECHANISM OF CONSCIOUSNESS AND HIGHER CEREBRAL FUNCTIONS IN MAN

Based on our observations made during functional neurosurgery for the relief of pain, epilepsy, and involuntary movements, we have developed a unitary hypothesis for the "how" and "why" of cerebral asymmetry in the localization of higher cerebral functions and the relation of this to the problem of consciousness. We postulate that instead of the current dualistic theories of left/right brain, apositional vs. prepositional functions, and similar language vs. visuospatial dichotomies, it is more parsimonious to conceive of the linguistic mode of cognition as being the externally dominant mode of motor expression, which in turn can only function optimally when complemented by the internally dominant mode of "gnostic" cognition, which sets the stage as it were for the analytic linguistic mode to function in the proper synthetic contexts provided by the gnostic mode. This complementarity is provided by a unitary mechanism which evolves to allow progressively increasing abstraction from sensory reality in order to free the brain from the essentially "hard-wired" reflexive behavior of bilaterally symmetric brains by increasing asymmetry of functions. The signal benefit of this development in phylogeny is that such an asymmetry enables a much larger variety of motor programs to be internally rehearsed without any obligatory motor output linkage as required by the more primitive bilaterally symmetric brains. This step permits the formation of what is best called "the critical attitude," which is considered to be analogous to increasing the *content* of consciousness. This development in phylogeny enhances individual survival directly rather than simple survival of the species, an effect which is quite adequately supported by the bilaterally symmetric brain. The evidence and arguments for this hypothesis and its development as an experimentally testable theory are to be published elsewhere (8).

THE BOUNDARY BETWEEN RESEARCH AND PRACTICE IN FUNCTIONAL NEUROSURGERY

It is appropriate that in reviewing how our work as neurosurgeons can contribute at the growing edge of medicine, we should consider the problem of defining, if possible, the boundary between what research is and what practice in functional neurosurgery is. This question was one of the issues faced by the National Commission for the Protection of Human Subjects of Biomedical and Behavioral Research (7). I had the good fortune to serve as one of the consultants to the Scientific Advisory Board for Psychosurgery to this Commission, and the following is my understanding of what is a reasonable approach to this matter.

The field of functional neurosurgery may be loosely defined as consisting of a set of neurosurgical procedures that are aimed not at directly removing or structurally improving existing lesions in the nervous system, but rather by positive interventions of an often indirect nature to attempt to so alter the abnormal functioning of a disturbed nervous system as to restore or create a degree of normality. The first area in which functional neurosurgery may be said to have been born was the introduction of operations on the frontal lobes for the relief of certain psychoses and abnormal mental functioning. As in so many definitions in medicine, careful examination shows that there is no precise line that can be drawn between what may be called on the one hand, *functional neurosurgery,* and on the other, for lack of a better term, *structural neurosurgery.* Thus, the initial hope voiced by Sir Victor Horsley that the surgical treatment of epilepsy would consist ultimately of focal removals of epileptogenic sources produced by abnormal structure in the brain has not been supported. The pioneering work by Penfield, Rasmussen, and their colleagues at the Montreal Neurological Institute has shown that the actual treatment of patients with epilepsy ranges from the classical removal of focal lesions to more extensive removals aimed at reducing the volume of potentially epileptogenic tissue. The more strictly functional procedures range from splitting of the corpus callosum and stereotactic lesions in the Fields of Forel to recent attempts to control epilepsy by stimulation of the cerebellum as described earlier. Similar examples of the overlap between structural and functional methods can also be derived from the management of pain where classical surgical procedures designed to block the perception of pain from a diseased segment of the body are conceptually quite different from techniques that combine stimulation and lesion making to modify the perception of pain at a higher level of neural integration.

One of the problems faced by the National Commission was to consider, within the context of the use of such methods, whether it was possible to define a boundary between what constitutes biomedical research on the one hand and the practice of medical therapies on the other. Although it is always somewhat artificial and difficult to establish such a boundary between the two distinct activities of research and practice, it is extremely important to understand their radically different goals. Biomedical research involving human subjects refers to activities designed to produce generalized knowledge, i.e., data, on which theories, principles, or relationships can be developed and corroborated with accepted scientific observation and inferences. Although only neurosurgeons can define the criteria for evaluating research in their own area, some components are common to all research, e.g., (a) explicit objectives and (b) formal procedures for investigation designed to reach those objectives. Both of these components are commonly written in a protocol and difficulties in the field of functional neurosurgery, particularly with reference to psychosurgery, have arisen and will continue to arise when the intent to do research is not expressed formally in a suitable protocol. It is important, therefore, to ensure that formal mechanisms exist within institutions and that these should continuously survey their own activities so as to establish whether an activity is research even in the absence of a formal protocol or other acknowledgment of an investigative aim. This attitude to biomedical research is very different from that involved in the practice of medicine and surgery, whether it be aimed at the removal of lesions or at improving the behavior of an individual by a variety of methods. The goal in medical practice is solely to enhance the well-being of an individual. The customary standard for routine and accepted practice ensures a reasonable expectation of success. It cannot be sufficiently emphasized that even if such an expectation is not valid or is only imprecisely valid, this does not in and of itself define the clinical activity in question as research.

As clinicians, we can testify to the constant uncertainty inherent in therapeutic practice because of the variability of physiological and behavioral human responses to any intervention. In addition to such routine and accepted uncertainties, further uncertainties may be introduced when a new procedure that deviates from the common practice is introduced. We may call such new therapies innovative therapy, but they do not as such constitute research unless we formally structure them as a research project in a protocol, as previously described. Because of the natural enthusiasm of practitioners and the constant need of patients for treatment, there is always reason for concern that innovative therapies may be applied as part of practice and achieve an undeserved approved position in our armamentarium without valid testing. Significant innovations and therapies should therefore be always incorporated into a research project in order to establish their true efficacy and safety while retaining the therapeutic objectives from which they were originally developed.

Failure to incorporate these innovations and therapies has resulted in the retention of outmoded and inefficient procedures time and time again in medicine and particularly in surgical practice. For example, the use of radical mastectomy in the treatment of breast cancer is a case in point. Properly controlled trials of this procedure have only recently been completed after decades of the application of what is now realized to be an unnecessarily extensive procedure. A key factor separating research and practice is therefore the aim, purpose, goal, or intent for which the maneuver is undertaken. In some instances, examination of the facts will reveal that the intent of the professional as expressed to the patient or to his colleagues is not consistent with what is actually done or proposed. In other instances, research and practice may coexist. For example, a research component may be added to a standard maneuver such as monitoring the changes in blood flow in order to ascertain the effectiveness of microvascular shunting procedures in the treatment of transient ischemic attacks. In other cases, the therapeutic procedure itself may be the focus of research (for example, varying the parameters of stimulation or of lesion placement and size in the development of stereotactic procedures in the treatment of pain). Even in the delivery of standard service procedures, changes may be introduced in the mode of operation which even though considered as being within the legal or customary latitude for change enjoyed by the practitioner will constitute research to the extent that they are either introduced as a trial and then evaluated for possible application on a broader scale, or, incorporated into a design which includes some data collection and analysis to determine its effectiveness.

In all these situations, concern may arise because of the possibility that the research may interfere with the treatment given to the individual patient or that the patient may not be certain as to which of the procedures are a necessary part of the treatment and which are introduced solely for increase of knowledge, which would of course not be applied to his own case but to some later patient. Although it would seem unnecessarily bureaucratic to describe specific guidelines and procedures, the necessity for doing so has arisen because of the failure by some individuals and such bodies as the hospital board, tissue and medical practice committees, and professional societies to understand fully and exercise the duty that they have to identify significant deviations in the practice of medicine which have not been sufficiently validated and either to restrict their use or to require that they be applied only in the context of properly designed research and under the supervision of an in-house research board. Although the intent of the practitioner to conduct research may be sufficient to make the determination that research is in fact being conducted, other factors may produce the same result in the absence of such intent or even in the face of an intent to remain in the realm of practice. These factors include the presence of maneuvers, data collection, or analysis which are different from or in addition to those required to enhance the well-being of an individual, deliver a service, or to conduct routine administrative monitoring of operations. They also include the application of procedures that constitute a significant departure from routine or accepted practice. In the first instance, a research component is clearly involved. In the second instance, research may not be involved but it is reasonable to suggest that it should be. In such cases, appropriate action should be initiated by the practitioner working with the bodies empowered with the authority of setting and enforcing professional standards, and these bodies should always consist primarily of his peers. If there are separate committees that regularly monitor practice and research, they should communicate with each other regarding the procedures and techniques that seem unacceptable but they should retain final authority over their own respective jurisdictions. It is the duty of such bodies to develop mechanisms for the systematic appraisal of techniques and procedures in current practice. The role of the Federal Government should be only to provide support for such systematic evaluations and never to interfere by conducting the evaluations directly or indirectly.

I believe that this approach to defining the boundary between biomedical research and practice may be of some use in ensuring that useful knowledge gained by research in the course of practice is not dissipated or lost. Although good medical practice so often mixes attempts to cure the patient with research so closely that it is often quite artificial to separate them, failure to do so will in specific instances lead to the loss of useful data and what is worse the perpetuation of ineffective or unnecessarily invasive procedures. It should be emphasized that this approach in no way restricts the individual practitioner from developing innovative therapies. It is only after the pilot study of the innovation has been completed that the protocol-controlled studies should begin.

REFERENCES

 1. Blakemore, W. F. (1977): Remyelination of CNS axons by Schwann cells transplanted from the sciatic nerve. *Nature (Lond.)*, 266:68–69.
 2. Cooper, I. S. (1973): Chronic stimulation of the paleocerebellar cortex in man. *Lancet*, 1:206.
 3. Drachman, D. A., and Arbit, J. (1966): Memory and the hippocampal complex: Is memory a multiple process? *Arch. Neurol.*, 15:52–61.
 4. Drachman, D., and Ommaya, A. K. (1964): Memory and the hippocampal complex. *Arch. Neurol.*, 10:411–425.
 5. Gol, A., and Fabish, G. M. (1967): Effects of human hippocampal ablation. *J. Neurosurg.*, 26:390–398.
 6. Kao, C. C., Chang, L. W., and Bloodworth, J. M. B., Jr. (1977): The mechanism of spinal cord cavitation following spinal cord transection. III. Delayed grafting with and without spinal cord retransection. *J. Neurosurg.*, 46:757–766.
 7. National Commission for the Protection of Human Subjects of Biomedical and Behavioral Research (1977): *Report and Recommendations: Psychosurgery*. DHEW Publication No. (OS)77–0001, U.S. Government Printing Office, Washington, D.C.
 8. Ommaya, A. K. (1978): Cerebral asymmetry and human consciousness: A unitary hypothesis. *(manuscript in preparation)*
 9. Ommaya, A. K., and Fedio, P. (1972): The contribution of cingulum and hippocampal structures of memory mechanisms in man. *Confin. Neurol.*, 34:398–411.
10. Ommaya, A. K., and Gennarelli, T. A. (1974): Cerebral concussion and traumatic unconsciousness. *Brain*, 97:633–654.
11. Teuber, H. L., Corkin, S. H., and Twitchell, T. E. (1977): Study of cingulotomy in man: A summary. In: *Neurosurgical Treatment in Psychiatry, Pain, and Epilepsy*, edited by W. H. Sweet, S. Obrador, and J. G. Martin-Rodriguez, pp. 355–362. University Park Press, Baltimore, London, Tokyo.
12. Van Buren, J., Wood, J. H., Oakley, J., and Hambrecht, F. (1977): Preliminary evaluation of cerebellar stimulation in the treatment of epilepsy by double-blind stimulation and biological criteria. *J. Neurosurg. (in press)*.
13. Wood, J. H., Poplack, D. G., Bleyer, W. A., and Ommaya, A. K. (1977): Primate model for long-term study of intraventricularly or intrathecally administered drugs and intracranial pressure. *Science*, 195:499–501.

Functional Neurosurgery, edited by T. Rasmussen
and R. Marino. Raven Press, New York © 1979.

The Use of Pacemakers (Electrical Stimulation) in Functional Neurological Disorders

Philip L. Gildenberg

*Department of Surgery, Division of Neurosurgery, The University of Texas Medical
School at Houston, Texas 77030*

A revolutionary change took place in the field of functional neurosurgery with the advent of electronic stimulators that could be implanted within the body. Previously, the only procedures providing long-term effective therapy were those which produced lesions to ablate a structure or interrupt a pathway. Stimulation could be performed only for brief periods during stereotactic procedures or other surgery performed under local anesthesia. At best, leads could be left emerging through the skin for only several days or weeks.

The electronics of cardiac pacemakers was borrowed and improved upon. Because external control of stimulation parameters was necessary, only part of the stimulating device could be implanted. This led to the development of a passive or nonpowered internal stimulator consisting of a radio receiver connected by leads to electrodes which could be applied to nervous tissue. The external control device consists of a power supply and a control unit which regulates the radiofrequency signal transmitted from an external antenna taped to the skin over the internalized radio receiver. Sufficient power is transmitted through the skin to provide a stimulus so that it is not necessary to implant a power supply. Thus, the internalized apparatus is completely passive.

This new technique then went in search of indications. It seemed reasonable to assume that it would be safer to apply chronic stimulation, which could be discontinued at any time, than to perform a destructive or ablative procedure, which is irreversible. Nevertheless, it was necessary first to consider whether chronic stimulation causes any permanent damage to nervous tissue. This question has not been completely resolved even at the present time.

SAFETY

It has long been recognized that excessive stimulation, particularly monophasic, of central nervous tissue can eventually lead to tissue damage (53). The electrolytic effect of direct coupled monophasic stimulation can be partly avoided by the use of capacitative coupling. Ideally, biphasic stimulation should be used with the charges in each half of the stimulating pulse balanced (82,83). There is no evidence that repeated momentary stimulation, as used in electrocorticography (79), or stimulation during brief stereotactic procedures, causes any neural damage if properly applied (82).

Chronically implanted electrodes must be biologically inert (8–10,47,82, 83,108) so that they do not deteriorate in tissue or polymerize to the extent that they might impart an electrolytic charge to the surrounding tissue. It has been recognized that electrodes placed in the subarachnoid space or in the subdural space to stimulate the dorsal columns and the spinal cord may lose their effectiveness after a time because they become surrounded by scar tissue (11,81,90). Fortunately, this effect is minimized when the electrodes are placed within the dura (11) or epidurally (34).

After it had been reported that stimulation of the cerebellum might control convulsive seizures or abnormal movements in patients (20–23,25,26), concern was raised that such stimulation might cause damage to the cerebellum. In one study to evaluate the safety of chronic stimulation, electrode arrays were placed over the cerebellar hemispheres in monkeys (35) and stimulation applied to some of those arrays for periods up to a month. At autopsy, all except one unstimulated electrode array and cable were found densely embedded in connective tissue. Changes in Purkinje cells were noted in the area beneath the electrode or beyond the electrode site, depending on the amount of stimulation applied.

Question was raised whether the disproportionately large size of the electrode in the small posterior fossa of the monkey may have contributed to the damage. Also, cerebellar damage can be seen in patients with epilepsy, even without stimulation (24).

Later studies (7,88) demonstrated that although there was some meningeal thickening associated with the mere presence of the electrodes in the posterior fossa of monkeys, effective stimulation parameters could be found which were below the level at which any cerebellar injury was demonstrated, indicating that safe parameters for human stimulation could be obtained (88).

The question of mechanical and electronic efficiency of stimulation devices is critical, especially since these devices must perform flawlessly for years or essentially for the life of the patient. A review of complications with implanted devices (97) reveals that the most complex part of the system, the implanted radio receiver, is so well encapsulated and the components so reliable that less than a 0.5% receiver failure for a series of 218 devices was found. The major cause for electronic failure of the internal components is failure of insulation of the conducting lead wires; this occurs in 10% of the devices over a 6-year period (97) and it appears to be caused by mechanical factors involved with continuous motion of lead wires within the tissue as the patient moves. Also, microscopic failures in insulation within the hostile biological environment of the body can progress to become major pores. At present, there is no way to test for such minute failures or to repair them, so that if they occur it is necessary to replace the entire internalized system.

Likewise, the most common site of failure of the externalized portion of the system is in the antenna wires, and these must be replaced at least annually. Failure of the electronic transmitter is also not uncommon (approximately a 12% failure rate per year), often presumably the result of mishandling or trauma to the control box (97).

PAIN

Coincident with the development of electronic circuitry which could be implanted for chronic nervous system stimulation came the gate theory of pain, as outlined by Melzack and Wall (64). Despite some inconsistencies in this theory, it provided a theoretical framework for new pain treatments.

According to the theory, a gating mechanism exists in the area of the substantia gelatinosa. If firing occurs predominantly in the large low-threshold nerve fibers, the substantia gelatinosa cells likewise fire to inhibit transmission along the pathways subserving the sensation of pain. On the other hand, as the intensity of stimulation increases to become nociceptive, the higher threshold small fibers begin to fire, inhibiting the substantia gelatinosa cells, and, in turn, allowing those cells conducting pain information to fire and transmit a pain message to higher centers. One can see that the gate might be closed by increasing the firing of the large fibers, in effect "shutting off" the pain. The large fibers are those which conduct sensation other than pain and temperature from the periphery, with collaterals ascending in the dorsal columns of the spinal cord to higher centers.

A common physiological demonstration of the closure of the pain gate by stimulation of large fibers can readily be seen by rubbing a painful area with your hand to "make it feel better." This nonpainful mechanical stimulation of the large fibers at the periphery in effect tips the balance toward the large fibers to "close the gate."

Continuous mechanical stimulation, however, might be cumbersome, especially depending on the painful area of the body. Also, such a stimulation might be more efficiently applied by some sophisticated electronic device. Indeed, one such device was patented in 1908 as the Electreat (Electreat Inc., Minneapolis, Minnesota) and was the first device used by Shealy (89) in his search for a nondestructive pain treatment. Since 1973, there have been a number of more sophisticated transistorized transcutaneous stimulators commercially available (91).

The history of transcutaneous stimulation, however, goes back quite a while further. In about 15 A.D., a freed man of the Emperor Tiberius was suffering from gout. He stepped on a torpedo-fish, which resulted in a sudden shock, and subsequently his pain was cured. Scribonius, the local physician, thereafter recommended torpedo shocks both for gout and as an analgesic for headache (98).

Present-day transcutaneous stimulators are not nearly as impressive. Generally, they consist of a small transistorized battery-operated control unit to which are attached two leads connected to flat electrodes, frequently of carbonized silicone (91).

The electrodes are applied to the skin in the area of pain. The application and contact of the electrodes remains the most cumbersone problem with this type of stimulation. Alternative methods of applying electrodes are being sought, such as application without electrode paste (42), so-called epiductive paste (13), local modification of skin resistance (42), or solvent-activated current-passing tape electrodes (14). The patient himself controls the voltage so that he is able to adjust it to the point at which he feels a cutaneous sensation that is not painful, that is, the voltage at which the large fibers are stimulated, but which is below the voltage to fire the small fibers.

It was during a screening procedure for the use of implanted stimulating devices for the treatment of pain when transcutaneous stimulation became recognized as a pain treatment in its own right (56). Since then there have been numerous other series indicating generally good long-term relief in 12 to 25% of patients, with an additional 50% of patients obtaining partial relief (48,54, 56,89). Transcutaneous stimulation has also been found effective in the treatment of migraine and other headaches (2).

In attempts to use transcutaneous stimulation to decrease pain after various types of surgery, it has been serendipitously found that transcutaneous stimulation also significantly decreases the incident of postoperative atelectasis and ileus after thoracic or abdominal surgery, but the mechanisms for this have not yet been determined.

If pain is secondary to injury to a single peripheral nerve, the pain syndrome may be confined to the distribution of that nerve or its component roots. More efficient stimulation of the large fibers from a large portion of the painful area might be obtained by stimulating the peripheral nerve itself, rather than the cutaneous afferents. Indeed, in 1967 Wall and Sweet (106) noted that temporary low-threshold stimulation by a subcutaneous electrode at a peripheral nerve in five patients and cauda equina rootlets in three others relieved their clinical pain. Sweet (99) later reported on 69 patients over a 10-year period who had permanently implanted peripheral nerve stimulators. Seventeen individuals maintained relief until death or to the time of the report, and 13 others had weeks or months of temporary relief.

Temporary stimulation of peripheral nerves by means of percutaneously inserted electrodes has been used either as a treatment modality (65,75) or to screen patients prior to implantation of a permanent peripheral nerve stimulator (15,56,80). With attention to proper patient selection, various series have reported a long-term success rate of peripheral nerve stimulation generally of about 50% (15,48,55,80). As with other pain-relieving procedures, the initial success rate is not always maintained, but for pain originating from peripheral nerve injury, stimulation by means of an implanted peripheral nerve stimulator appears to be justifiable. Of significance is the fact that patients with pain of lumbar radiculopathy have as poor a success rate with this as with most other procedures.

The cause for the frequently observed transient nature of pain relief from peripheral nerve stimulation was not apparent. It does not seem that the formation of scar tissue is as significant a factor in peripheral nerve stimulation as in spinal cord stimulation (67,101,106). However, once the relief has faded, attempt at revision is frequently unsuccessful. Nielson et al. (74) recorded two cases where the peripheral nerve appeared to be damaged from insertion of an implanted stimulating device with scarring and hyperemia noted at surgery.

As one reviews the original concept of the Melzack-Wall gate theory, one is struck by the anatomical accident in which collaterals from the large fibers ascend in the dorsal columns to provide to consciousness sensation other than pain and temperature. Thus, the dorsal columns of the spinal cord consist of a compact array of only large fibers. One might consider that stimulation of the dorsal columns at any given level of the spinal cord will influence large fibers from most or all of the segmental levels below the level of stimulation, thus providing an extremely efficient means of pure large-fiber stimulation (32).

Indeed, Shealy et al. (94) noted that dorsal column stimulation totally abolished the prolonged small-fiber afterdischarge uniquely related to nociceptive stimulation in the experimental animal. This led this same group (93) to implant a dorsal column stimulator in the first patient in 1967. Although the patient who was suffering from widespread metastatic disease died 1½ days after the procedure, of problems unrelated to the dorsal column stimulation, both the incisional pain of the implantation and the pain of the metastatic disease were effectively controlled by electrical stimulation of the dorsal columns. This led Shealy (90,92), and soon after Sweet and Wepsic (100,101), to use a fully implantable device to stimulate the dorsal columns in a series of patients. This was followed by other authors as well (4,11,12,33,46,48,49,57,68,72,73,81), and it has now been estimated that over 3,000 patients have been treated with dorsal column stimulation (102).

Most series report short-term relief of 65 to 80% and long-term pain relief of approximately 50%. Again, patients who have experienced multiple surgical operations on the lower back appear to be in a less favorable category, especially when one considers the multitude of psychological, drug, and compensation factors. Nevertheless, this appears to be one of the most satisfactory pain-relieving procedures in that group of patients.

Dorsal column stimulation, as generally described, involves a laminectomy with the surgical implantation of the electrode posterior to the dorsal columns of the spinal cord. A subcutaneous pocket is made at a site convenient for the implantation of the radio receiver, usually below the clavicle over the chest or along the side of the abdomen. A subcutaneous tunnel is made from that incision to a midline dorsal incision at a convenient level above the level of the pain. A laminectomy is performed. Originally, the dura and the arachnoid were opened, and the electrodes were implanted in the subarachnoid space. In attempts to avoid late failures caused by scarring around the electrode, the position of the electrode was later modified to the subdural space, and then to a pocket formed within the dura (11), or to the epidural space (34). The electrode is sutured in place and the incision closed.

When this is performed under general anesthesia, it is not possible to test the effectiveness of stimulation until after the patient awakes, a decided disadvantage. However, Sweet (101) reports implantation under local or short-acting anesthesia so that the placement of electrodes can be tested while it can still be modified in the operating room.

One of the most common causes for failure of dorsal column stimulation is the failure of the induced sensation to project into the area of pain. Curiously, patients may have excellent stimulation sensation, frequently described as a vibration or tingling sensation over most of the body below the level of stimulation, with the sole exception of the area of pain, a phenomenon which has not thus far been explained.

Pineda (81) has plotted the time course of dorsal column stimulator failure and relates this to the type of electrode. In 11 unipolar implants, failures began at the end of the first month and were completed by the seventeenth in those patients who did not have sustained relief. Other authors have reported late failures in almost all the patients who were originally implanted with the tinsel wire type of unipolar electrode. With an improved bipolar electrode, failure generally began a bit later, if at all, at the end of three months. By the end of 20 months, 7 of 23 implanted bipolar electrodes had failed despite initial excellent relief in 14, which he relates to thickening of arachnoid membranes with prolonged stimulation.

In an attempt to screen patients more efficiently preoperatively, electrodes have been inserted percutaneously either into the subarachnoid space (12,17, 34,46) or epidurally (75). Such percutaneous stimulating electrodes were first used to screen patients with torticollis (34). As these electrodes were developed, they proved to be quite helpful in evaluating patients for dorsal column stimulators for pain as well. Generally, a needle is inserted from laterally at the C_{1-2} level, as in percutaneous cervical cordotomy, except that the needle is inserted dorsal to the dentate ligament. Initially, every effort was made to manipulate the electrode so that it lay behind the spinal cord, but often it had a tendency to emerge between the attachments of the dentate ligament to come to rest anterior to the cord. It later became apparent that the effect of the stimulation and the sensation were essentially the same whether the electrode lay behind or in front of the cord, which opens the door for considerable discussion about whether the effectiveness of this prodecure is really a result of stimulation of the dorsal columns or not.

One disadvantage of the use of subarachnoid stimulating electrodes is that the sensation varies as the patient moves about or turns his head. The electrode may come into contact with a cervical nerve root so that the patient has pain along distribution of that root at voltages too low to afford projection of the sensation to the rest of the body.

The distribution of stimulation, however, can be more effectively controlled if the electrodes are implanted in the epidural space (75). The procedure was modified so that the percutaneously inserted epidural electrodes can be attached to a radio receiver implanted under local anesthesia, obviating the necessity for surgical laminectomy (75). In addition, since the procedure is performed under local anesthesia, it is possible to modify the placement of the electrodes until satsifactory distribution of sensation is obtained. It is still somewhat early to evaluate the long-term effects of such percutaneously inserted epidural stimulators. In my own experience, I have had some difficulty in obtaining a strong enough stimulation with this technique but still prefer it as a screening procedure for the surgical implantation of a dorsal column stimulator.

In a significant modification of the technique of dorsal column stimulation, Larson (50,52) employ a system wherein one electrode is placed dorsal and one electrode ventral to the spinal cord, so that the stimulating current theoretically passes through the cord. His results are comparable to or better than the classical dorsal column stimulating techniques, but he has reported primarily patients with metastatic disease whose life expectancy is short, so that late failures may not yet have become apparent.

Other stimulation techniques for the treatment of pain involve stimulating the internal capsule (45) or thalamus (45,60) or the periaqueductal gray, so-called stimulation-produced analgesia (1,44,59,63,66,84–87), and will be discussed in a later chapter.

Of considerable historical interest is the experience of Heath (41) and later of Gol (38), who stimulated the septal area in patients with the pain of metastatic disease. Techniques at that time necessitated direct connection to a stimulator. The stimulation site was selected to conform to a reward site, that is, an area that would promote lever-pressing activity in rats when such lever-pressing resulted in stimulation. Although the patients had no particular sensation that would be related to such a drive in experimental animals, they experienced significant reduction in their pain.

MOTOR DISORDERS

Stimulation techniques have been employed for the treatment of movement disorders as well as pain. In a project which began in 1972, dorsal column stimulation has been employed for the treatment of spasmodic torticollis (34). Patients were selected who were emotionally stable and able to tolerate the stimulation apparatus. The screening procedure involved first transcutaneous stimulation and to date 3 out of 24 patients responded well enough to that modality so that no other treatment was necessary. Those patients who tolerated stimulation but still did not have sufficient relief from transcutaneous stimulation were screened for dorsal column stimulation with a subarachnoid dorsal column stimulating electrode. Six of the 17 torticollis patients thus evaluated showed significant improvement in their spasmodic torticollis, so that permanent dorsal column stimulating electrodes were inserted at the C_{1-2} level. Five of those patients experienced significant improvement which lasted for as long as a 3½ year follow-up.

Interestingly, optimal relief was obtained at frequencies much higher than those generally employed for pain. As the frequency was first increased, initially there was an increase in the sensation projected to the body. As the frequency was increased above 800 Hz, the sensation gradually disappeared. It was only then that the most significant improvement in the torticollis was noted, with optimal effects seen generally at 1,100 Hz. The major improvement was in the distressing and disabling pulling and painful sensation of the muscles, even though the position of the head might not return to normal.

The theoretical consideration which led to this project was the possibility that torticollis might present an imbalance of tonic neck reflexes, from whatever central cause. It was anticipated that the addition of afferent input to the cervical roots might lessen the vigor of these reflexes to afford relief.

The availability of implantable electronic stimulating devices has opened the possibility of stimulating peripheral nerves to induce movement of paralyzed extremities. Leaders in this application have been at the Rancho Los Amigos Rehabilitation Engineering Center (62), where they have investigated improvement of ambulatory function through functional replacement or neurological retraining in hemiplegia, treatment of scoliosis in idiopathic and spinal-injured patients, and provision of sensory feedback in below-elbow amputees using a myoelectric hand. The primary use has been for dropfoot (61,107). Thirty-one units have been implanted, one for as long as 7.3 years, and 18 are still implanted. Some problems were encountered with the buildup of scar tissue around the nerve or edema of the nerve at the implant site.

One of the major problems with implantation of such stimulating devices in footdrop is graded control of muscle contraction. One might theoretically consider the possibility of a feedback system so that as the patient's heel strikes the floor a graded stimulus is initiated to allow the ankle to dorsiflex during the appropriate part of the gait. Although considerable developmental work must still be done, such techniques of peripheral nerve stimulation suggest exciting possibilities for the future (16).

One nerve which particularly lends itself to life-saving electronic stimulation is the phrenic nerve (36,37,105). Patients with lesions or transection of the upper cervical spinal cord with resultant ventilatory paralysis or patients with sleep-induced apnea, so-called Ondine's curse, from high cervical cordotomy or congenital etiology have been treated with such stimulating devices. The electrode is applied to each phrenic nerve in the lower neck or upper chest. Generally, two separate receivers are employed. In the adult, it is possible to obtain sufficient ventilation by stimulating a single phrenic nerve, so that the nerves may be stimulated alternately to minimize fatigue. In the infant, it is necessary to stimulate both phrenic nerves simultaneously to obtain adequate ventilation because of the mechanical factors involved with paradoxical movement of the mediastinum. In order to avoid a sudden hiccup type of contraction of the diaphragm, intermittent ramp stimulation may be employed.

Another use of implanted electronic stimulators has been the control of bladder evacuation. Initially, attempts were made to stimulate the muscles of the bladder directly (5). This led to problems with incomplete emptying and mechanical fatigue of the electrodes from the repeated contraction of the muscle into which they were implanted.

However, Nashold (69–71) developed a technique whereby a specific locus within the conus medullaris can be stimulated to give a much smoother and complete contraction of the bladder, so that the urinary evacuation can be controlled by the use of the external control unit. A cystometrogram is performed during laminectomy at which the conus is exposed. Fine wire electrodes are used to probe the lower end of the spinal cord to identify those loci that cause the bladder to contract. The electrodes are secured in place with a band around the conus and led to a radio receiver control unit implanted subcutaneously in a convenient location. Not only does this technique provide a needed prosthetic function, but the prospect of identifying other specific loci within the spinal cord which control organized activity may provide additional future opportunities for the use of similar implanted stimulating devices. One might speculate that there would be an artificial gait by the sequential stimulation of loci within the lumbar cord.

Hoppenstein (42; R. Hoppenstein, *personal communication*) has an interesting group of five elderly female patients treated for pain with dorsal column stimulation. In what may be a significant advance in the use of dorsal column stimulation, he reports that all had significant sexual arousal on using the stimulator. In fact, one patient could frequently produce an orgasm by manipulating her stimulation parameters.

Implanted stimulators have also been used for the treatment of other motor disorders. Patients with spasticity may note a significant decrease in abnormal muscle tone and improvement of voluntary function with the use of dorsal column stimulation (18,29,96). Cook (18) has had a large series of patients with multiple sclerosis whose spasticity has been treated with this technique. My own experience is quite limited, but initial results have been impressive. In addition, Dooley (29) has treated other demyelinating disease such as olivo-pontocerebellar atrophy, amyotrophic lateral sclerosis, and Friedreich's ataxia, as well as spinal cord injury. Some patients had diminution of ataxia and were better able to perform such tasks as feeding themselves, buttoning their clothes, and, significantly, turning the dials of the transmitter, which they had not been able to do without stimulation. Most patients had an increase in voluntary function in one or more extremities which enabled them to walk with less support. Dooley (29) coincidentally noted improvement in various modalities of sensation, such as proprioception, vibratory sensibility, and ability to distinguish between sharp and dull stimuli. Frequently, the beneficial effect outlasts the duration of stimulation, which has been observed in patients using stimulation for other indications as well.

Dooley (29) also made the observation that patients with transcutaneous or dorsal column stimulation had an increase in blood flow in the adjacent nerve root distribution. He and others (78) have used transcutaneous electrical stimulation to treat vascular ulcers of lower extremities with favorable results. He also used transcutaneous stimulation of the cervical and thoracic regions in 96 patients with vasospastic disorders of the upper extremities. Cook (17) has used epidural dorsal column stimulation of the spinal cord for long-term treatment of this group of patients.

Spasticity has also been treated by chronic stimulation of the anterior lobe of the cerebellum. As early as 1897, Lowenthal and Horsley (58) and Sherrington (95) demonstrated that stimulation of the cortex of the anterior lobe of the cerebellum resulted in inhibition of extensor hypertonus resulting from decerebrate rigidity. The decrease in muscle tone by stimulation of the paleocerebellum was later documented in other experimental circumstances (31). This technique was adopted by Cooper (20–23,103) and later by Davis (25,26) and Larson (51,88) for the treatment of spasticity in patients with cerebral palsy. In addition, Davis (25,26) also treated spasticity caused by stroke, head injuries, carbon monoxide poisoning, and hypoxia secondary to anesthetic arrest.

It was found that such electronic stimulation of both anterior lobes of the cerebellum may also result in an improvement in athetosis. A decrease in spasticity was usually noticed within minutes after turning on the stimulator, and this was documented by a reduction in the electrophysiological H-reflex response, (23,26,103) such cerebellar stimulation being primarily inhibitory. Although the maximum improvement in spasticity was noted fairly soon after the use of the stimulator was begun, the improvement in athetosis occurred gradually over a period of weeks and did not reach its maximum in some cases for as long as 6 months. One must interpret carefully the improvement in voluntary movement in patients with cerebral palsy, since they have not had the opportunity to learn movements and coordination prior to the treatment, so that cerebellar stimulation must be employed along with a program of training and physical therapy.

EPILEPSY

Stimulation of the anterior lobe of the cerebellum has also been used in the treatment of epilepsy by Cooper (20,21). Such stimulation is based on the experimental evidence that it inhibits electrically induced cerebral discharges (19), although there is also experimental evidence to the contrary (3,30,39).

This group reported a good clinical response to cerebellar stimulation in 18 of 32 patients. They indicated that in these patients seizures were reduced at least by 50%, with other significant evidence of clinical improvement (21), including patients with both partial and generalized seizures. Virtually all of the patients reportedly had a sensation of increased alertness as well as improved ability to concentrate and improved performance in daily function of living (21), and significant EEG improvement was noted in some (20,87). Other investigators, however, have not yet confirmed the beneficial effect of cerebellar stimulation on epilepsy. This may be in part a result of the significant difficulties in evaluating the effectiveness of any procedure on the incidence of seizures (77). As an example of this, Van Buren (104) implanted cerebellar stimulators in patients with epilepsy, but his protocol indicated that the stimulator would not be turned on until the patient returned to the presurgical seizure frequency. The time it took varied considerably, and, indeed, one patient was seizure-free for months, even though the stimulator had not been turned on.

THE FUTURE

The future of the use of electronic stimulating devices in functional neurosurgery represents perhaps the most exciting field in all of neurosurgery. Treatment of epilepsy, for instance, may become more sophisticated now that implanted microprocessors are available. These miniature computers can be programmed to recognize preclinical seizure activity and to turn on the appropriate inhibitory stimulation only when needed. In fact, Delgado's experiments (27) suggest that such computer-controlled stimulation can be used to condition the brain to modify EEG activity. For instance, with the aid of a computer and an external stimoceiver, he demonstrated the possibility of pattern recognition of brain waves anatomically localized in the amygdala. Detection of such waves serves as a triggering device for contingent stimulation of the reticular formation in order to inhibit the waves and to modify related behavior.

Ojemann (76) has demonstrated an increased learning ability during stimulation of certain areas of the thalamus. One can envision an implanted device that can be turned on during study periods to enhance learning, perhaps to make smarter and smarter neurosurgeons.

It has been recognized that stimulation of points on the visual cortex results in the visualization of phosphenes, a subjective visual sensation of discrete points of light at specific loci within the visual field (6). This information was used by Brindley to develop an electrode array which was implanted over the visual cortex of a blind patient; by stimulating the discrete electrode sites, patterns of phosphenes could be seen. The ultimate goal, of course, would be for a miniature television camera to "see" for a blind patient. By means of a microcomputer, the image seen by the television camera might be converted into the appropriate stimulation of multiple sites in the visual cortex so the patient might "see" a pattern which would represent what the television camera sees, the ultimate visual prosthesis (28,40).

Additional work involves the development of an auditory prosthesis as well. It has been demonstrated that stimulation of the auditory nerve or cochlea can allow some deaf patients to hear sounds. One can likewise anticipate that, as the appropriate stimulation parameters evolve, a miniature computer inserted beneath the scalp might "hear" and convert the sounds to the appropriate stimulation parameters to simulate the sounds for the patient.

REFERENCES

1. Akil, H., and Richardson, D. E. (1974): Electrophysiological correlates of stimulation produced analgesia, morphine analgesia, and their blockade by naloxone. *Proceedings of the Society for Neuroscience, Annual Meeting,* St. Louis, Missouri. p. 114.
2. Appenzeller, O., and Atkinson, R. (1975): Transkutane Nervenreizung zur Behandlung der Migraine und anderer Kopfschmerzen. *Munch. Med. Wochenschr.,* 117:1953–1954.
3. Babb, T. L., Mitchell, A. G., Jr., and Crandall, P. H. (1974): Fastigiobulbar and dentatothalamic influences on hippocampal cobalt epilepsy in the cat. *Electroencephalogr. Clin. Neurophysiol.,* 36:141–154.
4. Blair, R. D. G., Lee, R. G., and Vanderlinden, G. (1975): Dorsal column stimulation: Its effect on the somatosensory evoked response. *Arch. Neurol.,* 32:826–829.
5. Bradley, W. E., Chou, S. N., and French, L. A. (1963): Further experience with radio transmitter receiver unit for the neurogenic bladder. *J. Neurosurg.,* 20:953–960.
6. Brindley, G. S., and Lewin, W. S. (1968): The sensations produced by electrical stimulation of the visual cortex. *J. Physiol. (Lond.),* 196:479–493.
7. Brown, W. J., Babb, T. L., Soper, H. V., Lieb, J. P., Otting, C. A., and Crandall, P. H. (1977): Tissue reactions to long-term electrical stimulation of the cerebellum in monkeys. *J. Neurosurg.,* 47:366–379.
8. Brummer, S. B., and Turner, M. J. (1977): Electrochemical considerations for safe electrical stimulation of the nervous system with platinum electrodes. *IEEE Trans. Biomed. Eng.,* 24:59–63.
9. Brummer, S. B., and Turner, M. J. (1977): Electrical stimulation with Pt electrodes: Part I. A method for determination of "real" electrode areas. *IEEE Trans. Biomed. Eng.,* 24:436:439.
10. Brummer, S. B., and Turner, M. J. (1977): Electrical stimulation with Pt electrodes: Part II. Estimation of maximum surface redox (Theoretical non-gassing) limits. *IEEE Trans. Biomed. Eng.,* 24:440–443.
11. Burton, C. (1975): Dorsal column stimulation: Optimization of application. *Surg. Neurol.,* 4:171–176.
12. Burton, C. V. (1977/78): The safety and clinical efficacy of implanted neuroaugmentive spinal devices for the relief of pain. *Appl. Neurophysiol.,* 40:175–183.
13. Burton, C., and Maurer, D. D. (1974): Pain suppression by transcutaneous electronic stimulation. *IEEE Trans. Biomed. Eng.,* 21:81–88.
14. Burton, C., and Maurer, D. D. (1976): Solvent-activated current passing tape electrode for transcutaneous electrical stimulation of the peripheral nervous system. *IEEE Trans. Biomed. Eng.,* 23:346–347.
15. Campbell, J. N., and Long, D. M. (1976): Peripheral nerve stimulation in the treatment of intractable pain. *J. Neurosurg.,* 45:642–699.
16. Childress, D. S. (1973): Neural organization and myoelectric control. In: *Neural Organization and Its Relevance to Prosthetics,* edited by W. S. Fields, pp. 117–130. Intercontinental Medical Book Corp., New York.
17. Cook, A. W., Oygar, A., Baggenstos, P., Pacheco, S., and Kleriga, E. (1976): Vascular diseases of the extremities: Electric stimulation of spinal cord and posterior roots. *N.Y. State J. Med.,* 76:366–368.
18. Cook, A. W., and Weinstein, S. P. (1973): Chronic dorsal column stimulation in multiple sclerosis. *N.Y. State J. Med.,* 73:2868–2872.
19. Cooke, P. M., and Snider, R. S. (1955): Some cerebellar influences in electrically induced cerebral seizures. *Epilepsia,* 4:19–28.
20. Cooper I. S. (1973): Effect of chronic stimulation of anterior cerebellum on neurological disease. *Lancet,* 1:206.

21. Cooper, I. S., Amin, I., Upton, A., Riklan, M., Watkins, S., and McLellan, L. (1977/78): Safety and efficacy of chronic cerebellar stimulation. *Appl. Neurophysiol.,* 40:124–134.
22. Cooper, I. S., Cringhel, E., and Amin, I. (1973): Clinical and physiological effects of stimulation of the paleocerebellum in humans. *J. Am. Geriatr. Soc.,* 21:40–43.
23. Cooper, I. S., Riklan, M., Amin, I., Waltz, J. M., and Culliman, T. (1976): Chronic cerebellar stimulation in cerebral palsy. *Neurology (Minneap.),* 26:744–753.
24. Dam, M. (1970): Number of Purkinje cells in patients with grand mal epilepsy treated with diphenylhydantoin. *Epilepsia,* 11:313–320.
25. Davis, R., Cullen, R. F., Duenas, D., and Engle, H. (1976): Cerebellar stimulation for cerebral palsy. *J. Med. Assoc.,* 63:910–912.
26. Davis, R., Cullen, R. F., Jr., Flitter, M. A., Duenas, D., et. al. (1977/78): Control of spasticity and involuntary movements. *Appl. Neurophysiol.,* 40:135–140.
27. Delgado, J. M. R. (1978): Instrumentation, working hypotheses and clinical aspects of neurostimulation. *Appl. Neurophysiol.,* 40:88–110.
28. Dobelle, W. H., Mladejovsky, M. G., Evans, J. R., Roberts, T. S., and Girvin, J. P. (1976): "Braille" reading by a blind volunteer by visual cortex stimulation. *Nature (Lond.),* 259:111–112.
29. Dooley, D. M., and Sharkey, J. (1977/78): Electrostimulation of the nervous system for patients with demyelinating and degenerative diseases of the nervous system and vascular diseases of the extremities. *Appl. Neurophysiol.,* 40:208–217.
30. Dow, R. S., Fernandez-Guardiola, A., and Manni, E. (1962): The influence of the cerebellum on experimental epilepsy. *Electroencephalogr. Clin. Neurophysiol.,* 14:383–398.
31. Dow, R. S., and Moruzzi, G. (1958): *The Physiology and Pathology of the Cerebellum,* pp. 113–137, 151–159, 311–327. University of Minnesota Press, Minneapolis.
32. Emmers, R. (1974): Inhibition of the T-cells of the spinothalamic tract: A neurophysiological basis for electrically induced analgesia. *Proc. Soc. Exp. Biol. Med.,* 145:1310–1316.
33. Fox, J. L. (1974): Dorsal column stimulation for relief of intractable pain: Problems encountered with neuropacemakers. *Surg. Neurol.,* 2:59–64.
34. Gildenberg, P. I. (1978): Treatment of spasmodic torticollis by dorsal column stimulation. *Appl. Neurophysiol. (in press).*
35. Gilman, S., Dauth, G. W., Tennyson, V. M., and Kremzner, L. T. (1975): Chronic cerebellar stimulation in the monkey. *Arch. Neurol.,* 32:474–477.
36. Glenn, W. W. L., Holcomb, W. G., Gee, J. B. L., and Rath, R. (1970): Central hypoventilation: Long-term ventilatory assistance by radiofrequency electrophrenic respiration. *Ann. Surg.,* 172:755–773.
37. Glenn, W. W. L., Holcomb, W. G., Hogan, J., Matano, I., Gee, J. B. L., Motoyama, E. K., Kim, C. S., Poirier, R. S., and Forbes, G. (1973): Diaphragm pacing by radiofrequency transmission in the treatment of chronic ventilatory insufficiency: Present status. *J. Thorac. Cardiovasc. Surg.,* 66:505–520.
38. Gol, A. (1967): Relief of pain by electrical stimulation of the septal area. *J. Neurol. Sci.,* 5:115–120.
39. Grimm, R. J., Frazee, J. G., Bell, C. C., Kawasaki, T., and Dow, R. S. (1970): Quantitative studies in cobalt model epilepsy: The effect of cerebellar stimulation. *Int. J. Neurol.,* 7:126–140.
40. Hambrecht, F. T. (1973): Visual prostheses: Theoretical objectives, present status and future possibilities. In: *Neural Organization and Its Relevance to Prosthetics,* edited by W. S. Fields, pp. 281–292. Intercontinental Medical Book Corp., New York.
41. Heath, R. G., and Mickle, W. A. (1960): Evaluation of seven year's experience with depth electrode studies in human patients. In: *Electrical Studies on the Unanesthetized Brain,* edited by E. R. Ramey and D. S. O'Doherty, pp. 214–247. Hoeber, New York.
42. Hoenig, S., Gildenberg, P. L., and Murthy, K. S. K. (1978): Generation of permanent, dry, electrical contacts by tattooing carbon into skin tissue. *IEEE Trans. Biomed. Eng.,* 25:380–382.
43. Hoppenstein, R. (1975): Percutaneous implantation of chronic spinal cord electrodes for control of intractable pain: Preliminary report. *Surg. Neurol.,* 4:195–198.
44. Hosobuchi, Y., Adams, J. E., and Lynchitz, R. (1976): Pain relief by electrical stimulation of the central gray matter in humans. Proceedings of the 6th Annual Meeting, Society for Neuroscience, Toronto.

45. Hosobuchi, Y., Adams, J. E., and Rutkin, B. (1975): Chronic thalamic and internal capsule stimulation for the control of central pain. *Surg. Neurol.,* 4:91–92.
46. Hosobuchi, Y., Adams, J. E., and Weinstein, P. R. (1972): Preliminary percutaneous dorsal column stimulation prior to permanent implantation: Technical note. *J. Neurosurg.,* 37:242–245.
47. Johnson, P. F., and Hench, L. L. (1978): An *in vitro* analysis of metallic electrodes for use in the neurological environment. *IEEE Trans. Biomed. Eng. (in press).*
48. Kirch, W. M., Lewis, J. A., and Simon, R. H. (1975): Experiences with electrical stimulation devices for the control of chronic pain. *Med. Instrum.,* 9:217–220.
49. Krainick, J.-U., and Thoden, U. (1974): Indikationen Neurochirurgischer Schmerzoperationen. *Munch. Med. Wochenschr.,* 116:1973–1976.
50. Larson, S. J., Sances, A., Jr., Cusick, J. F., Meyer, G. A., and Swiontek, T. (1975): A comparison between anterior and posterior spinal implant systems. *Surg. Neurol.,* 4:180–186.
51. Larson, S. J., Sances, A., Jr., Hemmy, D. C., Millar, E. A., and Walsh, D. R. (1977/78): Physiological and histological effects of cerebellar stimulation. *Appl. Neurophysiol.,* 40:160–174.
52. Larson, S. J., Sances, A., Jr., Reigel, D. H., Meyer, G. A., Dallman, D. E., and Swontek, T. (1974): Neurophysiological effects of dorsal column stimulation in man and monkey. *J. Neurosurg.,* 41:217–223.
53. Lilly, J. C. (1961): Inquiry and excitation by electrical currents: A. The balanced pulse-pair waveform. In: *Electrical Stimulation of the Brain,* edited by D. E. Sheer, pp. 60–64. University of Texas Press, Austin.
54. Loeser, J. D., Black, R. G., and Christman, A. (1975): Relief of pain by transcutaneous stimulation. *J. Neurosurg.,* 42:308–314.
55. Long, D. M. (1973): Electrical stimulation for relief of pain of chronic nerve injury. *J. Neurosurg.,* 39:718–729.
56. Long, D. M. (1974): Cutaneous afferent stimulation for relief of chronic pain. *Clin. Neurosurg.,* 21:257–268.
57. Long, D. M., and Hagfors, H. (1975): Electrical stimulation in the nervous system: The current status of electrical stimulation of the nervous system for relief of pain. *Pain,* 1:109–123.
58. Lowenthal, M., and Horsley, V. (1897): On the relation between the cerebellar and other centers. *Proc. R. Soc. London (Biol.),* 61:20–25.
59. Mayer, D. J., and Hayes, R. L. (1975): Stimulation-produced analgesia: Development of tolerance and cross-tolerance to morphine. *Science,* 188:941–953.
60. Mazars, G. J. (1975): Intermittent stimulation of nucleus ventralis posterolateralis for intractable pain. *Surg. Neurol.,* 4:93–94.
61. McNeal, D. R., and Reswick, J. B. (1976): Control of skeletal muscle by electrical stimulation. In: *Advances in Biomedical Engineering,* Vol. 6, edited by J. H. U. Brown and J. F. Dickson, III, pp. 209–256. Academic Press, New York.
62. McNeal, D. R., Waters, R., and Reswick, J. (1977/78): Experience with implanted electrodes at Rancho Los Amigos Hospital. *Appl. Neurophysiol.,* 40:235–239.
63. Melzack, R., and Melinkoff, D. F. (1974): Analgesia produced by brain stimulation: Evidence of a prolonged onset period. *Exp. Neurol.,* 43:369–374.
64. Melzack, R., and Wall, P. D. (1965): Pain mechanisms: A new theory. *Science,* 150:971–979.
65. Meyer, G. A., and Fields, H. L. (1972): Causalgia treated by selective large fiber stimulation of peripheral nerves. *Brain,* 95:163–168.
66. Meyerson, B. A., Boëthius, J., and Carlsson, A. M. (1978): Percutaneous central grey stimulation for cancer pain. *Appl. Neurophysiol. (in press).*
67. Mortimer, J. T., Shealy, C. N., and Wheeler, C. (1970): Experimental nondestructive electrical stimulation of the brain and spinal cord. *J. Neurosurg.,* 32:553–559.
68. Nashold, B. S., Jr., and Friedman, H. (1972): Dorsal column stimulation for control of pain: Preliminary report on 30 patients. *J. Neurosurg.,* 36:590–597.
69. Nashold, B. S., Jr., Friedman, H., and Boyarsky, S. (1971): Electrical activation of micturition by spinal cord stimulation. *J. Surg. Res.,* 11:144–147.
70. Nashold, B. S., Jr., Friedman, H., Glenn, J. F., Grimes, J. H., Barry, W. F., and Avery, R. (1972): Electromicturition in paraplegia. *Arch. Surg.,* 104:195–202.
71. Nashold, B. S., Jr., Friedman, H., Grimes, J., and Avery, R. (1973): Electromicturition in the paraplegic: An electroneuroprosthesis to control voiding. In: *Neural Organization and*

Its Relevance to Prosthetics, eidted by W. S. Fields, pp. 349–368. Intercontinental Med. Book Corp., New York.

72. Nashold, S., Jr., Somjen, G., and Friedman, H. (1972): Paresthesias and EEG potentials evoked by stimulation of the dorsal funiculi in man. *Exp. Neurol.,* 36:273–287.

73. Nielson, K. D., Adams, J. E., and Hosobuchi, Y. (1975): Phantom limb pain: Treatment with dorsal column stimulation. *J. Neurosurg.,* 42:301–307.

74. Nielson, K. D., Watts, C., and Clark, W. K. (1976): Peripheral nerve injury from implantation of chronic stimulating electrodes for pain control. *Surg. Neurol.,* 5:51–53.

75. North, R. B., Fischell, T. A., and Long, D. M. (1977/78): Chronic dorsal column stimulation via percutaneously inserted epidural electrodes: Preliminary results in 31 patients. *Appl. Neurophysiol.,* 40:184–191.

76. Ojemann, G., and Fedio, P. (1968): Effect of stimulation of the human thalamus and parietal and temporal white matter on short-term memory. *J. Neurosurg.,* 29:51–59.

77. Ojemann, G. A., and Ward, A. A., Jr. (1975): Stereotactic and other procedures for epilepsy. *Adv. Neurol.,* 8:241–263.

78. Page, C., and Gault, W. R. (1976): Managing ischemic skin ulcers. *Ann. Fam. Pract.,* 22.108–114.

79. Penfield, W., and Jasper, H. (1954): *Epilepsy and the Functional Anatomy of the Human Brain.* Little Brown and Co., Boston.

80. Picaza, J. A., Hunter, S. E., and Cannon, B. W. (1977/78): Pain suppression by peripheral nerve stimulation: Chronic effects of implanted devices. *Appl. Neurophysiol.,* 223–234.

81. Pineda, A. (1975): Dorsal column stimulation and its prospects. *Surg. Neurol.,* 4:157–163.

82. Pudenz, R. H., Agnew, W. F., Yuen, T. G. H., Bullara, L. A., Jacques, S., and Sheldon, C. H. (1977/78): Adverse effects of electrical energy applied to the nervous system. *Appl. Neurophysiol.,* 40:72–87.

83. Pudenz, R. H., Bullara, L. A., and Talalla, A. (1975): Electrical stimulation of the brain: I. Electrodes and electrode arrays. *Surg. Neurol.,* 4:37–42.

84. Reynolds, D. V. (1969): Surgery in the rat during electrical analgesia induced by focal brain stimulation. *Science,* 164:445.

85. Rhodes, D. L. (1976): Ph.D. dissertation, UCLA, 1975. Cited by Liebeskind, J. C. Pain modulation by central nervous system stimulation. In: *Advances in Pain Research and Therapy,* edited by J. J. Bonica and D. Albe-Fessard, pp. 445–453. Raven Press. New York.

86. Richardson, D. E., and Akil, H. (1973): Acute relief of intractable pain by brain stimulation in human patients. *Proceedings of the Annual Meeting American Association Neurological Surgery.*

87. Richardson, D. E., and Akil, H. (1977): Pain reduction by electrical brain stimulation in man: II. Chronic self-administration in the periventircular gray matter. *J. Neurosurg.,* 47:184–194.

88. Sances, A., Jr., Larson, S. J., Myklebust, J., Swiontek, T., Millar, E. A., Cusick, J. F., Hemmy, D. C., Jodat, R., and Ackmann, J. J. (1977/78): Studies of electrode configuration upon cerebellar implants. *Appl. Neurophysiol.,* 40:141–159.

89. Shealy, C. N. (1974): Transcutaneous electrical stimulation for control of pain. *Clin. Neurosurg.,* 21:269–277.

90. Shealy, C. N. (1975): Dorsal column stimulation: Optimization of application. *Surg. Neurol.,* 4:142–145.

91. Shealy, C. N., (1976): External electrical stimulation: Types, techniques and results. *Neuroelectric News (Neuroelectric Soc.),* 6:4–9.

92. Shealy, C. N., Mortimer, J. T., and Hagfors, N. R. (1970): Dorsal column electroanalgesia. *J. Neurosurg.,* 32:560–564.

93. Shealy, C. N., Mortimer, J. T., and Reswick, J. B. (1967): Electrical inhibition of pain by stimulation of the dorsal columns. Preliminary clinical report. *Anesth. Analg. (Cleve.),* 46:489–491.

94. Shealy, C. N., Taslitz, N., Mortimer, J. T., and Becker, D. P. (1967): Electrical inhibition of pain: Experimental evaluation. *Anesth. Analg. (Cleve.),* 46:299–304.

95. Sherrington, C. S. (1897): Double (antidromc) conduction in the central nervous system. *Proc. R. Soc. London (Biol.),* 61:243–246.

96. Siegfried, J., Krainick, J. V., Hass, H., Adorjani, C., Meyer, M., and Thoden, U. (1978): Electrical spinal cord stimulation for spastic movement disorders. *Appl. Neurophysiol. (in press).*

97. Smith, C. (1977/78): Instrumentation problems with implanted neuroaugmentive devices. *Appl. Neurosphysiol.*, 40:218–222.
98. Stillings, D. (1971): The Medtronic Archive on Electro-stimulation. *Minn. Univ. Bill.* 2:83.
99. Sweet, W. H. (1975): Control of pain by direct electrical stimulation of peripheral nerves. *Clin. Neurosurg.*, 23:103–111.
100. Sweet, W. H., and Wepsic, J. G. (1973): Electrical stimulation for suppression of pain in man. In: *Neural Organization and Its Relevance to Prosthetics*, edited by W. S. Fields, pp. 219–240. Intercontinental Medical Book Corp., New York.
101. Sweet, W. H., and Wepsic, J. G. (1974): Stimulation of the posterior columns of the spinal cord for pain control: Indications, technique and results. *Clin. Neurosurg.*, 21:278–310.
102. Taub, A. (1975): Electrical stimulation for the relief of pain: Two lessons in technological zealotry. *Perspect. Biol. Med.*, 19:125–135.
103. Upton, A. R., and Cooper, I. S. (1976): Some neurophysiological effects of cerebellar stimulation in man. *J. Can. Sci. Neurol.*, 3:237–253.
104. Van Buren, J. M., Wood, H. H., Oakely, J., and Hambrecht, F. (1978): Preliminary evaluation of cerebellar stimulation in the treatment of epilepsy by doubleyblind stimulation and biological criteria. *J. Neurosurg. (in press)*.
105. Vanderlinden, R. G., Gilpin, L., Harper, J., McClurkin, M., and Twilley, D. (1974): Electro-phrenic respiration in quadriplegia. *Can. Nurse*, 70:1–4.
106. Wall, P. D., and Sweet, W. H. (1967): Temporary abolition of pain in man on stimulation of large diameter cutaneous afferent fibers. *Science*, 155:108–109.
107. Waters, R., McNeal, D., and Perry, J. (1975): Experimental correction of footdrop by electrical stimulation of the perineal nerve. *J. Bone Joint Surg. (Am.)*, 57A:1047–1054.
108. White, R. L., and Gross, T. J. (1974): An evaluation of the resistance to electrolysis of metals for use in biostimulation microprobes. *IEEE Trans. Biomed. Eng.*, 21:487–490.

Functional Neurosurgery, edited by T. Rasmussen and R. Marino. Raven Press, New York © 1979.

Computers in Functional Neurosurgery

Gilles Bertrand

Montreal Neurological Institute and Hospital, and Department of Neurology and Neurosurgery, McGill University, Montreal, Quebec, Canada H3A 2B4

Computers have become part of our everyday life. As they have become smaller, cheaper, and more sophisticated, they have found their way into every aspect of human endeavor—scientific, financial, even musical. In the medical field, they not only pay our fees but are also doing automatic biochemical analyses and are replacing conventional X-ray procedures. Functional neurosurgery has also benefited from this technological revolution. At the Montreal Neurological Institute, we have been interested over the last 6 or 7 years in the application of computer techniques to stereotactic procedures.

Stereotactic surgery, which involves the introduction of probes into deep, invisible, cerebral structures, uses various systems of cartesian or polar coordinates to relate the probe position to brain atlases and to radiographic landmarks. In the past, problems of X-ray magnification and distortion, morphological and dimensional discrepancy between the atlas and the patient, and obliquity of probe tracts to the atlas planes have been avoided when possible, simply ignored, or solved by using teleradiographic techniques or mobile image amplifiers, optical devices, mechanical analogs, or mathematical coefficients.

It soon became obvious that most of these problems, which involve complex projection geometry and multiple angles, were ideally suited to computer treatment. Once the rather formidable mathematical formulas were presented to the computer in a suitable language, the most difficult problems could be solved almost instantaneously. Bates and Brewer (1) and Peluso and Gybels (13,14) were among the first to make use of these possibilities in human stereotaxis.

Through a grant from the Medical Research Council of Canada, a Digital Equipment Corporation P.D.P. 12a computer was purchased for the research laboratories of the Montreal Neurological Institute. This computer is connected to a Tektronix Type 4002 Computer Graphics Terminal equipped with a Tektronix Type 4901 Interactive Graphics Unit and Joy Stick. An adequate interface and simple coaxial lines allow the terminal to be used 150 meters away from the main computer so that only a small mobile console supporting the viewing screen and the keyboard need to be taken into the operating room (Fig. 1). The apparatus also has facilities for using an 800-kW word cartridge disk, and the graphic displays can be produced in permanent form with a Tektronix

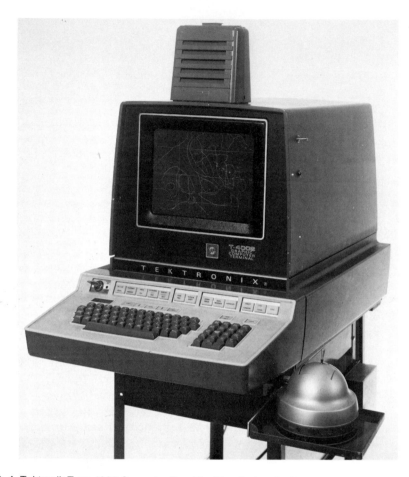

FIG. 1. Tektronik Type 4002 Computer Graphics Terminal and a Tektronix Type 4901 Graphics Unit and Joy Stick. Intercom provides voice connection with main computer.

4001 Hard Copy Unit, mounted under the terminal console or with a Hewlett-Packard X-Y Plotter.

With this equipment, our aim was to display and scale various stereotactic atlas maps in the three different planes, plot and outline probe and electrode tracts against these maps, and codify and store for future use the various physiological responses obtained at different points within the brain.

Most of the extensive programming was done by Christopher Thompson, and work started by digitizing 48 of the 52 maps available in the Schaltenbrand and Bailey atlas (15). To accomplish this, the outline drawings of the atlas were photographically enlarged. Each one was then traced over with the mechanical pen of a Hewlett-Packard X-Y Plotter. The varying voltages across the X and Y slide potentiometers of the plotter were then fed to two channels of the P.D.P. 12 analog-to-digital converter and the computer was instructed to store the X and Y coordinates of each point drawn. Programs were also written to allow proper labeling and identification of the various subdivisions of the thalamus, using a slightly abbreviated version of Hassler's nomenclature (3,17, 18).

This part of the work was carried out by Dr. André Olivier. Later, the atlas of Van Buren and Borke (19) was also digitized in a similar manner by Dr. David Duvoisin, so that one can now rapidly switch from one atlas to the other for comparison when using the program in the operating room or in the laboratories.

In the Schaltenbrand and Bailey atlas, the horizontal and the sagittal sections are from the two hemispheres of the same brain but the frontal sections are from a somewhat smaller brain and, in order to match the frontal sections with the others as best as possible, they were enlarged by 13%. The distance between sections was also increased by 13% and they were relabeled accordingly.

Allowances also had to be made for the fact that the atlas horizontal sections are angled 8° on the intercommissural plane. Programs were then written to allow scaling of any of these maps, expanding or shrinking them in one plane or the other to match the map's intercommissural distance and the thalamic height to the dimensions measured on the individual patient's ventriculogram (Fig. 2). It is also possible to shift the maps in the mediolateral plane to compensate for the variable width of the third ventricle as seen on the anteroposterior ventriculogram.

In practice, all this is made very easy even for someone with very limited knowledge of computers. When the program is loaded, a list of the available maps appears on the screen. This is followed by a set of simple questions which can be answered by typing the required dimensions in millimeters, as measured on the patient's X-rays (Figs. 3 and 4). The operator then types the distance from the midline at which he wishes the target to be. The computer immediately displays the nearest available sagittal map, properly scaled to the patient's dimensions.

The angle made by the intercommissural plane and the horizontal base of the instrument, the angle of tilt of the head to right or left in the frame, easily measured on the X-rays, and the angle of rotation, a little more difficult to ascertain (6), are also typed on the keyboard in answer to specific questions appearing on the terminal screen. The target is selected on the ventriculogram and its coordinates relative to the stereotactic frame are plotted by the method described by Leksell (8,9).

The stereotactic probe is then introduced toward the chosen target as it would be without the computer, but the angles of approach of the probe, relative to the frame, as read on the instrument protractors, are fed to the computer. Cross hairs, visible on the screen, can be moved by manipulating the joy stick to coincide with the target selected on the ventriculogram. Pressing a key will then display the probe correctly oriented toward the target, corrections having

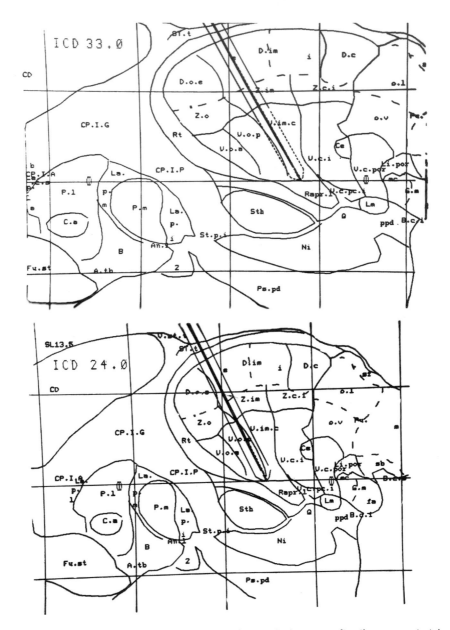

FIG. 2. Sagittal maps **(left)** as they appear on the terminal screen after they were stretched or compressed to match the patient's intercommissural distance as measured on a positive contrast ventriculogram **(right).** In the case at the top, intercommissural distance (middle of commissures) was 33 mm; in the case below, it was only 24 mm.

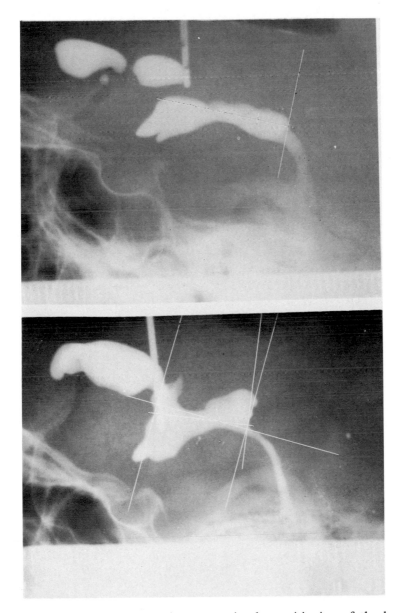

been made for the tilt and rotation errors in the positioning of the head in the frame.

The position of the probe can be displayed against other sagittal maps by simply requesting them on the keyboard. Any part of the probe projected medial to the plane displayed then appears with a dotted outline, indicating clearly the point at which it penetrates that given plane.

```
***** MAP VERSION 100 24 DEC/74 *****
ELECTRODE TIP POSITION X=  7.1 Y=  2.5 Z=  13.7
PROBE TIP POSITION X=  3.7 Y=  2.5 Z=  13.0


IDENTIFY PATIENT   (I)

CHANGE BRAIN SIZE AND ANGLES   (A)

MOVE PROBE OR CHANGE ELECTRODE   (C)

CHANGE CRITERIA FOR DISPLAY OF UNITS   (U)

IDENTIFY UNIT AT ELECTRODE TIP   (E)

DISPLAY PROBE ON MAPS (DISPLAY UNITS ON MAPS)

REDRAW MAP
```

FIG. 3. Option table as it is displayed on the computer terminal allowing a choice of various sets of questions and instructions by typing on the keyboard the character in parentheses.

By moving the horizontal and vertical cross hairs with the joy stick and pressing the key "H" or "F," the available horizontal or frontal section nearest to the corresponding cross hair will be displaced, properly scaled, as well as the probe in its new projection. If other than straight probes are used—curved side-protruding, stimulating, or recording electrodes for instance, or leuko-tomes—the computer is informed by typing the serial number of the probe used in answer to a question on the screen, since the particular geometry of each probe used has been stored on the computer disk memory. The probe can be displayed correctly on the screen after also feeding in other necessary information concerning the distance of the probe tip from the target, the direction around the axis of the probe in which the electrode is extruded, and how far it protrudes (Fig. 5).

During the exploration with electrical stimulation and microelectrode record-ing, preliminary to the making of the therapeutic lesions, a number of responses are obtained that are of great value in ascertaining the target location for each patient, but they also represent useful information for our understanding of the physiological anatomy of the region. Each significant response, positive or negative, can be given a code and the coordinates of its locus; that is, the position of the electrode tip at that moment with respect to the point of origin of the map (the midcommissural plane at the midline) can be displayed immedi-ately or stored on the disk memory (Fig. 6). The present disk, which also contains the data for the two atlases, has enough space for 200 cases, providing 512 "words" for each patient. The first 160 of these 512 words are used for identification of the patient, scale factors, probe angles, etc. The remaining 352 words are used to store unit descriptors each requiring four 12-bit words to save the X, Y, and Z coordinates, information on whether it is from stimulation or recording, the side of the response (ipsilateral, controlateral, bilateral), the

```
***** MAP VERSION 111  27 MAR 1975  *****
TARGET      COORDINATES X=  0.0 Y=  0.0 Z=  0.0
ELECTRODE TIP POSITION X=  0.0 Y=  0.0 Z=  0.0
PROBE    TIP    POSITION X=  0.0 Y=  0.0 Z=  0.0
NO. OF UNITS STORED= 0
```

A 1   RETURN TO OPTION TABLE

A 2   CHANGE INTERCOMMISSURAL DISTANCE FROM: 23.5 TO::

A 3   CHANGE THALAMIC HEIGHT FROM: 19.5 TO::

A 4   CHANGE THIRD VENTRICLE WIDTH FROM: 2.0 TO::

A 5   CHANGE A-P ‹X› OFFSET FROM: 0.0 TO::

A 6   CHANGE VERTICAL ‹Y› OFFSET FROM: 0.0 TO::

A 7   CHANGE HORIZONTAL ‹Z› SCALE FACTOR FROM: 10.0 TO::

A 8   CHANGE FRAME SKEW ‹LATERAL› ANGLE FROM: 0 TO::

A 9   CHANGE FRAME TILT ‹FRONTAL› ANGLE FROM: 0 TO::

A 10 CHANGE ROTATION ANGLE OF BRAIN IN FRAME FROM: 0 TO::

A 11 CHANGE A-P ANGLE OF PROBE FROM: 0 TO::

A 12 CHANGE LATERAL ANGLE OF PROBE FROM: 0 TO::

A 13 CHANGE A-P TARGET ‹ *P* › POSITION FROM: 0.0 TO::

A 14 CHANGE VERTICAL TARGET ‹ *H.V.* › POSITION FROM: 0.0 TO::

A 15 CHANGE LATERAL TRAGET ‹Z› POSITION FROM: 0.0 TO::

A 16 IDENTIFY TARGET ON SAGITAL SECTION

A 17 REDRAW MAP

FIG. 4. List of directions, as they appear on the computer terminal, allowing for the scaling of maps to the patient's dimensions, correction of tilt, rotation errors, and display of probe tract to target. The target can be selected by pointing at it with cross hairs and a joy stick on the sagittal map, or by typing its coordinates.

type of response, and a code indicating one of three levels of confidence. High levels of confidence are given to units precisely identified during recording, such as cells responding to a light touch of small skin areas or responses to low-voltage stimulation—less than 1 V for motor, less than 0.5 V for sensory responses. Units less clearly identified or doubtful, and responses to higher voltages, are given lower levels of confidence.

Hardy (6) has recently carried out a retrospective analysis of some 275 operations and selected 130 for which adequate stimulation and recording protocols, as well as ventriculograms outlining both commissures and films of the probes in position, were available.

Data from all these patients have been entered on the computer disk memory, which now contains more than 2,000 responses of various types.

Simultaneous display of all these responses is not very useful except to outline

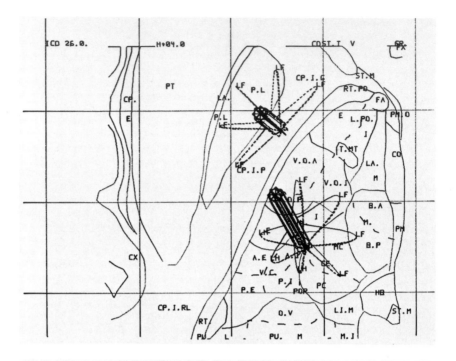

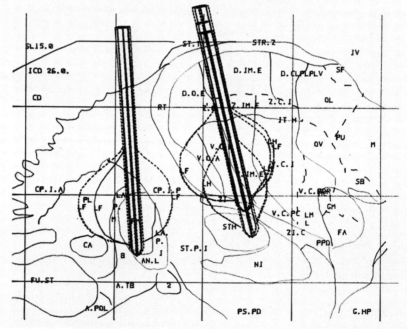

the general area which has been subjected to exploration, but the use of restrictor subroutines can determine which type of unit or motor response is to be displayed, restrictions regarding the level of confidence, laterality of the response, and one or more brain dimensions; the patient's age or diagnosis can also be imposed. Furthermore, the data can be displayed according to their real coordinates relative to the midline midcommissural point (MCP), as they are stored on the disk or with respect to maps scaled for each individual case as is usually done in the operating room. Each section shown on the screen represents a slice of brain within which responses are obtained. The thickness of these slices can be varied at will so that various strata of the brain can be examined in turn (18) (Figs. 7 and 8).

As can be seen, this computer program is a powerful tool that we find extremely useful in the operating room, since it allows us to keep track of the position of our probes at any time, to recall and compare the physiological data obtained, and to plan the location and shape of our therapeutic lesion accordingly. It is also a research instrument and a bank containing a wealth of information that would be very difficult and time-consuming to analyze otherwise. Similar computer displays are also being used in other centers. In Germany, Mundinger, Birg, and their collaborators (4,10) are using theirs. Tasker's group in Toronto is using a very elegant and illustrative method to display the responses to thalamic stimulations with Woolsey-type figurines on scaled maps (7,18). Others, such as Colloff and his collaborators in San Francisco (5), use the computer primarily to calculate the target coordinates from the ventriculogram, whereas in Tokyo, Ohye, Narabayashi, and Saito are applying the computer techniques to on-line automatic analysis of the unit discharges recorded from the thalamus during operations (11).

It is obvious that such sophisticated computer techniques are not within the reach of individual neurosurgeons, but nearly every large center, and particularly University Hospitals, now have some type of computer center and more importantly people capable of understanding the problems of stereotactic surgery and of programming their machines according to the specific needs of the surgeon and the stereotactic instrumentation.

Smaller and more powerful computers and microprocessors can now perform the functions I have described and more, for only a fraction of the cost of our original equipment. We are also hearing the first reports on what should be a happy marriage between stereotaxis and computerized axial tomography (2). Better definition and thinner "slices" now permit visualization of the outlines of the larger nuclear groups, caudate nucleus, globus pallidus, thalamus, amyg-

---

FIG. 5. Horizontal **(top)** and sagittal **(bottom)** representation of two leukotome tracts (separate procedures on same patient with dystonia musculorum deformans) and extent of lesions made each time. The horizontal map chosen is 4 mm above the commissural plane. All parts of the probes or leukotome wire loops below this plane appear in dotted lines. Solid lines are above the plane. The sagittal view illustrated is 15 mm from the midline. The dotted portion of the probes is medial to that plane.

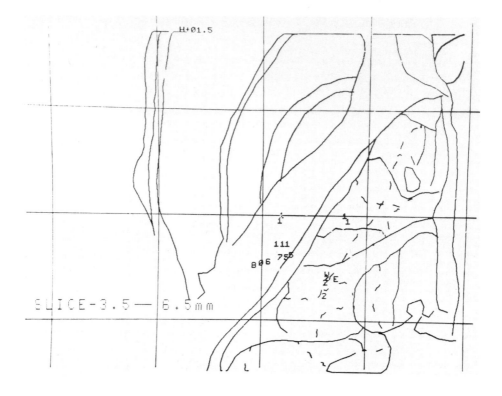

SLICE -3.5 — 8.5mm

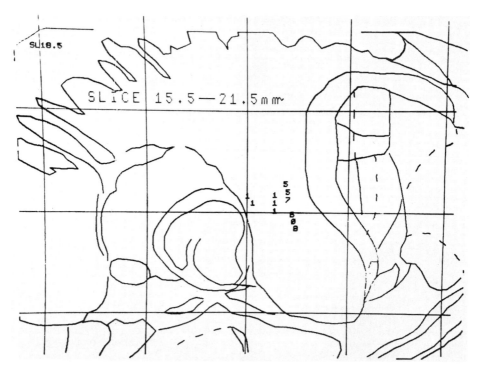

SLICE 15.5 — 21.5mm

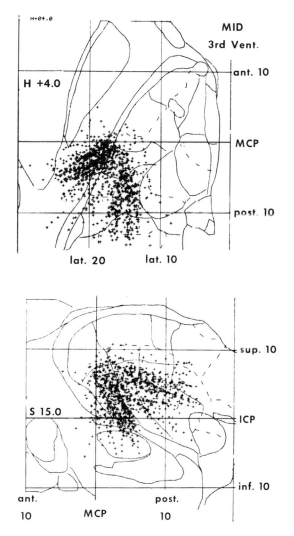

FIG. 7. Horizontal **(top)** and sagittal **(bottom)** representation of all points stimulated in 130 selected cases (number of units-1,264, slice thickness-40 mm). (From ref. 6.)

FIG. 6. Horizontal **(top)** and sagittal **(bottom)** (as they appear on terminal) displaying points stimulated with a side-protruding monopolar electrode. Only positive responses are shown. The horizontal map is the one at 1.5 mm above the intercommissural plane (ICP), but the responses are from a slice 10-mm thick, between −3.5 mm and +6.5 mm. The sagittal map **(bottom)** which is 18.5 mm from the midline outlines the responses within a 6-mm thick slice (15.5 to 21.5 mm from midline), so that only the capsular responses are seen where code 1 indicates tongue movements; (codes 5, 6, and 7 indicate finger, hand, and arm movements; and 0 and 8 indicate trunk and leg movements, respectively. Code letters in the thalamus on horizontal view refer to various sensory responses.

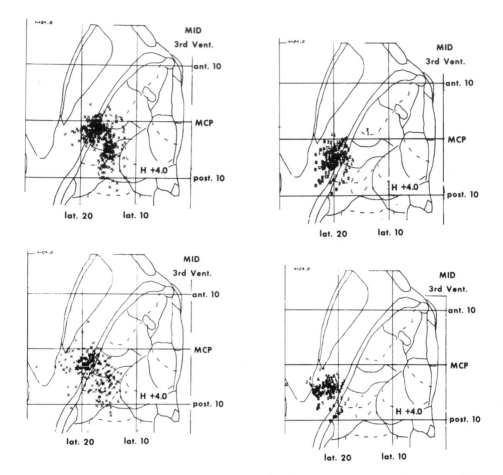

FIG. 8. Location of points where stimulation produced motor responses at low voltage (0.5 V or less; high level of confidence) and where no response was obtained with up to 2 V. **Top:** 71 cases with narrow third ventricle, 1–5 mm as measured on the anteroposterior ventriculogram. *(Left):* Negative responses; number of units-295, slice thickness-40mm. *(Right):* Positive motor responses; number of units-250, slice thickness-40 mm. **Bottom:** 58 cases with wide third ventricle, 6 to 14 mm. *(Left):* Negative responses; number of units-213, slice thickness-40 mm. *(Right):* Positive motor responses; number of units-190, slice thickness-40 mm. In cases with narrow third ventricle, the cluster of responses is centered 20 mm from the midline. In the wide ventricle group, the cluster centers at 22 mm and extends further laterally. MCP, midcommissural point. (From ref. 6.)

dala, and internal capsule, so that targets will become directly visible without the need for guidance by distant reference points, and the lesions themselves can be seen. This is only the beginning.

REFERENCES

1. Bates, J. A. V., and Brewer, A. (1968): Geometric Aspects of Stereotaxic Surgery. *(Manuscript in preparation.)*

2. Bergström, M. (1976): Stereotaxic computed tomography. *Am. J. Roentgenol.*, 127:167–170.
3. Bertrand, G., Olivier, A., and Thompson, C. J. (1974): Computer display of stereotaxic brain maps and probe tracts. *Acta Neurochir.*, 21 (Suppl.):235–243.
4. Birg, W., and Mundinger, F. (1974): Computer programmes for stereotactic neurosurgery. *Confin. Neurol.*, 36:326–333.
5. Colloff, E., Gleason, C. A., Alberts, W. W., and Wright, E. W., Jr. (1973): Computer-aided localization techniques for stereotaxic surgery. *Confin. Neurol.*, 35:65–80.
6. Hardy, T. L. (1975): Computer display of the electrophysiological topography of the diencephalon during stereotaxic surgery. M. Sc. Thesis, McGill University, Department of Neurology and Neurosurgery.
7. Hawrylyshyn, P., Rowe, I. H., Tasker, R. R., and Organ, L. W. (1976): A computer system for stereotaxic surgery *Comput. Biol. Med.*, 6:87–97.
8. Leksell, L. (1951): The stereotaxic method and radiosurgery of the brain. *Acta Chir. Scand.*, 102:316.
9. Leksell, L. (1971): *Stereotaxis and Radiosurgery: An Operative System.* Charles C Thomas, Springfield, Illinois.
10. Mundinger, F. (1974): Neuerungen der stereotaktische Operation durch den Einlezug von Computerverfahren. *Z. Allg. Med.*, 50:817–821.
11. Ohye, C., and Narabayashi, H. (1972): Activity of thalamic neurones and their receptive fields in different functional states in man. In: *Neurophysiology Studied in Man*, edited by G. G. Somjen, pp. 64–78. Excerpta Medica, Amsterdam.
12. Ohye, C., Saito, Y., Fukamachi, A., and Narabayashi, H. (1974): An analysis of the spontaneous rhythmic and non rhythmic burst discharges in the human thalamus. *J. Neurol. Sci.*, 22:245–259.
13. Peluso, F., and Gybels, J. (1969): Computer calculation of two-target trajectory with "center of arca target" stereotaxic equipment. *Acta Neurochir.* 21:173–180.
14. Peluso, F., and Gybels, J. (1970): Calculation of position of electrode point during penetration in human brain. *Confin. Neurol.*, 32:213–218.
15. Schaltenbrand, G., and Bailey, P. (1959): *Introduction to Stereotaxis with an Atlas of the Human Brain.* Grune & Stratton, New York.
16. Tasker, R. R., Rowe, I. H., Hawrylyshyn, P., and Organ, L. W. (1976): Computer mapping of brain stem sensory centers in man. *J. Neurosurg.*, 44:458–464.
17. Thompson, C. J., and Bertrand, G. (1972): A computer programme to aid the neurosurgeon to locate probes during stereotaxic surgery on deep cerebral structures. *Comput. Programs Biomed.*, 2:265–276.
18. Thompson, C. J., Hardy, T., and Bertrand, G. (1977): A system for anatomical and functional mapping of the human thalamus. *Comput. Biomed. Res.*, 10:9–24.
19. Van Beuren, J. M., and Burke, R. C. (1972): *Variations and Connections of the Human Thalamus.* Springer-Verlag, New York.

Functional Neurosurgery, edited by T. Rasmussen
and R. Marino. Raven Press, New York © 1979.

Functional Surgery of Abnormal Movements

P. Molina-Negro

*Department of Surgery, University of Montreal and Service of Neurosurgery,
Hôpital Notre-Dame, Montreal, Quebec, Canada H2L 1M4*

The particular agency by which the lesion is made appears to be of less importance than the precision of its placement.

—Russell Meyers, 1968

Surgery of abnormal movements is as old as neurosurgery. Indeed, in 1909,
Horsley (48) reported the relief of hemiathetosis by removal of the precentral
gyrus. The same technique was advocated by Bucy and Buchanan, who, in
1932 (22) described the procedure in detail and speculated about its mechanisms
of action. Foerster, in 1911 (29), published the result of posterior rhizotomy
on Parkinson's disease and in spasticity. Pollock and Davis in 1930 (72) also
reported on the role of posterior rhizotomy in the alleviation of parkinsonian
tremor and rigidity. Each of these techniques, cortical removal and posterior
root section, represents the two main currents of thought in the surgical treatment
of dyskinesias during the first half of this century. The first technique, according
to Bucy, is based on the belief that abolition of tremor necessarily depends on
the interruption of corticospinal projections, the final common path of both
normal and abnormal movements. Based on this same view, other techniques
were described that now have been abandoned, such as pedunculotomy (38,82),
and cordotomy (73). On the other hand, the practice of posterior rhizotomy
in Parkinson's disease is based on the assumption that physiopathology of tremor
and/or rigidity is related to proprioception, a view that seems to be right for
rigidity only, since it disappeared permanently after rhizotomy. Tremor, on
the other hand, recurs, although in a disorganized manner, after a short period.
Those who support ventro-intermedius nucleus (Vim) of the thalamus as the
stereotactic target for the arrest of tremor (11,25) follow the same line of thought.

Lesions of the corticospinal system and rhizotomies represent the prehistory
of functional neurosurgery. Both lack the essential prerequisite of techniques
of functional neurosurgery, namely, to be directed to a normal yet hyperfunction-
ing primitive structure, as a result of a loss of function of a new center directly
affected by the disease. Both techniques act on the two ends of the complex
reflex arch that represents the nervous system of mammals, leaving untouched
the intermediate integrative centers where motor functions are organized.

The fact that lesions of the corticospinal system affect only indirectly involuntary movements was remarked by James Parkinson, who reports in his "Essay
on the Shaking Palsy" the case of a patient suddenly paralyzed by what seems

to have been an ischemic cerebrovascular accident: " . . . during the time of their having remained in this state, neither the arm nor the leg of the paralytic side was in the least affected with the tremolous agitation; but as their paralysed state was removed, the shaking returned." (68). It is obvious that abnormal involuntary movements are organized in the core of the primitive motor centers and that precisely there, functional surgical techniques must be directed.

The first functional procedure directed to the basal ganglia seems to be the direct transventricular caudatotomy performed by Russell Meyers in 1939 and published in 1941 (62) in a parkinsonian woman in whom the undercutting of the premotor cortex failed to abolish the tremor. Little by little the target moved from the head of the caudate nucleus to the tip of the internal globus pallidus, a technique named ansotomy by Meyers, because it interrupts the final common efferent path of the basal ganglia, the ansa lenticularis. By 1949 Meyers had performed 22 ansotomies (64). It was precisely this last procedure that became the main and almost the unique treatment of parkinsonian tremor during the next decade.

The great morbidity rate of the open procedures of pallidotomy and ansotomy led Fenelon to perform cauterization of the globus pallidus with an electrode through a temporal burr hole (28). Although Fenelon used only external anatomical references, his operation was probably the first stereotactic procedure. The success of stereotactic surgery is related on the very first hand to the mapping of brains with precise references to internal anatomical landmarks which are easily identifiable. The first such atlas was published by Spiegel and Wycis in 1952 (75), and after this date, the development of modern stereotactic surgery really began. It was also Spiegel et al. (76) who in 1947 described the first apparatus for human stereotactic surgery. It is important to mention that an analogous instrument had already been described for the use in animals by Horsley and Clarke in 1908 (49).

The development of a new stereotactic atlas and instruments was paralleled by the application of neurophysiological methods of exploration during surgery. In 1949, Hayne et al. (47) published the first recording of the electrical activity of the basal ganglia. Hassler, in 1955 (42), proposed a physiopathological mechanism for the tremor at rest and, at the same time gave a detailed account of the result of stimulation and coagulation in the human thalamus. Following Hassler's point of view, the basal ganglia were soon abandoned in favor of different nuclei of the thalamus and the thalamo-subthalamic carrefour as the optimum targets for treatment of tremors and other kinds of hyperkinesia.

The introduction in 1961 of microelectrode recording as a routine technique during stereotactic surgery by Albe-Fessard et al. (1), together with precise mapping of sensory and motor responses to stimulation (8,14,37), have opened a new field of research concerning the physiopathology of abnormal movements. Neurophysiological methods of localization have also added precision and safety to stereotactic surgery of abnormal movements, which remains one of the most important fields of functional stereotactic neurosurgery.

GENERAL PRINCIPLES AND OUTLINE OF STEREOTACTIC PROCEDURES

Although the basic ideas that follow apply to all stereotactic procedures independent of the target, the anatomical landmarks, and the instruments employed, we will follow, step by step, the technique originally described in 1955 by Bertrand (7) and progressively perfected during the last 20 years in the performance of about 2,000 operations (8,9,12,16,17).

Indication for Surgery

The first condition is the existence of a precise indication for surgery. The fulfillment of this condition required first the presence of an abnormal movement disorder whose intensity justifies operative treatment. Second, the lack of efficiency of all known conservative procedures must be established after a reasonable trial period. Third, any possible contraindication should be ruled out. The contraindication can arise both from the presence of a systemic disease, such as malignant hypertension, uncontrolled diabetes, severe liver or kidney disease, or from the presence of advanced negative symptoms accompanying the positive ones.

To give two diametrically opposed cases of borderline indications for surgery, we can outline the case of a young right-handed cabinetmaker who suffered from predominant right-sided heredofamilial tremor of attitude of mild intensity. The opposite could be the case of a middle-aged housewife suffering from severe multiple sclerosis, with complete paraplegia, dysarthria, and with a violent movement or intention tremor, making any purposeful movement impossible. The risk of side effects can be justified if the first patient, the cabinetmaker, has the responsibility of providing for a family and if the second patient, the housewife, suffers physically or psychologically from the absolute dependence on others for everything.

Definition of a Target

There has been an era of empiricism in the choice of targets for the control of abnormal movements. Ligation of the anterior choroidal artery, accidentally performed by Cooper during the approach to the midbrain in a case of parkinsonism, produced necrosis of the globus pallidus, thus suppressing the tremor of the contralateral limbs without any major side effect (23). For a few years, this procedure became the technique of choice by Cooper and others. The same author reported in 1961 (24) how ventrolateral thalamotomy had been his new technique of choice since 1957, following an accidental thalamotomy while attempting a pallidotomy. The originality of the discovery is diminished by the fact that Hassler had already published in 1955 the rationale of the use of thalamotomy in the treatment of parkinsonian tremor (42). In the treatment of an abnormal movement, every surgical procedure must today be preceded by the choice of a precise target based on some anatomophysiological assumption regarding its mechanism of production. Little has been done in this regard since the publication by Hassler in 1959 of a review of all the types of dyskinesia with a discussion of their mechanism and the optimal targets for the alleviation of dyskinesia (45).

In the choice of targets one must keep in mind the surrounding structures. In functional surgery, side effects must be carefully prevented and avoided. It was almost 20 years ago that Hassler wrote: "It is also no longer necessary to create additional functional disturbances in exchange for the alleviated ones when the intervention is performed by way of the stereotaxic method. The only decisive problem is which neuron system is to be disrupted" (45).

Localization of the Target in a Stereotactic Atlas

One of the major advances in functional stereotactic surgery was a publication by Spiegel and Wycis in 1952 on the first stereotactic atlas of human brain (75), followed shortly afterward by publications of Talairach et al. (77) in 1957 and Shaltenbrand and Bailey in 1960 (74). In each atlas, careful measurements of the model brains were made in relation to three planes of Cartesian coordinates constructed over a base line. Spiegel and Wycis used the foramen of Monro–pineal gland line. Talairach and Shaltenbrand used the anterior-posterior bicommissural line (AC-PC) with minor variation. While Talairach employed a tangent to the upper limit of the anterior commissure and inferior limit of the posterior commissure, Shaltenbrand used the center of both commissures. Once the choice of the target has been made, its coordinates in relation to the three planes—vertical, parasagittal, and horizontal—are determined.

Transposition of the Cartesian System of Coordinates into the Patient's Brain

Once anatomical landmarks have been localized in the radiography, the base line is traced and measured. Then the coordinates of the target in the model brain are translated into the patient's brain. If one used absolute measurements, the distortion produced by the enlargement of the radiographic image must be carefully avoided by the use of teleradiography or else it must be corrected through mathematical calculation. The coordinates of the target must suffer further correction by comparison between the anthropomorphic type of skull of the patient and that of the model brain of the atlas. Most of the painstaking calculations described can be easily overcome with the use of proportional measurement, as will be discussed later.

Electrophysiological Analysis of the Trajectory from the Periphery to the Target

Electrical stimulation at different points within the trajectory and at the target point is an absolute requirement prior to making the lesion. It will provide confirmation of the accuracy of the trajectory with threshold intensity and information on surrounding structures with stronger stimuli.

Microelectrode recording is highly desirable, since it provides exact information about the function of each point of the trajectory. Upper and lower limits of the thalamus and/or the lenticular nucleus are very accurately determined. The choice of a subthalamic target demands almost of necessity microelectrode recording to permit the localization of the subthalamic nucleus and the medical lemniscus.

Making the Lesion

A last method of verification of the exactness of the localization and the efficacy of the lesion is to make a reversible lesion. That is possible with mechanical, physical, and chemical agents. If, for any reason, the temporary lesion is ineffective or provokes undesirable side effects, a new placement is made. As a rule, a perfect immediate effect must be obtained during surgery. Recurrence is the rule if the immediate result is only partial.

INDICATION FOR SURGERY IN ABNORMAL MOVEMENTS

General Discussion

Abnormal movements, like all other functional disorders of the brain, result from increased uncontrolled activity of certain primitive centers that have been deprived of the inhibitory action of newly developed centers, and have been affected directly by the disease. Negative manifestations of the latter are called "primary," in order to distinguish them from negative symptoms "secondary" to the positive ones.

Indications for surgery arise from positive symptoms and, occasionally from some of their negative consequences also. But a primary negative symptom will never be an indication for surgical treatment. Furthermore, primary negative symptoms constitute, as a rule, a contraindication. Indeed, they can only be increased by surgery, since every lesion, no matter how carefully planned and performed, will of necessity add some further negative effects.

It is therefore essential, before the choice of the target, to understand the basic physiopathological mechanism of the abnormal movement to be treated and, more precisely, the place where it originated, or at least the pathways through which it travels. These conditions are fulfilled only by three categories of abnormal movements: tremors, torsion dystonias, and some manifestations of cerebellar dyskinesia. The mechanism of production and the precise targets for the treatment of other abnormal movements such as choreas, athetosis, symptomatic dystonia, and hemiballism remain, at the present time, matters of speculation, and the results of treatment often poor and temporary.

Mechanism of Production of Parkinsonian Tremor and Optimum Target for Its Arrest

The first description of the pathology of Parkinson's disease was made by Trétiakoff in 1919 (78), about 100 years after the publication of the "Essay on the Shaking Palsy." Hassler in 1938 (41), Benda and Cobb in 1942 (6), and Greenfield and Bosanquet in 1953 (33) confirmed that depigmentation followed by degeneration of nigral cells was the essential feature. The same authors concluded that Lewy bodies and depigmentation can be found in all pigmented nuclei of the brain stem and particularly in the dorsal nucleus of the vagus nerve and in the locus ceruleus. Cases 3 and 6 of Benda and Cobb (6) served to demonstrate that the presence of tremor in only one side is related to degeneration of the opposite substantia nigra. A variable degree of pallidal and striatal involvement can be found in advanced cases of parkinsonism, but the same findings have been made in subjects of advanced age without Parkinson's disease. In cases of severe primary akinesia, degeneration of periaqueductal gray matter is prominent. Mental involvement seems to be correlated with premotor and frontal cortex degeneration. This was particularly evident in case number 6 of Benda and Cobb (6). In postencephalitic parkinsonism, the localization of lesions is essentially the same as in idiopathic disease, but instead of Lewy bodies, one finds neurofibrillary Alzheimer tangles.

A study of pathological conditions does not enable one to localize the place of origin of the tremor. It is nevertheless evident, according to Jackson's principle, that the centers primarily involved by the degeneration are not responsible for the positive symptoms.

The substantia nigra and the other pigmented nuclei can be reasonably excluded as candidates for the tremorogenic center. On the other hand, periaqueductal gray matter, reticular tegmentum, and frontal and premotor cortex become progressively involved as the disease progresses. And since it is well known that in advanced cases the tremor tends to become disorganized and diminished, parallel to the increase of akinesia, the hypothesis can be advanced that tremor is the positive symptom and akinesia the negative one resulting, respectively, from excess of function and loss of function of reticular tegmentum, periaqueductal gray, and possibly also of prefrontal and premotor cortex. Anatomical experiences have contributed decisively to the recognition of the centers where tremor originated.

In 1948, Ward et al. (83) produced for the first time, in the monkey, a parkinsonian-like tremor by placing small electrolytic lesions between the red nucleus and the substantia nigra. In 1953, Jenker and Ward (53), with electrical stimulation of the midbrain and upper pons reticular substance, in intact monkeys, produced rhythmical alternating activity analogous to the spontaneous tremor of the monkey with paranigral lesion. The same authors showed that the electrically induced tremor is abolished by intravenous injection of anticholinergic drugs. The work of Ward et al. (83) was confirmed by Poirier in 1960 (69), who showed that the tegmental lesion must provoke retrograde degeneration of the pars compacta of the substantia nigra in order to produce postural parkin sonian-like tremor. On the other hand, the hypothesis of Jenker and Ward (53) of a cholinergic tremorogenic center in the midbrain reticular tegmentum was confirmed by George et al. in 1962 (31). These authors demonstrated that oxi-tremorine, a powerful cholinergic drug, provokes a postural or resting tremor that is in turn abolished by electrolytic lesions in the midbrain tegmentum.

Biochemical experiments have also thrown some light on the problem of tremorogenesis. Ehringer and Hornykiewicz in 1960 (27) found in the striatum of patients with Parkinson's disease a decrease of dopamine and epinephrine. Poirier and Sourkes, on the other hand, described in 1965 (70), in the brain of monkeys with tremor after tegmented lesions, a decrease of striatal content of dopamine parallel to the loss of cells of the substantia nigra. In 1961, Barbeau (4) suggested a relation between the parkinsonian syndrome that follows prolonged administration of reserpine and the depletion of dopamine from the striatum. This hypothesis was reinforced by the discovery by Barbeau et al. in 1961 (5) of a diminution of urinary excretion of dopamine in parkinsonian patients. In the same year, McGeer et al. (61) based on the fact that tremors and rigidity diminished after administration of anticholinergic drugs, advanced the following hypothesis: In the brain, and particularly in the striatum, there exists an equilibrium between two groups of antagonistic substances; on one hand, the dopamine and the serotonin exert an inhibitory action; on the other hand, acetylcholine and histamine produce facilitory action. Parkinsonian syndrome would be characterized by the imbalance of this system, with predominance of acetylcholine and histamine over dopamine and serotonin.

Electrophysiological studies of human beings during stereotactic procedures have also contributed to the elucidation of the pathophysiology of tremors. In the thalamo-subthalamic junction, at the level of the prelemniscal radiations, there exists a minute area of a few millimeters where microelectrodes can record spontaneous 5-per-second autonomous rhythms, that is, a rhythm that is not provoked by the muscle contraction. The same type of rhythm has been recorded in a broader zone of the thalamus corresponding to the anterior half of the dorsal thalamic nucleus and the ventro-oralis anterior (Voa) (10,79). It is precisely in this critical zone that the introduction of both the recording microelectrode and the larger stimulating electrode provokes the arrest of tremor. This area is so sharply delimited that a deviation of 2 mm in any direction is sufficient for the persistence of the tremor. The same type of rhythmic cellular activity has been recorded by Velasco *(personal communication)* in the motor area of the cortex of monkeys with tremor produced by midbrain tegmental lesions. Finally, although autonomous rhythms have not been recorded from the pallidum, this nucleus remains a good target for the arrest of tremors.

Based on these premises, we postulate the existence of a tremorogenic circuit in which the main relays are the midbrain reticular tremorogenic center, the globus pallidus, the Voa nucleus of the thalamus, and the premotor frontal cortex (Fig. 1). This circuit employs acetylcholine as the main neurotransmitter. The tremorogenic center corresponds to the ascending activating reticular system of Moruzzi and Magoon (67) or to part of it. Rhythmic motor activity in primitive vertebrates and in man originates in this circuit. We postulate that the level of activation of the circuit in relation to motor function is regulated by the substantia nigra, through its cholinergic efferents from the big pigmented cells of the pars compacta that project monosynaptically to the reticular cells of the midbrain, the pallidum, the Voa nucleus of the thalamus, and probably also to the premotor frontal cortex (65). There exists a feedback mechanism that controls the level of activity of the substantia nigra, through strionigral projections to the pars reticulata; also it probably employs GABA as its neurotransmitter (3,55). The existence of a tremorogenic circuit with acetylcholine as transmitter, would explain the disappearance of tremor during sleep and its diminution with cholinergic drugs. On the other hand, association of levodopa with anticholinergic drugs reinforced the antitremorogenic action of the latter, since it acts in opposition to the basic biochemical disequilibrium underlying the parkinsonian syndrome.

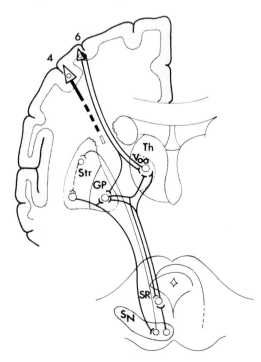

FIG. 1. The tremorogenic circuit of the brain, overactive because of lesions of the subtantia nigra (SN) in parkinsonism and of the striatum (Str) in heredofamilial tremor of attitude (th, thalamus; Voa, ventro-oralis anterior; GP, globus pallidus; SR, reticular substance).

The optimum physiological target for the arrest of tremor is the posterior part of the zona incerta, usually called prelemniscal radiations, probably because it corresponds to the upper limit of the tremorogenic center, where the bulk of the fibers connect it with the other relay of the tremorogenic circuit.

Hassler (45), following Jung (54), affirms that "tremor at rest is a pathophysiological phenomenon arising from the internuncial neurones of the spinal cord." Although we don't agree with such a statement, it appears from our personal studies with the recovery curve of the H reflex in parkinsonian patients that the rhythm of the tremor depends upon the refractory period of the alpha motoneurons. Indeed, in patients with postural tremor, and in the same side in cases with unilateral tremor, there exists, following an absolute refractory period of normal duration, a period of hyperexcitability between 150 and 250 msec demonstrated by an effect of overshoot, characterized by a higher value of the second H reflex. This phenomenon disappears immediately after a successful operation. That may explain the rhythm of parkinsonian tremor that varies from 4 to 7 cps, and also may explain the disorganization of the tremor after posterior rhizotomy (72). The Voa nucleus, where the pallidothalamic bundle ends, is the second most important target, followed by the pallidum internus (GPI) and the ansa lenticularis. It is the author's opinion that ventro-oralis posterior (Vop) and Vim nuclei, terminations, respectively, of cerebello-rubro-thalamic and vestibulo-thalamic pathways, are not involved in the generation of tremors and are not ideal targets for tremor. Those who sustain the contrary view agree that recurrence is very high with lesions located entirely above AC-PC line. The results are, on the contrary, better when the lesion encroaches on the zona incerta and on Forel's field.

Pathophysiology of Heredofamilial Tremor of Attitude and Target for Its Arrest

The tremor of attitude, usually called (from Critchley) essential or heredofamilial tremor, is related to striatal disease. Transmitted as an autosomal dominant character, sometimes related to sex, it appears as an isolated phenomenon. In about 5 to 10% of the cases, one can find in the family of a patient with spasmodic torticollis another case of a well-known striatal disease. Hassler (43) described the "état pré-criblé" of the striatum as the main pathological feature of tremor of attitude. Further evidence of involvement of the striatum is the appearance of tremor of attitude following invasion of the putamen by tumors of the frontal or temporal lobes. I have personally studied five cases of astrocytoma of the caudate or putamen. In another personal case, a lesion placed in the anterior limb of the internal capsule because of an unusually important dilatation of both lateral ventricles in a case of intractable pain accidentally encroached on the caudate nucleus. Forty-eight hours later the patient developed a bilateral tremor of attitude of both upper limbs that remained unchanged until the patient died 2 weeks later *(unpublished cases)*. The infrequent observation of tremor of attitude in cases of tumoral invasion of the basal ganglia is explained by the fact that when the ganglia are involved, the thalamus and/

or the internal capsule are also involved, and that prevents the appearance of the tremor.

We do not know with certainty the place where tremor originates, but it is the author's opinion that the tremorogenic center and circuit are the same as in Parkinson's disease. The underlying biochemical mechanism and the structure acting as the circuit's control are different. The target for the arrest of tremor described for the parkinsonian tremor is exactly the same, that is, the prelemniscal zona incerta or Voa nucleus.

Pathophysiology of Spasmodic Torticollis and Target for Its Alleviation

In accordance with the Jackson's principle, torticollis represents an exaggeration of the head's function of rotation resulting from a lesion of a structure which, normally, inhibits this movement. In order to explain the mechanism of the torticollis' production, one must first determine which are the anatomical centers and pathways involved in transmission of impulses responsible for the turning movement of the head and then identify the inhibiting structures controlling those centers.

The principal source of stimuli responsible for the rotatory motions of the head is the vestibular system. Indeed, in two patients with paroxysmal vertigo secondary to a labyrinthine fistula, ipsilateral caloric stimulation induced adversive conjugate deviation of eyes and head *(unpublished case)*. Frequently, in patients with spasmodic torticollis, caloric stimulation on both sides, but particularly on the opposite side, induces dramatic and maintained accentuation of the torticollis. On the other hand, there are certain cases in which irritation of the vestibular nerve seems to be the cause of the torticollis. This was the case of a 37-year-old female patient, treated for a cochleovestibular syndrome for 6 years, to which was added in the past 2 years a spasmodic torticollis with rotation of the head toward the left. Audiometry and ENG suggested a right retrocochlear lesion. In addition, trigeminofacial and facial reflexes supported this hypothesis. Finally, angiography of the posterior cranial fossa showed a vascular anomaly close to the internal auditory meatus. Surgical exploration disclosed an arterial loop firmly adherent to the acousticofacial complex. Release of the loop resulted in progressive diminution and disappearance of the vestibular syndrome within a few weeks. At the same time, the rotary motions of the head progressively disappeared.

Nevertheless, one should not exaggerate the part taken by the vestibular system in the production of the spasmodic torticollis. Indeed, this case is an exception, and one should not confuse a real spasmodic torticollis with abnormal postures of the head found in some patients suffering vestibular syndrome and without involuntary movements of the head. In those cases, careful examination shows that the abnormal posture represents a defense mechanism, often unconscious, positioning the head in a most advantageous posture in order to prevent vertigo. I had the occasion to study a patient with permanent tilting and slight rotation of the head where a trial of head-straightening, either by the patient or the observer, started a paroxysmal vertigo with nausea. It is not surprising, therefore, that trials of torticollis treatment by surgery at the peripheral vestibular system level were progressively abandoned because of inconstant and transitory results.

Vestibular impulses nevertheless do not constitute the only source of the rotary movements of the head. Indeed, auditory and tactile impulses coming from the side opposite to the direction of the movement can increase the rotary motions of the head. Where we study the blink reflex obtained with electrical stimulation of the trigeminal nerve in patients with torticollis, we can observe occasionally, and particularly when stimulations are made without previous notice, the accentuation of the turning movements of the head. In view of this result, we placed the recording electrodes not only in the orbicularis oculi but also in the sternocleidomastoid. The electrical stimulations of the trigeminal nerve produces a bilateral response with a latency of about 50 msec which is more prominent ipsilaterally. This response probably represents an archaic polysynaptic trigeminospinal reflex that we do not find in normal persons and that manifests the hyperexcitability of the rotary centers of the head.

Experimental physiological and anatomical studies on the vestibular nucleus and its projections related almost exclusively the function of the vestibular nucleus in relation to equilibrium and postural tonus. It is not the time to insist on the description of connections of the vestibular nucleus with the cerebellum and spinal cord. The role of the vestibular system in relation to the turning movements of the body and head has on the contrary been neglected. This is probably because this system constitutes an acquisition of superior mammals, particularly developed in humans. We owe to Hassler the systematic description of central tracts of vestibular projection (44). The principal thalamic relay of ascendant vestibular pathways is the Vim nucleus. This nucleus shows a somatotropic characteristic of the thalamus with a medial cephalic projection and lateral limbs projection. During stereotactic procedures, microelectrode recording shows cells firing in response to movements of the limbs in the lateral part of the Vim nucleus and to contralateral ocular movements close to the middle line. It is precisely at this level that we record rhythmic discharges evoked by peripheral tremor in cases of Parkinson's disease or attitudinal tremor. The extremely short latency of evoked potentials in response to movements suggests the possibility of a projection of proprioceptive pathways directly to the thalamus without passing by the cerebellum.

The Vim nucleus would therefore play a role of integration of proprioceptive and vestibular impulses in relation to equilibrium and orientation. The cortical projection of the Vim nucleus seems to correspond to the sensitive and motor areas, and particularly to the four and three in the Brodmann's nomenclature. The vestibular nucleus has, on the other hand, ascendant connections with the oculomotor nuclei and the Cajal interstitial nucleus. When trying to reproduce postural tremor by tegmental mesencephalic lesion on the monkey, a spasmodic torticollis can occasionally appear with turning the head on the same side of the lesion. This torticollis is joined sometimes by dystonic movements of contra-lateral limbs. Anatomical study shows a tegmental lesion encroaching in the interstitial nucleus. The interstitial nucleus represents, therefore, a reticular center specialized in movements of rotation of the head. Besides the descendant projection constituted by the interstitiospinal bundle, this nucleus sends ascendant projections to the ventro-oralis internus nucleus (Voi). This nucleus represents the central part of the Voa, which receives pallidal projections through the pallidothalamic bundle and the Vop, site of the termination of cerebello-thalamic projections, through the brachium conjunctivum. The Voi nucleus probably receives cephalic projections of the same bundles. It realizes, therefore, the integration of the vestibular and cerebellar impulses. Its fundamental role in the rotatory movements is confirmed by the fact that during the recordings with microelectrodes a 3- to 4-cps rhythmic spontaneous activity has been found that desynchronized while the patient moved his eyes in the contralateral direction. The passage of the Voi nucleus by the microelectrode or stimulation electrode can be enough temporarily to stop the EMG discharges recorded on the ipsilateral sternocleidomastoid or contralateral splenius-complexus group in patients suffering spasmodic torticollis. Hassler (46) reported that Voi stimulation in cases of spasmodic torticollis induces slow tonic rotation of the head toward the opposite side with a peculiar dystonic spasm of the contralateral arm. We have not been able to reproduce this phenomenon. The only response obtained at this level has been the result of spread of stimulus toward the internal capsule. Finally, the Voi nucleus projects to the area 8 of Brodmann, the cortical center responsible for the lateral gaze and rotation of the head.

The pallidum represents among the basal ganglia the motor center of automatic movements. Among the efferent projections toward mesencephalic tegmentum figures the interstitial nucleus. On the other hand, the internal pallidum projects to the Voa and Voi nuclei. The role of the pallidum in movements of rotation of the head is confirmed by repeated observation during stereotactic surgery at the ansa lenticularis level of a transitory palsy of the contralateral gaze. It is not exceptional, on the other hand, to observe temporarily during surgery for spasmodic torticollis at the pallidum level a change of direction of the torticollis.

The spasmodic torticollis would then be similar to the tremor, the result of the uncontrolled activity of a reticulo-pallido-thalamo-cortical circuit, in which the relays would be the interstitial nucleus, the internal pallidum, the Voi nucleus, and the area 8 of Brodmann (Fig. 2). The level of activity of this circuit would be enhanced by vestibular afferents and by multiple sensory afferents through the collaterals of the specific projection systems, ending in the Cajal interstitial nucleus and other surrounding reticular centers.

This circuit is inhibited by the activity of the striatum through its projections to the pallidum. Indeed, the only lesions reported to this date in the cases of spasmodic torticollis are foci of degeneration in the putamen (2,84). On the other hand, in families who present typical heredofamilial tremor, the association

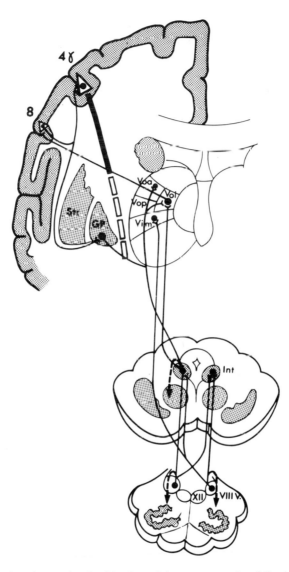

FIG. 2. Anatomical pathways involved in the rotatory movements of the head. This circuit becomes overactive in spasmodic torticollis because of lesions of the inhibitory striatum (Vest, vestibular nucleus; Int, interstitial nucleus of Cajal; Vim, nucleus ventro-intermedius; Voi, nucleus ventro-oralis internus).

of cases with spasmodic torticollis is usually noticed. Even more noticeable is the frequent association, in the same patient, of dystonic movements, torticollis type, with a real tremor of the head.

The target for the treatment of spasmodic torticollis is constituted by the Voi nucleus and its afferent projections coming from the interstitial nucleus. This lesion is sometimes adequate to stop the movements of the torticollis completely, but often an additional lesion of the internal pallidum is required. In advanced cases, with hypertrophy of the SCM, the section of the peripheral branch of the spinal nerve destined to this muscle is required either prior to or after the thalamotomy (18).

Physiopathology of Cerebellar Dyskinesia

An apparent contradiction exists between the results of experimental work in animals and the clinical symptoms observed in man following cerebellar lesions. From the experiences of Lange in 1891 (58), it is known that strong extensor hypertonia follows acute and chronic ablation of the anterior lobe of the cerebellum in avians. Thus, this lobe exerts a powerful tonic inhibition of extensor antigravity muscles. Moreover, the extensor decerebration hypertonia that follows intercollicular midbrain section is increased by a selective anterior lobe lesion (20) or by the total anemic cerebellectomy described by Pollock and Davis in dogs (71).

On the other hand Luciani, in 1891 (59), described ipsilateral extensor hypotonia after unilateral cerebellar lesion in dogs. This experience, apparently contradictory with Lange's observation, confirmed what is a constant law in man, that permanent hypotonia follows cerebellar dysfunction.

The study of comparative anatomy and physiology helps with the understanding of the apparent complexity of cerebellar function. Bremer, in 1935 (21), explained that extensor antigravity mechanisms are tonically inhibited, via cerebelloreticulo spinal pathways, by the paleocerebellum. The neocerebellum exerts, on the contrary, a facilitatory influence over the cerebral cortex through the cerebello-thalamo-cortical projections. In birds, the bigger development of paleocerebellum conditions an inhibitory bias, whereas in upper mammals and in man, the relatively higher development of neocerebellum is responsible for the tonic extensor facilitation. For this reason, hypotonia and loss of postural adjustment between agonist and antagonist muscles are the constant result of loss of cerebellar function. But there exists also in man positive symptoms caused by loss of inhibition resulting from paleocerebellar lesions. In a systematic review of mechanically and electrically induced reflexes in all types of motor disorders, I found, not without surprise, that in most of the cases with cerebellar lesions, there exists an increase of the H/M index and a shortening of the absolute and relative refractory periods of the recovery curve of the H reflex. This constitutes a sure sign of hyperexcitability of alpha motoneurons. Eccles et al. wrote in 1967: "It is generally believed that in some way, the cerebellum functions as a type of computer that is particularly concerned with the smooth and effective control of movement. It is assumed that the cerebellum integrates and organizes the information flowing into it along the various neural pathways and that the consequent cerebellar output either goes down to the spinal cord to the motoneurons and so participates in the control of movement or else is returned to the basal ganglia and the cerebral cortex, there to modify the control of movement from these higher centers" (26). Explaining the dual nature of cerebellar impulses, the same authors wrote: "The intermediate zone of the anterior lobe projects by the interpositus nucleus to the red nucleus and so down the rubrospinal tract and also to the VL nucleus of the thalamus and so to the cerebrum. The pathway from the interpositus nucleus to the VL nucleus has feed-forward inhibitory connections. Evidently this intermediate part of the cerebellar cortex has a dual role and may be thought of as mediating some kind of coordinative function between that part of the cerebellum solely oriented to the spinal cord and that part solely oriented to the cerebrum" (26). Therefore, at the level of the nucleus VL, there is a convergence of facilitatory stimuli coming from the globus pallidus via the pallidothalamic fasciculus and of inhibitory impulses from the anterior part of the cerebellar cortex and the dentate nucleus. Lesions of the latter result in overfunction of the pallidothalamocortical circuit, manifested clinically by the movement or intention tremor, the first type of cerebellar hyperkinesia.

The second type of cerebellar hyperkinesia is myoclonus. Hammond in 1867 was probably the first to establish a relation between myoclonus and cerebellar dysfunction (39). Later, in 1914, when Hunt published his work "Dyssynergia Cerebellaris Myoclonica: A chronic Progressive Form of Cerebellar Tremor" (50), this relation became evident. It was Hunt himself who in 1921 reported the first pathological study with a primary atrophy of the dentate nucleus (51). This finding has been confirmed in all the cases described thereafter in the literature. Among the various forms of cerebellar myoclonus, palatal myoclonus, described originally by Küpper in 1873 (57), occupied a privileged place. Guillain and Mollaret, in 1931 (34), gave a detailed description of the clinical picture characterized by rhythmic contraction of the larynx, the pharynx, the diaphragm, and, occasionally, the muscles of the neck, the shoulders, and the abdominal wall, at a frequency varying from 1.5 to 3 cps. The pathologic condition found is pseudohypertrophy of the olive resulting from retrograde transneuronal degeneration. The lesion responsible can be located in the ipsilateral central tegmental tract or the contralateral dentate nucleus of brachium conjunctivum relative to the altered olive. The clinical symptoms are contralateral to the olive. Olivocerebellar projections reach the Purkinje cells of cerebellar cortex via the climbing fiber system, in a one-to-one correlation between every olivary and Purkinje cell. Degeneration of olivary neurons would provoke the loss of excitatory input to the Purkinje cells, thus determining a disinhibitory input both to the spinal motoneurons, via the dentatorubrospinal pathways, and to the motor cortex via the dentatorubrothalamic pathways. The former would be responsible for the myoclonic contraction, whereas the latter is probably at the origin of the EEG polyphasic potentials that frequently accompany the myoclonus.

The optimal target for the control of movement or intention tremor and of the myoclonus is the posterior part of the ventrolateral nucleus or Vop (Fig. 3). The suppression of uncontrolled cerebellar impulses serves to abolish the manifestation of overfunction leaving unchanged the negative aspect resulting from the loss of function.

THE PROBLEM OF ANATOMICAL INDIVIDUAL VARIATION AND THE USE OF THE ATLAS OF STEREOTACTIC ANATOMY

Variation of the form and size of the human skull has been the object of a great number of publications (74,75,77). The reader can find a detailed analysis of different factors conditioning the shape of the skull in the article by Gerlach in the atlas of Shaltenbrand and Bailey (32). Race, and particulary immediate heredity, seem to be the main determining factors. It appears that cranial landmarks are useless as reference points for any brain structure, unless it has an immediate relation with a particular point of the endocranium. Moreover, the two reference points necessary for the construction of the base line in a system of coordinates must belong to structures ontogenetically related and, phylogenetically, as old as possible. The reason is that structures with these characteristics vary less from one individual to another. Finally, the closer the target and base line the better. Spiegel and Wycis proposed the foramen of Monro and the pineal shadow as reference points (75). The choice was unfortunate because both points are subject to the influence of variation of size of the ventricular system. I suspect that many early failures of pallidal surgery were a result of these inaccurate reference points. Talairaich et al. proposed in 1957 (77) the intercommissural line, tangent to the upper limit of the anterior commissure (AC) and to the inferior border of the posterior commissure (PC). Its length is measured between two vertical lines, respectively, posterior to AC and anterior to PC. Shaltenbrand and Bailey (74) measure the intercommissural line between the center of both commissures.

The intercommissural line (AC-PC) possesses the two conditions required for targets located within the thalamus and basal ganglia. The anterior commissure, located immediately in front of the columns of the fornix, connects the oldest telencephalic structures: the olfactory bulb, the archistriatum, the claustrum, and the middle temporal gyrus of both sides. It sharply delimits the frontier between the thalamus and the hypothalamus. The posterior commissure marks the limit between the diencephalon and the mesencephalon. It interconnects the superior colliculi, the pretectal nuclei of Edinger-Westphal, the interstitial nuclei of Cajal, and the nuclei of Darkshevich. Finally, the intercommissural line coincides almost exactly with the sulcus hypothalamicus of Hiss, which separates the midbrain and the fourth ventricle from the diencephalon and

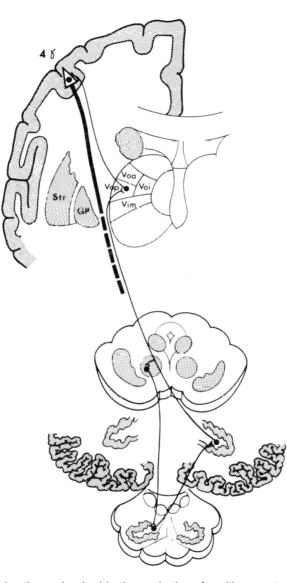

FIG. 3. Anatomical pathways involved in the production of positive symptoms of cerebellar dysfunction, movement or intention tremor, and myoclonus. A lesion within the triangle formed by dentato-rubral, rubro-olivary, or olivo-cerebellar projections will leave the nucleus ventro-oralis posterior (Vop) liberated from the inhibitory outflow of the cerebellum, and submitted exclusively to the excitatory impulses from the globus pallidus.

the third ventricle. Moreover, the hypothalamic sulcus is the natural continuation of the sulcus limitans, which divides the primitive neural tube in the two primitive plates: the basal plate, from which the motor centers derive, and the alar plate, origin of sensory centers.

Soon after its appearance, at the end of the tenth week, the telencephalic vesicle starts to grow, pushing in a rostrocaudal direction with a movement of rotation precisely around the axis constituted by the mesodiencephalic sulcus. When the first sulcus, the Sylvian fissure, appears toward the nineteenth week, as the result of growth of the cortex, the thalamic nuclei develop in a parallel way and both commissures are pushed apart progressively. But the axis of rotation of the telencephalon remains in the same position. At term, the hypo-thalamic sulcus and AC-PC line are parallel to the Forel's axis, that is, the longest fronto-occipital diameter. Wahren and Braintenberg (81) call the *encephalometric center* the junction between the axis of the brain stem, also called Meynert's axis and the Forel's axis. This point is always located in the posterior half of the intercommissural line, 6 mm behind its center on the average. The same authors demonstrate that after superimposing the center of AC-PC line in 20 brains, the plotting of the primary sulci—that is, the Sylvian sulcus, the central sulcus, and the calcarine fissure—shows a variation below 15 mm. The variation increases to 30 mm for the secondary sulci. Needless to say, the variation diminishes as the structures compared lie closer to the base line. What actually varies from one individual to another is the vertical, anteroposte-rior, and lateral diameters of the head, but, at the level of the intercommissural line, the variation is minimal. The telencephalic vesicle provokes with its growth the dilatation of cranial sutures and the growth of the skull. At the same time, the shape of the skull, which is partially predetermined by heredity, forces the telencephalon to embrace its contours. The brain mantle progressively folds and at the end of the second year, 75% of its surface is hidden in the depth of sulci. This process will necessarily influence the relative position of sulci but not the size of the diencephalic centers.

We have approached the problem of individual variations in two different ways. First, taking for granted that individual differences in absolute size will respect the relative situation of diencephalic structures in relation to one another, we decided to stretch out or to compress all the AC-PC lines to a common standard model in which one-tenth of the total length of the AC-PC line was the unit of base in all three planes of the Cartesian system of coordinates. Then we plotted on this standardized model the corrected coordinates of the points where the tremor stops suddenly at the mere impact of the tip of recording or stimulating electrodes. Without surprise, we realized that, even though this point is in one case 18 mm behind AC and 24 mm in another, it is in all cases located in a very minute zone immediately below the eight-tenth point of the AC-PC line (10) (Fig. 4). Plotting in the standardized model localized motor or sensory responses to threshold stimuli permitted us to realize that the relative position of each point varies less than 10%. The variation is slightly bigger in a lateral sense (79). The second approach was to measure the radio-

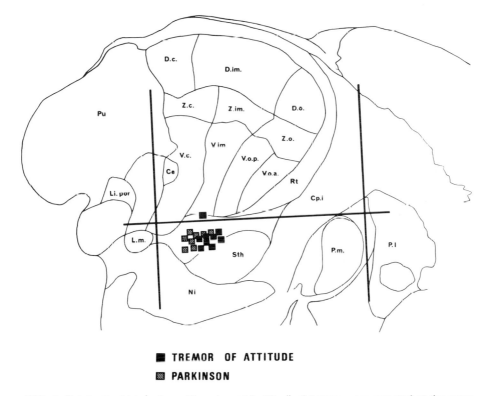

■ TREMOR OF ATTITUDE

▨ PARKINSON

FIG. 4. Points at which both parkinsonian and attitudinal tremor were arrested at the mere impact of the stimulating electrode. The points were plotted in a standardized model according to the principle of proportional measurements.

graphic length of the AC-PC line in 400 cases. The length was on the average 24 mm: the shortest, in a 12-year-old child, was 20 mm; the longest, belonging to a patient with the so-called normal pressure hydrocephalus, was 32 mm. We realize that in any patient more than 15 years old, a length inferior to 20 mm indicates a severe deformity resulting from craniostenosis or microcephaly. A length over 30 mm means pathological hydrocephalus. Within these limits, it is possible to predict the point at which tremor will stop at the passage of the electrode in every case. More than 200 cases have been tested since this study was started and in every instance when the tremor stopped the trajectory was correct with a variation of less than 5%, in the anteroposterior axis, and of 7% on the lateral axis. Conversely, if the tremor did not stop, we can affirm that the trajectory is deviated in one or another sense. In no single instance did a correct trajectory fail to stop the tremor, or did a deviated one stop it.

In conclusion, for structures located close to the AC-PC line, according to the method of proportional measurement and within the limits explained above, individual variations can be neglected, and that is precisely the case for all the targets for abnormal movements. I recently had the opportunity to make the following observation. In a parkinsonian patient operated on by left thalamotomy 11 years previously, the AC-PC line measured 24 mm. The size and shape of the ventricles were at the time normal and symmetrical. Eleven years later, a right subthalamotomy was proposed in order to suppress a violent postural tremor on the right side. Ventriculography showed marked dilatation of both lateral ventricles, more pronounced on the left. The diameter of the III ventricle increased from 6 to 11 mm. Yet the AC-PC line measured exactly 24 mm on both occasions. Atrophy of the brain will provoke modification of the shape and size of the ventricles and, because of the secondary atrophy of cortical-related thalamic nuclei, modification of the diameter of the third ventricle also. But the remaining thalamic nuclei are not pushed apart; they stay in the same position in relation to the midline. In the patient referred to above, the introduction of the stimulating electrode at 12 mm from the midline, that is five-tenths of the total length of this AC-PC line, suddenly stopped the tremor of the left limbs, exactly as was the case on the right side 11 years before, despite the fact that the distance of the target point to the wall of the third ventricle was 9 mm the first time and 6.5 the second.

On the other hand, mechanical dilatation of the ventricles secondary to hydrocephalus can obviously increase the length of the AC-PC line.

Therefore, it appears that, for target points located around AC-PC line, as is the case for abnormal movements, the use of proportional measurements make the use of teleradiography to avoid magnification of the introduction of complex mathematical calculations unnecessary in order to rectify the position of the target according to the shape and the size of the skull. These precautions on the contrary became essential, if instead of proportionate, one uses absolute measurements. A last concrete example could perhaps help in understanding this apparent complex problem: The AC-PC line measures in one patient 22 mm and 28 mm in another. Looking to the sagittal projections of the atlas of Shaltenbrand and Bailey, in which the length of AC-PC line is 20 mm (74), we realize that the target point for the arrest of tremors is located 16 mm behind AC. We must obviously make a lot of calculations before finding out where the target must be sited in both patients if we refuse to consider the three thalami as proportionate, but if we transform all the previous measurements in units corresponding to one-tenth of the total length of the time AC-PC line, then the target point will be found in all three cases at the level of the eight-tenth behind AC, that is, 16 mm in the atlas, 17.5 mm in the case of a 22 mm AC-PC line, and 22.5 mm in the case of a AC-PC line of 28 mm. The parameter for the laterality will be, respectively, of 10, 11, and 14 mm, but five-tenths of the AC-PC line in all three cases.

ELECTROPHYSIOLOGICAL STUDIES

Two electrophysiological methods are currently in use during stereotactic surgery: the recording of electrical activity and electrical stimulation. The first provides information about the structures the electrode passes through. Threshold stimulation provides the same type of information as the microelectrode recording. With higher-intensity electrical stimulation, important information is provided regarding the location and proximity of important structures in the neighborhood of the target.

Microelectrode Recording

The use of the bipolar concentric electrode originally described by Albe-Fessard et al. in 1961 (1) provides useful information regarding both cellular unitary and background activity. Since its introduction by Hardy in 1962, this technique has been used routinely at Notre-Dame Hospital in more than 700 cases, and the results have been the object of different publications (16,17,40,60,80). The descriptions of recordings in previous publications portray mainly the trajectories usually employed for the arrest of tremor and the tentative trajectory for alleviation of chronic persistent pain. These trajectories traverse first the nucleus dorso-oralis anterior (Doa) and penetrate the ventral thalamus at the level of the nuclei Voa, Vop, Vim, or ventro-caudalis (Vc). A brief account of the main information will be summarized here.

The anterior half the dorsal thalamus (Doa) is characterized by the presence of rhythmic cellular activity at a frequency of 4.5 to 5 cps. This type of activity is present in patients with or without tremor and it cannot be modified by any activity of the patient or by any external stimulus of any kind. It is therefore an antonomous idiopathic rhythm. (Fig. 5).

The Voa nucleus is characterized by the same type of rhythmic activity previously described. This rhythm seems to be more easily and constantly recorded in patients with parkinsonian or attitudinal tremor. The Voa nucleus is the main end of the pallidothalamic bundle.

The Vop nucleus is characterized by the presence of rhythmic slow oscillation of the background activity at a frequency of 18 to 22 cps. This activity behaves exactly as the alpha activity of the EEG recording in the scalp: it is desynchronized with any tentative focusing of either the gaze or the mind. It becomes more organized with closing of the eyes and with relaxation, both mental and physical. Vop nucleus is the termination of the dentatorubrothalamic projections.

The Vim nucleus is characterized by a dense cellular activity of higher amplitude, according to the larger size of its cells. This activity is modified by muscle activity according to a double somatotropy. In its anterior half, movement is the specific stimulus. In the posterior half, the cells respond best to pressure on the muscle. In a mediolateral direction, as in the rest of the thalamus, the face is located medially, the upper limb intermediate, and the lower limb laterally. The neck and the upper extremity seem to possess a broader representation. Rhythms, evoked by the tremor, can be recorded. It is often possible artificially to reproduce a rhythmic cellular activity either by repetitive articular movements in front, or muscle pressure behind. Vim is the terminal station of vestibulo-thalamic pathways (Fig. 2).

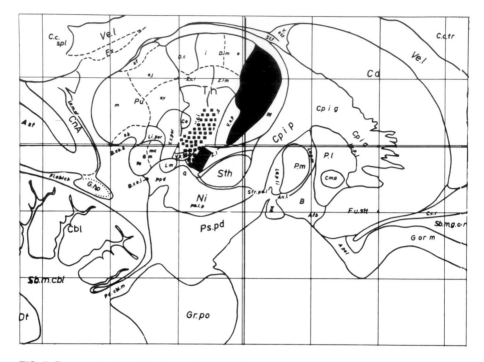

FIG. 5. Representation of the thalamic and subthalamic areas where different kinds of rhythmic cellular activity are recorded. The black area corresponds to the zones where autonomous 5-cps rhythms are recorded at the level of the nucleus dorso-oralis anterior, (Doa), ventro-oralis anterior (Voa), and in the prelemniscal radiation of the posterior subthalamic region. The dotted areas represent the zone where rhythms evoked by tremor were recorded: the nucleus ventro-intermedius (Vim) and the anterior part of the medial lemniscus.

The Vc nucleus is characterized by high-voltage, dense cellular activity that is increased with fine tactile stimulation of the skin. Besides, triphasic slowly evoked potentials can be recorded with a very precise somatology; this is well described by Guiot et al. (35,36) and by Jasper and Bertrand (52). The Vc nucleus is the thalamic end of the medial lemniscus.

The activity recorded in the caudate nucleus and in the pallidus has been described in relation with stereotactic anterior capsulotomy for the treatment of chronic persistent pain (60). Slow waves of 10 to 14 cps are recorded as a background activity of the caudate nucleus. Cellular activity appears in bursts at a frequency of about 2 cps. Corresponding to the two different types of cells in the striatum, there exist two types of cellular spikes: big spikes of 50 to 80 mv appear in a proportion of about 1 to 20 in relation with smaller 10 to 20-mv spikes. The globus pallidus is characterized by low-voltage background and cellular activity without any rhythm.

In the more medial and anterior trajectories used for spasmodic torticollis, the target point is the Voi nucleus. Voi corresponds to the cephalic representation of both Voa and Vop. It receives pallidal, interstitial, and cerebellar influences. Its electrical activity is characterized at rest, the patient lying with eyes closed, by an autonomous rhythm of 3 to 4 cps. This activity is desynchronized when the patient directs his gaze in the opposite direction.

In the posterior part of the zona incerta, called "prelemniscal radiations," autonomous rhythms of cellular activity at a frequency of 4.5 to 5 cps are occasionally recorded. When this happens, the tremor of the contralateral extremities disappears as the tip of the electrode passes through (Fig. 5).

If the electrode traverses the subthalamic nucleus, high-voltage rhythmic activity of the background at a frequency of 12 to 14 cps is recorded. Sparse high-voltage cellular activity is characteristic of this nucleus.

Medial lemniscus is characterized by the presence of slow triphasic potentials evoked respectively by joint movement, muscle pressure, or touch of the skin in an anteroposterior direction. The polarity of the lemniscal potentials is always inverted in relation to that of the Vc nucleus.

Electrical Stimulation

The results of monopolar electrical stimulation have been described by Bertrand et al. on different occasions (9,12). The most recent analysis of our material was done by Velasco in 1970, and the results were published in 1973 by Bertrand et al. (17). The following paragraphs are taken from this publication. A detailed study of tremor in Parkinson's disease (75 cases) and of tremor of attitude (46 cases) has been made. There was a total of 190 trajectories, and the cases were divided into two groups according to the distance of the electrode from the midline: the first one included electrode placements at 11 to 13 mm (45 times); and the other, electrode placements at 14 to 16 mm (145 times) from the midline. The results were as follows:

1. In reviewing the results of all stimulations, either a motor or a sensory response was obtained from contact No. 1, motor response being further anterior, as might be expected. From contact No. 2, a sensory response was obtained only with posterior trajectories or when the contact was below the inferior border of the thalamus. Motor responses occurred only when the electrode was too far lateral. No response was ever obtained from the highest contact, No. 3.

2. Sensory responses were obtained at 11 to 13 mm from the midline, with 0.5 V or less, at 60 cps only below the AC-PC line (Fig. 6A). In the more lateral placements (14 to 16 mm from the midline), responses were obtained both above and below the AC-PC line (Fig. 6B). Above it, responses were localized to the hand or arm, the latter being below the former. Below the AC-PC line, responses were referred either to the entire contralateral side of the body or at times to a localized body segment.

3. Motor responses obtained at frequencies of 60 cps and up to 2 V affected

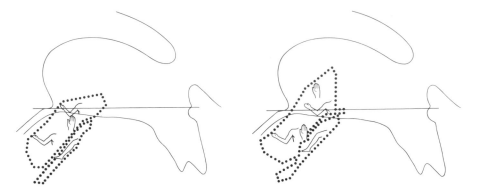

FIG. 6. (A, left) Sensory responses were obtained below the AC-PC line when the electrode was 11 to 13 mm from the midline, probably from stimulation of the medial lemniscus. (**B,** right) Sensory responses were obtained below and above the AC-PC line when the electrodes were 14 to 16 mm from the midline, the latter probably from stimulation of nucleus ventrocaudalis (Vc) (VPL of Walker). (From ref. 10.)

large segments of the body, as might be expected, and they were more numerous in the group 14 to 16 mm from the midline. With low-voltage stimulation, motor responses were obtained only from the lowest contact and had a definite topographical arrangement. Those of the upper extremities were located above and in front of the response seen in the lower extremities. The areas representing the foot and the hand were considerably larger than those of the rest of the body; responses from the face area were located more anteriorly (Fig. 7A and B)

4. Increase or decrease of tremor from stimulation was seen only occasionally, and it was difficult to assess the importance of other factors, such as an emotional response to a sensory stimulus or a motor response. It was much more common

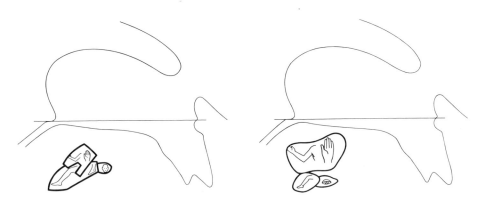

FIG. 7. Motor responses were obtained with low-voltage stimulation from contact No. 1 with the following topographical arrangement: (**A,** left): 11 to 13 mm from midline. (**B,** right): 14 to 16 mm from midline. (From ref. 10.)

and consistent to obtain an arrest of tremor from the mechanical trauma of the electrode penetrating the target point. The last 15 mm of penetration is carried out very slowly so as to detect the depth at which tremor stops. When arrest of tremor is sudden and complete, low-voltage stimulation at the lowest contact produces a sensory response, but there is no response from the intermediate contact which is situated at the target point (Fig. 8A). With a higher voltage, there might be a motor as well as a sensory response from contact No. 1 and a sensory response in the arm from contact No. 2 (Fig. 8B).

From these results, it may be inferred that the sensory responses obtained 8 mm below the AC-PC line are derived from the lemniscus, and those at the intermediate contact from the Vc nucleus (VPL of Walker). The topographical arrangement in the lemniscus was such that the representation of the arm was posterolateral to that of the leg, with that of the face situated in between; this may be a result of the curving pattern that these fibers describe as they ascend and then turn back toward the sensory nucleus; however, this point needs to be documented further.

Higher-voltage stimulation at 60 cps was most useful to detect the proximity of sensory fibers or cells and corticospinal fibers, but primarily that of the corticobulbar tract, which must be avoided. During stimulation at contact No. 2, the patient is asked to protrude and withdraw his tongue rapidly and to count clearly, so that dysarthria may be detected. Since, with these stimulus parameters, the current usually spreads more than 3 mm, the extent of the proposed lesion may be estimated. Even if no response has been elicited, this is verified again when the leukotome is gradually opened laterally. A similar procedure is followed posteriorly, in case of borderline sensory response, to see if mechanical stimulation will produce tingling before we go on with placing the lesion.

In summary, in our experience, low-voltage monopolar stimulation is suffi-

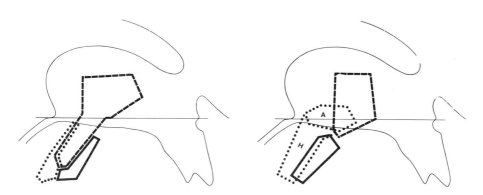

FIG. 8. (**A,** left): Result of stimulation of trajectories passing through the target point with low-voltage current (0.5 V). There is no response to stimulation at the target point. (**B,** right): At the same locus, a higher-voltage stimulus (up to 2 V) evokes sensory and occasionally motor responses. A, contralateral arm; H, contralateral half of the body. (From ref. 10.)

ciently precise to identify motor and sensory structures around the target point; and higher voltages at 60 cps help to indicate adjacent structures situated more than 3 mm away, which should be avoided. Stimulation has been of little value in identifying the target point; this is detected by the mechanical penetration trauma of the electrode.

THE LESION

All the available methods—chemical, physical, or mechanical—are good. But certainly some are better than others. The following are qualities of the ideal instrument: (a) ductility, that is the possibility of making a lesion of the desired size and shape; (b) selectivity, in order to destroy nervous substance and spare blood vessels; and (c) reversibility, which permits the placement of temporary lesions. Needless to say, none of the instruments available at the present time completely fulfills the above-mentioned requirements. Cryosurgery permits temporary lesions, but their size is necessarily spherical. Radiofrequency seems to be the best instrument regarding selectivity, but again the size is always spherical or elliptical. The blunt fine-wire leukotome originally described by Bertrand in 1955 (7) possesses the possibility of making a lesion of any size and shape (Fig. 9) and, by the mere opening of the wire, of making a temporary suppression of the function of the target point. These two qualities make it the best instrument available, in our opinion. Unfortunately the leukotome cannot make a lesion involving exclusively nervous cells or fibers. By making small, half-sized, pear-shaped lesions, important blood vessels would probably be spared but the possibility of section of a small atheromatous artery remains. Implantation of radioactive substances is surely the least satisfactory of the present methods of making a lesion. The use of ultrasound introduced in stereotactic surgery by Fry et al.

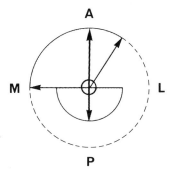

FIG. 9. Schematic illustration of the various possibilities afforded by merely opening a fine-wire leukotome. These possibilities include: (a) Opening in any direction around its axis *(arrow)* to produce temporary suppression of function. (b) Small quadrantic quarter or half-sized pear-shaped lesions in any desired direction. (c) Lesion 12 mm in diameter produced by repetitive opening and turning the wire-loop about the shaft of the leukotome, 15° on each side of the opening position. (From ref. 17.)

in 1960 (30), especially using high-frequency and high-directional ultrasound beams, can assure better results, but whatever method is used, it is worthwhile to quote one of the pioneers of stereotactic surgery: "The particular agency by which the lesion is made appears to be of less importance than the precision of its placement" (63).

RESULTS AND SIDE EFFECTS

In other fields of neurosurgery, the results depend on the experience and the technical skill of the surgeon. In functional, and particularly in stereotactic neurosurgery, good results are primarily dependent on the accuracy of choice of the right target. The careful planning and execution of the procedure have less influence. Table 1 summarizes an up-to-date survey of a series of 605 consecutive cases operated on at Notre-Dame Hospital between 1967 and 1976. In parkinsonism, where the target remained the same during this period, the results are stabilized. Thus, these results are quite similar to an initial evaluation made by Bertrand and Martinez in 1962 (15) on a series of 250 cases, and to a later evaluation made by Botana-Lopez in another series of 140 consecutive cases in 1967 (19). The choice of patients is more selective, we understand better what we do, the lesions are smaller, and yet the results are practically the same, except for the side effects. This is also the case for operations carried out for tremor of attitude and cerebellar dyskinesia.

On the contrary, in spasmodic torticollis, our approach has been progressively modified during the past 10 years. The results given in Table 1 include all the cases operated upon during this period. A recent survey of the last 40 cases (66) shows much better results.

In functional neurosurgery, the old sentence *primum non nocere* acquires a particular importance. Since in functional disorders of the brain, the aim is to improve function by suppressing an overfunction, we must consider a failure in any case in which the function is not improved even if we succeed in suppress-

TABLE 1. *Results of sterotactic surgery at Notre-Dame Hospital in 605 cases over a 10-year period (1967–1976)*

Condition	Parkinsonism	Tremor of attitude	Cerebellar dyskinesia	Spasmodic torticollis	Total
Excellent	137 (36%)	76 (52%)	12 (50%)	23 (43%)	248 (41%)
Good	118 (31%)	39 (28%)	7 (29%)	12 (22%)	176 (29%)
Fair	95 (25%)	22 (15%)	2 (8%)	7 (13%)	126 (21%)
Unimproved	19 (5%)	5 (3%)	3 (13%)	3 (5%)	30 (5%)
Worse	12 (3%)	3 (2%)	0	7 (13%)	22 (3%)
Death	1 (0.26%)	0	0	2 (4%)	3 (0.5%)
Total	382	145	24	54	605

Surgery was performed by C. Bertrand, S. N. Martinez, and J. Hardy, in collaboration with the author.

ing a particular positive symptom. For this reason, parkinsonian rigidity in itself is no longer an indication for surgery, nor is akinesia. The suppression of the former is followed often by loss of postural adjustment. The latter is either unaltered or increased by surgery.

Side effects are far more frequent in spasmodic torticollis than in any other abnormal movements. Seven cases were worse after surgery: in one instance, a pyramidal syndrome appeared after a left thalamotomy. All the others were cases with pseudobulbar palsy. As is shown in Fig. 10, the corticobulbar pathways lay immediately lateral to the target for the torticollis.

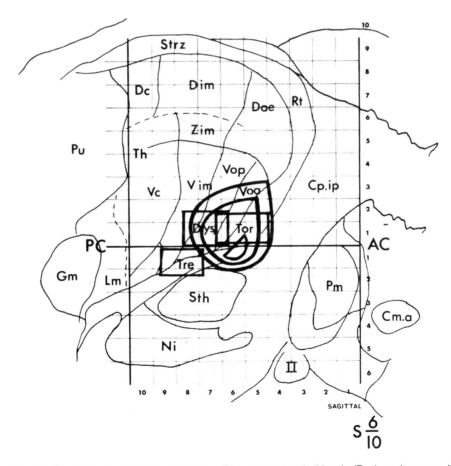

FIG. 10. The three target points for tremor (Tre), cerebellar dyskinesia (Dys), and spasmodic torticollis (Tor), as represented superimposed in a sagittal section of the brain six-tenths from the middle line, according to the method of proportional measurements. The two concentric pear-shaped images correspond to the area of overlap of 83 and 92%, respectively, of the lesion that provoked permanent pseudobulbar symptoms in 12 cases. The smaller half-circle-shaped area corresponds to the 100% area of overlap. The target points are located medially in relation to these areas.

Hemiballismus is a most feared complication in some centers. There is no single instance of postoperative hemiballismus in our series of more than 1,500 cases. The reason is probably the coronal parasagittal approach used at Notre-Dame. In the rare instances in which the lesion encroaches upon the subthalamic nucleus, it is its posteromedial part that is involved. Hemiballismus appears when the lesion touches the anteroexternal part of the nucleus.

There were three postoperative deaths. The first occurred in a patient with spasmodic torticollis with severe hypertension who sustained a massive intraventricular hemorrhage on the first postoperative day. The second occurred in a young girl with progressive dystonia in whom a unilateral thalamotomy and pallidotomy with partial result were followed by an intradural cervical rhizotomy. In the postoperative period, the patient died of severe meningitis. The third death occurred in a parkinsonian patient who had been operated upon on one side 10 years before, and for whom a second thalamotomy was decided upon because of a violent tremor on the second side. Some hours after an uneventful operation, the patient developed a small hematoma along the trajectory and died of an unexplained respiratory arrest. In the first and in the third cases, the operation was proposed after a long hesitation.

We said at the beginning of this section that the results were not too different from the previous series at least in parkinsonism and heredofamilial tremor of attitude, except in regard to side effect. It is worth mentioning that today a bilateral procedure is seldom performed and often regretted. All but one of the permanent pseudobulbar palsies appeared after a second side thalamotomy in which the localization was carefully planned so as to avoid corticospinal fibers. The first side, because of an excessively lateral placement of the lesion, is responsible in these cases, even if only a minimal transitory dysarthria appeared after the first lesion. Therefore, although in our statistics the incidence of speech disorders is by far less frequent than the 60% reported by Krayenbühl et al. (56), we agree that bilateral thalamotomy is at the present time indicated in only exceptional cases.

At the end of this discussion about the result, a word must be said regarding the possible modification of the natural history of the disease by surgery. This is a question that will probably never be answered with certainty. Yet we examine patients who have been operated upon by pallidotomy or ansotomy 10, 15, or even 20 years before with still a complete suppression of tremor and rigidity and only a moderate akinesia; often there is excellent mental drive. Inversely, a patient suffering from parkinsonism for more than 10 years, that is, before the introduction of levodopa, will be today in a far worse condition. I have the same impression with cases treated precociously with levodopa more than 5 years ago. Did the suppression of symptoms, and particularly the tremor, modify the natural course of the disease? There exists this possibility. It is reasonable to think that the nervous cells of the tremorogenic and tonigenic centers could become extenuated by its continuous overfunction; that is, what happened after an epileptic discharge or even after an excess of physical and even mental work or psychological tension. But leaving the speculation, there is a practical question to be answered concerning the timing of the surgical treatment. It is my personal conviction that medical treatment must be started as soon as the diagnosis is made. Surgery can be considered as soon as the quality of life of a patient both from the physical and psychical point of view starts to deteriorate because of a lack of efficiency of the conservative treatment. A good result will be certainly better if it arrives sooner.

CONCLUSION

A quarter of a century has passed since the beginning of stereotactic surgery in man. Enough anatomical and physiological data are now available in order to make a rational choice of the target before making a lesion. A critical analysis of success and failures will orient the surgeon as to the best direction. In particular, failures must be carefully recorded and reported and the reason of every failure must be found, because there is always a reason. Anatomical individual variations and particularities of an individual clinical picture have been in the past the scapegoat for bad results and side effects. It appears nevertheless that lack of precision, both in the choice of the target and in the actual surgical procedure, can more simply explain the failures of stereotactic surgery.

REFERENCES

1. Albe-Fessard, D., Arfel, G., Guiot, G., Hardy, J., Vourc'h, G., Hertzog, E., and Aleonard, P. (1961): Identification et délimitation précise de certaines structures sous-corticales de l'homme par l'électrophysiologie: Son intérêt dans la chirurgie stéréotaxique des dyskinésies. *C. R. Acad. Sci. (Paris),* 253:2412–2414.
2. Alpers, B. J., and Drayer, C. S. (1973): The organic background of some cases of spasmodic torticollis: Report of a case with autopsy. *Am. J. Med. Sci.,* 193:378–384.
3. Bak, I. J., Hassler, R., and Kim, J. S. (1972): Fine localization of dopamine and other chemical transmitter substances in basal ganglia and possible roles in akinesia. In: *Parkinson's Disease,* pp. 151–161. Hans Huber, Bern Stuttgart, Vienna.
4. Barbeau, A. (1961): Dopamine and basal ganglia diseases. *AMA Arch. Neurol.,* 4:97–102.
5. Barbeau, A., Murphy, G. F., and Sourkes, T. L. (1961): Excretion of dopamine in diseases of the basal ganglia. *Science,* 133:1706.
6. Benda, C. E., and Cobb, S. (1942): On the pathogenesis of paralysis agitans. (Parkinson's disease). *Medicine,* 21:95–142.
7. Bertrand, C. (1958): Une nouvelle modification technique pour la chirurgie des mouvements involontaires. *Union Med. Can.,* 84:150–154.
8. Bertrand, C. (1958): A pneumotaxic technique for producing localized cerebral lesions. *J. Neurosurg.,* 15:251–264.
9. Bertrand, C. (1966): Functional localization with monopolar stimulation: 2nd Symposium on Parkinson's Disease, part II. *J. Neurosurg.,* 14:403–409.
10. Bertrand, C., Hardy, J., Molina-Negro, P., and Martinez, S. N. (1973): Optimum physiological target for the arrest of tremor. In: *3rd Symposium on Parkinson's Disease,* Vol. 2, pp. 65–71. Hans Huber, Bern Stuttgart, Vienna.
11. Bertrand, C., and Jasper, H. (1965): Microelectrode recording of unit activity in the human thalamus. *Confin. Neurol.,* 26:205–208.
12. Bertrand, C., and Martinez, S. N. (1958): Pneumotaxic localization, recording, stimulation and section of basal brain structures in dyskinesia. *Neurology (Minneap.),* 8:783–786.

13. Bertrand, C., and Martinez, S. N. (1959): An apparatus and technique for surgery of dyskinesia. *Neurochirurgia (Stuttg.),* 2:35–46.
14. Bertrand, C., and Martinez, S. N. (1961): Basal ganglia versus corticospinal tract: Their relative importance in the relief of tremor and regidity. *Rev. Can. Biol.,* 20:365–375.
15. Bertrand, C., and Martinez, S. N. (1962): Localization of lesions, mostly with regard to tremor and rigidity. 1st International Symposium on Stereoencephalotomy. *Confin. Neurol.,* 22:274–282.
16. Bertrand, C., Martinez, S. N., and Hardy, J. (1963): Electrophysiological studies on the human thalamus and adjoining structures. *J. Neurol. Neurosurg. Psychiatr.,* 26:552.
17. Bertrand, C., Martinez, S. N., Hardy, J., Molina-Negro, P., and Velasco, F. (1973): Stereotaxic surgery for parkinson: Recording, stimulation and oriented microelectrode section with a leukotome. *Prog. Neurolog. Surg.,* 5:78–112.
18. Bertrand, C., Molina-Negro, P., and Martinez, S. N. (1977): Combined stereotaxic and peripheral surgical approach for spasmodic torticollis. 7th Symposium of the World Society for Stereotaxic and Functional Neurosurgery, Sao Paulo, Brazil. *Appl. Neurophysiol. (in press).*
19. Botana-Lopez, C. (1969–70): La cirugía estereotáxica en el tratamiento de las disquinesias. *Rev. esp. Oto-neuro-oftalmol. neurocir.,* 28:95–109 and 153–168.
20. Bremer, F. (1922): Contribution à l'étude de la physiologie du cervelet: La fonction inhibitrice du paleocerebellum. *Arch. Int. Physiol.,* 19:189–226.
21. Bremer, F. (1935): Le cervelet. In: *Traité de physiologie normale et pathologie,* Vol. 10, edited by G. H. Roger and L. Binet. Masson, Paris.
22. Bucy, P., and Buchanan, D. N. (1932): Athetosis. *Brain,* 55:479–492.
23. Cooper, I. S. (1954): Surgical occlusion of the anterior choroidal artery in parkinsonism. *Surg. Gynecol. Obstet.,* 99:207–219.
24. Cooper, I. S. (1961): *Parkinsonism: Its Medical and Surgical Therapy.* Charles C Thomas, Springfield, Illinois.
25. Cooper, I. S. (1973): Cryogenic technique of thalamic surgery for parkinsonism. *Prog. Neurol. Surg.,* 5:159–188.
26. Eccles, J. C., Ito, M., and Szentagothai, J. (1967): *The Cerebellum as a Neuronal Machine.* Springer-Verlag, New York.
27. Ehringer, H., and Hornykiewicz, O. (1960): Verteilung von Noradrenalin und Dopamin (3-hydroxytyranmin) in Gehirn des Menschen und ihr Verhalten bei Erkraukungen des extrapyramidalen Systems. *Klin. Wochenschn.,* 38:1236.
28. Fennelon, F. (1950): Essai de traitement neurochirurgical du syndrome parkinsonnien par intervention directe sur les voies extrapyramidales (anse lenticulaire). *Rev. Neurol.,* 83:437–440.
29. Foerster, O. H. (1911): Resection of the posterior spinal nerve roots in the treatment of gastric crises and spastic paralysis. *Proc. R. Soc. Med.,* 3:226–254.
30. Fry, W. J., Fry, F. J., Meyers, R., and Eggleton, R. J. (1960): The use of ultrasound in neurosurgery. Proceedings of the 3rd International Conference on Medical Electronics, London, pp. 453–458.
31. George, R., Haslett, W. L., and Jenden, D. J. (1962): The central action of a metabolite of tremorine. *Life Sci.* 1:361–363.
31a. George, R., Haslett, W. L., and Jenden, D. J. (1966): The production of tremor by cholinergic drugs: Central sites of action. *Int. J. Neuropharmacol.* 5:27–34.
32. Gerlach, J. (1959): Variations of the human skull. In: *Introduction to Stereotaxis with an Atlas of the Human Brain,* edited by G. Spaltenbrand and P. Bailey, pp. 29–41. Grune & Stratton, New York.
33. Greenfield, J. G., and Bosanquet, F. D. (1953): The brain stem lesions in parkinsonism. *J. Neurol. Neurosurg. Psychiatr.,* 16:213–226.
34. Guillain, G., and Mollaret, P. (1931): Deux cas de myoclonies synchrones et rythmées vélopharyngo-laryngo-oculo-diaphragmatiques: Le problème anatomique et physiopathologique de ce syndrome. *Rev. Neurol.,* 2:545–566.
35. Guiot, G., Derome, P., Arfel, G., and Walter, S. (1973): Electrophysiological recordings in stereotaxic thalamotomy for parkinsonism. *Prog. Neurol. Surg.,* 5:189–221.
36. Guiot, G., Hardy, J., and Albe-Fessard, D. (1962): Délimitation précise des structures souscorticales et identification des noyaux thalamiques chez l'homme par électrophysiologie stéréotaxique. *Neurochirurgie,* 5:1–18.
37. Guiot, G., Hertzog, E., Rondot, P., and Molina, P. (1961): Arrest and acceleration of speed

evoked by thalamic stimulation in the course of stereotaxic procedures of Parkinson. *Brain,* 84:363–380.
38. Guiot, G., and Pecker, J. (1949): Tractotomie mésencéphalique antérieure pour tremblement parkinsonien. *Rev. Neurol.,* 81:387–388.
39. Hammond, W. A. (1867): On convulsive tremor. *NY State J. Med.* 5:185–198.
40. Hardy, J. (1966): Electrophysiological localization and identification. *J. Neurosurg. (Suppl.),* January, part II, pp. 410–414.
41. Hassler, R. (1938): Zur Pathologie der Paralysis agitans und des post-encephalitischen Parkinsonismus. *J. Psychol. Neurol.,* 48:387–476.
42. Hassler, R. (1955): The influence of stimulations and coagulations in the human thalamus on the tremor at rest and its physiopathologic mechanism. Proceedings of the 2nd International Congress on Neuropathology, London. 2:637–642.
43. Hassler, R. (1955): The pathological and pathophysiological basis of tremor and parkinsonism. Proceeding of the Second International Congress on Neuropathology, London. 1:29–40.
44. Hassler, R. (1957–58): Functional anatomy of the thalamus. *Physiol. Exptl. Med. Sci.,* pp. 56–91.
45. Hassler, R. (1959): Stereotactic brain surgery for extrapyramidal motor disturbance: In: *Introduction to Stereotaxis with an Atlas of the Human Brain,* edited by G. Shalternbrand and P. Bailey., 472–488. Georg Thiem Verlag, Stuttgart.
46. Hassler, R. (1970): Stereotactic treatment of different kinds of spasmodic torticollis. *Confin. Neurol.,* 32:135–143.
47. Hayne, R. A., Meyers, R., and Knott, J. (1949): Characteristics of electrical activity of human corpus striatum and neighboring structures. *J. Neurophysiol.,* 12:185–195.
48. Horsley, V. (1909): The function of the so-called motor area of the brain. *Br. Med. J.,* 2:125–132.
49. Horsley, V., and Clarke, R. H. (1908): The structure and function of the cerebellum examined by a new method. *Brain,* 3:45–124.
50. Hunt, J. R. (1914): Dyssynergia cerebellaris myoclonica: A chronic progressive form of cerebellar tremor. *Brain,* 37:247–268.
51. Hunt, J. R. (1921): Dyssynergia cerebellaris myoclonica. Primary atrophy of the detate system: A contribution to the pathology and the symptomatology of the cerebellum. *Brain,* 44:499–538.
52. Jasper, H. J., and Bertrand, G. (1966): Thalamic units involved in somatic sensation and voluntary and involuntary movements in man. In: *The Thalamus,* edited by D. P. Purpura and L. Yahr, pp. 365–384. Columbia University Press, New York.
53. Jenker, F. L., and Ward, A. A., Jr. (1953): Bulbar reticular formation and tremor. *A.M.A. Arch. Neurol. Psychiatr.,* 70:489–502.
54. Jung, R. (1941): Physiologische Untersuchungen Über den Parkinson tremor und andere Zitter formen beim Menschen. *Z. Neurol.,* 173:263–322.
55. Kim, J. S., Bak, I., Hassler, R., and Okada, Y. (1971): Role of GABA in the extrapyramidal motor system. Some evidence for the existence of a type of GABA-side strionigral neurons. *Exp. Brain Res.,* 14:35–104.
56. Krayenbühl, H., Siegfried, J., and Yasargil, M. G. (1963): Late results of stereotaxic operations in the treatment of Parkinson's disease. *Rev. Neurol.,* 108:485–494.
57. Küpper, M. (1873): Ueber Klonische Krämpfe der Schlingmuskeln. *Arch. Ohrenh.,* 1:296–297.
58. Lange, B. (1891): Inwiewiet sind die Symptome welche nach Zerströng des Kleinhirns beobachtet Werden, anf Verlet zungen des Acousticus zuruckführen? *Arch. Ges. Physiol.,* 50:615–625.
59. Luciani, L. (1891): Il cervelletto: Nuovi studi di fisiologia normale e pathologica. Le Monnier, Florence.
60. Martinez, S. N., Bertrand, C., Molina-Negro, P., and Perez-Calvo, J. M. (1975): Alteration of pain perception by stereotaxic lesions of frontothalamic pathways. *Confin. Neurol.,* 37:113–118.
61. McGeer, P. L., Boulding, J. E., Gibson, W. C., and Foulkes, R. G. (1961): Drug-induced extrapyramidal reactions: Treatment with diphenhydramine hydrochloride and dihydroxyphenylalanine. *J.A.M.A.,* 177:665.
62. Meyers, R. (1941): The modification of alternating tremors, rigidity and festination by surgery of the basal ganglia. *Res. Publ. Ass. Nerv. Ment. Dis.,* 21:602–665.

63. Meyers, R. (1975): Surgery of hyperkinesias. In: *Handbook of Clinical Neurology,* edited by P. J. Vinken and G. W. Bruyn, p. 860. Elsevier, New York.
64. Meyers, R., Sweeney, D. B., and Schwidde, J. T. (1950): Hemiballismus: etiology and surgical treatment. *J. Neurol. Neurosurg. Psychiatr.,* 13:115–126.
65. Molina-Negro, P. (1969): Connexiones nigro-corticales: Un estudio en el gato con el método de la degeneracion retrograda. *Ann. Anat.,* 18:285–354.
66. Molina-Negro, P., Bertrand, C., Martinez, S. N., and Hardy, J. (1974): Controlled lesion of Voi and adjoining structures in stereotaxic surgery of spasmodic torticollis. Presented at the Congress of American Association of Neurological Surgeons. St. Louis, Missouri.
67. Moruzzi, G., and Magoun, H. W. (1949): Brain stem reticular formation and activation of the EEG. *Electroencephalogr. Clin. Neurophysiol.,* 1:455–473.
68. Parkinson, J. (1917): *Essay on the Shaking Palsy,* p. 16. Sherwood, Neely, and Jones, London.
69. Poirier, L. J. (1960). Experimental and histological study of midbrain dyskinesias. *J. Neurophysiol.,* 23:534–551.
70. Poirier, L. J., and Sourkes, T. L. (1965): Influence of the substantia nigra on the catecholamine content of the striatum. *Brain,* 88:181.
71. Pollock, L. J., and Davis, L. E. (1923): Studies in deccrebration. 1. A method of decerebration. *Arch. Neurol. Psychiatr.,* 10:391–398.
72. Pollock, L. J., and Davis, L. (1930): Muscle tone in parkinsonian states. *Arch. Neurol. Psychiatr.,* 23:303–319.
73. Putnam, T. J. (1933): Treatment of athetosis and dystonia by section of the extrapyramidal motor tracts. *Arch Neurol. Psychiatr.,* 29:504–521.
74. Shaltenbrand, G., and Bailey, P. (1960): Introduction to stereotaxis with an atlas of the human brain. Georg Thieme Verlag, Stuttgart.
75. Spiegel, E. A., Wycis, H. T. (1952): Stereoencephalotomy. In: *Method and Stereotaxic Atlas of Human Brain,* Vol. 8, p. 176. Grune & Stratton, New York.
76. Spiegel, E. A., Wycis, H. T., Marks, M., and Lee, A. J. (1947): Stereotaxic apparatus for operation on human brain. *Science,* 106:349.
77. Talairach, J., David, M., Tournoux, P., Corredor, H., and Kvasina, T. (1957): *Atlas D'anatomie Stéréotaxique.* Masson, Paris.
78. Trétiakoff, C. (1919): Contribution à l'étude de l'anatomie pathologique du Locus niger. Thesis, Paris.
79. Vealasco, F., Molina-Negro, P., Bertrand, C., and Hardy, J. (1972): Further definition of the subthalamic target for the arrest of tremor. *J. Neurosurg.,* 35:184–191.
80. Velasco, F., and Molina-Negro, P. (1973): Electrophysiological topography of the human diencephalon. *J. Neurosurg.,* 38:204–214.
81. Wahren, W., and Braintenberg, V. (1959): The brain as a whole. *J. Neurosurg.,* 1:42–64.
82. Walker, E. (1929): Cerebral pedunculotomy for the relief of abnormal movements: Hemiballism. *Acta Neurol. Psychiatr.,* 24:723–729.
83. Ward, A. A., Jr., McCulloch, W. S., and Magoun, H. W. (1948): Production of tremor at rest in monkeys. *J. Neurophysiol.,* 11:317–330.
84. Wimmer, D. (1929): Le spasme de torsion. *Rev. Neurol.,* 36:904–915.

Functional Neurosurgery, edited by T. Rasmussen and R. Marino. Raven Press, New York © 1979.

Neurosurgical Treatment of Spasticity

Jean Siegfried

Department of Neurosurgery, University of Zürich, Zürich, Switzerland

In the last 15 years, the introduction of new techniques has resulted in renewed interest in the neurosurgical treatment of pyramidal spasticity. Two types of neurosurgical procedures are employed today: the destruction of a brain target—of a medullary pathway or of a nerve root—and the electrical stimulation of nervous structures. A review of these methods will be made with objective long-term observations of the destructive procedures and first results for the techniques of stimulation.

DESTRUCTIVE METHODS

Stereotactic Dentatotomy

The first trial of selective destruction of the dentate nucleus was made by Delmas-Marsalet and van Bogaert in 1935 (6). The indication was not spasticity, but parkinsonian symptomatology. The denate nucleus was destroyed by means of a hook introduced through a small burr hole. Unfortunate complications of myoclonus, nystagmus, severe swallowing difficulty, right-sided hemiplegia and anesthesia, aggravation of tremor, and finally the death of the patient on the ninth postoperative day discouraged further new approaches to this nucleus for several years.

The first article on results obtained by stereotactic dentatotomy (the first case having been operated on in 1963) was published by Heimburger in 1965 (13). This resulted in a renewal of interest in the stereotactic approach to this nucleus in the treatment of certain functional disorders, particularly spasticity resulting from cerebral palsy. Between 1965 and 1969, there were many publications on this topic, but dentatotomy never became as popular as thalamotomy in cases of tremor. In recent years, interest in dentatotomy has declined markedly. Long-term assessment of the results obtained in several large series of patients now permits a reasonable evaluation of the effectiveness of this operation.

In one of his most recent articles, Heimburger (11) reports the results observed in a series of 64 patients, with an overall improvement of moderate degree in 46 cases. The patients with spastic diplegia (Little's disease) and hemiplegia provided the most impressive successes. Fraioli and Guidetti (9) observed moderate to good lessening of spasticity in about the half of their series of 47 patients operated on, but no long-term follow-up results were presented. In our previous papers, we reported encouraging results on spasticity (for instance, 29,30,31), but in 1975 (35) we analyzed in detail the long-term follow-up results, 3 to 8 years after operation, in a series of 50 patients. In 30% of the cases, a clear improvement in the spasticity was obtained, and in 50% of all cases nursing and rehabilitation were facilitated. We came to the conclusion that stereotactic dentatotomy never completely cured the spasticity and that spectacular therapeutic results were never observed. Stereotactic dentatotomy, however, provides moderate success in alleviating spasticity, particularly in cases of cerebral palsy, but its effectiveness decreases over the years. The operation can be performed, however, without complications or creating an unexpected neurological deficit. It retains limited usefulness today, although its long-term place in the future of functional neurosurgery may be questionable.

Stereotactic Pulvinarotomy

Our knowledge concerning the function of the pulvinar is very minimal. Nevertheless, it has been a neurosurgical target since 1966, when it was shown that this structure could play a role in the process of pain perception (18,26). In 1971, evidence was presented by Cooper et al. that the pulvinar contributes to motor function (5). In this first extensive clinical study, Cooper reported the results of 10 operations for spasticity resulting either from a cerebral vascular or traumatic lesion. Four of these patients had previously undergone ventrolateral nucleus surgery, two had cerebellar decortication and dentate nucleus ablation, and two had LP surgery prior to or in addition to the pulvinectomy. Seven of these 10 patients showed marked relief of spasticity. None of them was rendered hypotonic. Three failed to improve (4). This series, however, seems difficult to interpret, since most of the patients underwent other stereotactic operations as well. Fraioli, with a limited experience with spastic cases, did not report very encouraging results (9). Other reports on stereotactic pulvinarotomy alone for spasticity and with long-term follow up are rare, suggesting that this procedure has limited usefulness. In addition, in a series of 22 patients operated on by us between 1969 and 1972 with stereotactic pulvinarotomy in the treatment of intractable pain (34), we never observed a diminution of muscular tonus postoperatively.

Longitudinal Myelotomy

Since the intrathecal injection of phenol and alcohol, which has been widely used in selected cases with spasticity, affects the sensory and motor pathways and disturbs the function of the urinary bladder, more selective operations on the spinal cord have been tried. Cordotomy with transection of the anterior column (28) and of the posterior column (25) have been employed, with only minimal or transient beneficial effect.

In 1951, Bischof proposed the procedure of longitudinal myelotomy, in which the so-called Kölliker's anastomoses between the posterior and anterior horns are severed within the thoracolumbar spinal cord (2). The objective of this operation is to interrupt the connections between the anterior and posterior horns of the spinal cord bilaterally in order to prevent the transmission of the reflex arc. Good results in all types of spasticity of the legs were later reported (19,21,36,37), but the number of patients operated on is small. The spasticity disappears immediately after operation; the muscles become hypotonic and in the absence of articular contractures, active movements are possible. Residual motility may suffer from this type of myelotomy, but in some instances motility hidden behind severe spasticity may be regained to a more or less useful functional level. In patients in whom no sensory disturbances were present before operation, the sensation of temperature and pain may become reduced from L_1 distally, usually somewhat more pronounced on one side. Bladder disturbances are also reported to be observed postoperatively. In order to lessen the risk of increasing paresis as a result of injury to the pyramidal tract, the myelotomy can be done by carrying out a T-section through a commissural approach (19,27).

Rhizotomy

Anterior spinal rhizotomy for severe spasticity of the legs in patients with maximum paralysis of the legs was described by Munro (22), who advocated division of all anterior spinal nerve roots from the eleventh thoracic to the first sacral segments, inclusive. The remaining anterior roots were spared in order to avoid interference with the reflex arc for the urinary bladder. Kerr (15) modified the operation by preserving the lower thoracic anterior roots, thus allowing voluntary and reflex contractions of the abdominal muscles to assist in the emptying of the bladder; however, this method is applicable only in patients in whom maximum paralysis of the legs is already present.

Posterior spinal rhizotomy for the relief of spasticity was introduced by Foerster in 1908 (8). Foerster advocated division of the posterior roots of L_2, L_3, L_4, L_5, and S_1 in order to interrupt the afferent sensory component of the reflex arc for the lower extremities. This operation, or the partial, so-called selective posterior rhizotomy (9,10), was usually followed by relief of spasticity, but in some cases the spasticity eventually returned. This presumably resulted from the ability of some afferent impulses to find their way to the anterior horn cells via the extensive collateral nerve fiber systems.

Posterior rhizotomy of the cervical spinal nerve roots was proposed by Kottke (16) to abolish tonic neck reflexes in cases of cerebral palsy. This has resulted in a modest, but not dramatic, decrease in spasticity of the neck, spine, arms, and legs (12).

TECHNIQUES OF ELECTROSTIMULATION

The use of electrical stimulation in the treatment of paralyzed muscles and spasticity is an old method and was particulary recommended by Duchenne more than 100 years ago (7). Electrotherapy has since then been widely used by physiotherapists (14). In the past 10 years, however, the use of electrical stimulation for the control of pain and the development of implantable neurological stimulating systems has led to a resurgence of interest in the use of electrical stimulation of the afferent nervous system pathways for symptomatic relief of a variety of conditions.

"Gait-stimulators" were developed for transcutaneous stimulation and an improvement in spastic-paraparetic patients was achieved (23). In 1973, Cook and Weinstein observed striking improvements in voluntary motor control and sensory appreciation in a patient with multiple sclerosis who was treated by dorsal column stimulation for intractable back pain (3). After prolonged observation of this patient, four additional patients with multiple sclerosis, in whom pain was not a complaint, were subjected by these authors to dorsal column stimulation. A significant modification of abnormal neurological signs and dysfunction was reported:

1. Lessening of extensor spasticity of a leg and flexor spasticity of an arm.
2. Progressive improvement in synergy of movement of parts not paralyzed, including mechanisms for articulating speech.
3. Return of voluntary motor control in parts previously without such control.
4. Lowering of the threshold for various types of sensory stimuli below the level of stimulation.

Since February 1975, we have implanted a stimulating system (Medtronic) in eight patients with spasticity, among them six cases of multiple sclerosis. Tinsel monopolar electrodes were placed between two sheets of the dura (endodural) at C3/C4 level in three cases and at C1/D2 in five cases. The receiver was fixed in a subcutaneous infraclavicular pocket, with the cable between electrode and receiver lying in a subcutaneous tunnel above the clavicle. Before the operation, a test with a floating electrode introduced percutaneously from the lumbar region into the subarachnoidal space up to D_1 was performed. Intermittent stimulation of dorsal column during 36 hours showed in all cases a striking reduction of the spasticity of the legs. Such tests with a floating electrode have been used to date in a total of 17 patients with spasticity and have given the best objective indication of the potential therapeutic benefit. Two cases of cerebral palsy did not respond as well as the other cases and were deemed not suitable for operation with definitive implantation of a stimulating device. Eight patients have been operated on: six cases of multiple sclerosis, one case of a vascular lesion of the cord, and one posttraumatic case. The best results were observed in almost all cases of multiple sclerosis, and were verified by recording the muscle cell activity during passive movements (recording of the stretch reflex) (1). The patient with a vascular lesion of the cord was moderately improved. The patient with an almost complete traumatic section of the cord C_5 level, however, showed very little reduction of his very severe spasticity.

The physiological mechanisms of spinal cord stimulation on spasticity have not been elucidated, and thus we do not know in detail what neuronal structures or systems we are stimulating. Spasticity is caused by an exaggeration of the myotatic reflexes: the muscle spindle is stimulated abnormally because the gamma fibers are released from descending inhibition (27). An inhibition of the H reflex was found in pain patients with implanted spinal electrodes (17). Does stimulation inhibit the gamma-fibers or enhance descending inhibition? Nevertheless, despite the absence of a satisfactory neurophysiological explanation, the clinical observations of electrical spinal cord stimulation on spastic movement disorders have given promise of significant potential value of the method.

SUMMARY

Conservative treatment of spasticity is disappointing in severe cases. Drugs and occupational and physical therapy have demonstrated only limited benefit. Cerebral operations, particularly stereotactic dentatotomy seem to have some value in cases of cerebral palsy, but long-lasting successes are seen only in 30 to 50% of the cases. Operations on the spinal cord have not been widely used, because it is difficult to relax muscles without paralyzing them. Longitudinal myelotomy may nevertheless be a valuable operation in spastic paraplegia. Spinal cord stimulation seems the most promising technique to reduce spasticity, but the experience to date is too small to permit definitive evaluation of this new nondestructive method.

REFERENCES

1. Adorjani, L., Meyer, M., and Siegfried, J. (1977): Die Untersuchung des tonischen Dehnungsreflexes in der Klinik: Eine Methode zur Verbesserung der Diagnostik und der Quantifizierung von pathologischen zentralen Tonuserhöhungen der Muskulatur. *Méd. Hyg.,* 35:2038–2046.
2. Bischof, W. (1951): Die longitudinale Myelotomie. *Zentralbl. Neurochir.,* 11:79–88.
3. Cook, A. W., and Weinstein, S. P. (1973): Chronic dorsal column stimulation in multiple sclerosis. *New York State J. Med.,* 73:2868–2872.
4. Cooper, I. S., Amin, I., Chandra, R., and Waltz, J. M. (1974): Clinical physiology of motor contribution of the pulvinar in man: A study of cryopulvinectomy. In: *The Pulvinar-LP Complex,* Vol. 1, edited by I. S. Cooper et al., pp. 220–232. Charles C Thomas, Springfield, Illinois.
5. Cooper, I. S., Waltz, J. M., Amin, I., and Fujita, S. (1971): Pulvinectomy: A preliminary report. *J. Am. Geriatr. Soc.,* 19:553–554.
6. Delmas-Marsalet P., and van Bogaert, L. (1935): Sur un cas de myoclonies rythmiques continues déterminées par une intervention chirurgicale sur le tronc cérébral. *Rev. Neurol. (Paris),* 64:728–740.
7. Duchenne, G. B. (1855): *De l'électrisation localisée et de son application à la pathologie et à la thérapeutique.* J. B. Baillière, Paris.
8. Foerster, O. (1908): Ueber eine neue operative Methode der Behandlung spastischer Lähmungen durch Resektion hinterer Rückenmarkwurzeln. *Z. Orthop. Chir.,* 22:202–223.
9. Fraioli, B., and Guidetti, B. (1976): Problèmes cliniques et possibilités neurochirurgicales actuelles dans les syndromes d'hypertonie et de dyskinesie. *Neurochirurgie,* 22:557–567.
10. Gros, C., Ouakhine, G., Vlahovitch, B., and Frerebeau, P. (1967): La radicotomie sélective postérieure dans le traitement neurochirurgical de l'hypertonie pyramidale. *Neurochirurgie,* 13:505–518.
11. Heimburger, R. F. (1970): The cerebellum and spasticity. *Int. J. Neurol.,* 7:232–243.

12. Heimburger, R. F., Slominski, A., and Griswald, P. (1973): Cervical posterior rhizotomy for reducing spasticity in cerebral palsy. *J. Neurosurg.*, 39:30–34.
13. Heimburger, R. F., and Whitlock, C. C. (1965): Stereotaxic destruction of the human dentate nucleus. *Confin. Neurol.*, 26:346–358.
14. Hufschmidt, H. J. (1968): Die Elektrotherapie der Spastik. *Med. Welt*, 47:2613–2616.
15. Kerr, A. S. (1966): Anterior rhizotomy for the relief of spasticity. *Paraplegia*, 4:154–160.
16. Kottke, F. J. (1970): Modification of athetosis by denervation of the tonic neck reflexes. *Develop. Med. Child Neurol.*, 12:236–237.
17. Krainick, J. U., Thoden, U., Strassburg, H. M., and Wenzel, D. (1977): The effect of electrical spinal cord stimulation on spastic movement disorders. *Neurochirurgia (Stuttg.) (in press)*.
18. Kudo, T., Yoshii, N., Shimizu, S., Aikawa, S., and Nakahama, H. (1966): Effects of stereotaxic thalamotomy to intractable pain and numbness. *Keio J. Med.*, 15:191–194.
19. Laitinen, L., and Sigounas, E. (1971): Longitudinal myelotomy in the treatment of spasticity of the legs. *J. Neurosurg.*, 35:536–540.
20. Malmros, R. (1962): Neurosurgical possibilities in the treatment of spasticity. *Acta Neurol. Scand.*, 38 (Supp. 3):103–109.
21. Moyes, P. P. (1969): Longitudinal myelotomy for spasticity. *J. Neurosurg.*, 31:615–619.
22. Munro, D. (1945): Anterior rhizotomy for spastic paraplegia. *N. Engl. J. Med.*, 233:453–461.
23. Pateisky, K., Wessely, P., and Kifhtreiber, G. (1976): Zur Elektrobehandlung der spastischen Gangstörung mit einem "Schrittstimulator." *Fortschr. Neurol. Psychiatr.*, 14:21–33.
24. Pourpre, H. (1960): Traitement neuro-chirurgical des contractures chez les paraplégiques post-traumatiques. *Neurochirurgie*, 6:229–236.
25. Puusepp, L. (1933): *Chirurgische Neuropathologie*, Vol. 2, *Tartu Dorpat Pub.*, pp. 619–622.
26. Richardson, D. E. (1967): Thalamotomy for intractable pain. *Confin. Neurol.*, 29:139–145.
27. Rushworth, G. (1960): Spasticity and rigidity: An experimental study and review. *J. Neurol. Neurosurg. Psychiatry*, 33:99–118.
28. Schürmann, K. (1949): Die Durchschneidung der Pyramidenvorderstränge und benachbarter extrapyramidaler Bahnen bei spastischen Zuständen und unwillkürlichen Bewegungen. *Zeutralbf. Neurochir.*, 9:136–141.
29. Siegfried, J. (1971): Stereotaxic cerebellar surgery. *Confin. Neurol.*, 33:350–360.
30. Siegfried, J. (1972): Stereotactic treatment of hypertonicity. In: *Present Limits of Neurosurgery*, Vol. 1, edited by J. Fusek and Z. Kunc, pp. 549–550. Avisenum, Prague.
31. Siegfried, J. (1974): Methods and results in spasticity and hyperkinesias. In: *Recent Progress in Neurological Surgery*, Vol. 1, edited by K. Sano and S. Ishii, pp. 251–255. Excerpta Medica and Elsevier, Amsterdam.
32. Siegfried, J. (1976): Traitement neurochirurgical de quelques symptômes de la sclérose en plaques. *Méd. Hyg.*, 34:901–903.
33. Siegfried, J. (1977): Deux aspects différents du traitement neurochirurgical de la spasticité: Interventions cérébrales et stimulation des cordons postérieurs de la moelle. *Neuro-Chirurgie*, 23:344–347.
34. Siegfried, J. (1977): Stereotactic pulvinarectomy in the treatment of intractable pain. *Prog. Neurol. Surg.*, 8:104–113.
35. Siegfried, J., and Verdie, J. C. (1977): Long-term assessment of stereotactic dentatotomy for spasticity and other disorders. *Acta Neurochir. (Wien), (in press)*.
36. Tönnis, W., and Bischof, W. (1962): Ergebnisse der lumbalen Myelotomie nach Bischof. *Zeutralbl. Neurochir.*, 23:120–132.
37. Weber, W. (1955): Die Behandlung der spinalen Paraspastik unter Berücksichtigung der longitudinalen Myelotomie (Bischof). *Med. Monatsschr.*, 9:510–513.

Functional Neurosurgery, edited by T. Rasmussen
and R. Marino. Raven Press, New York © 1979.

Functional Surgery of the Trigeminal Nerve: Treatment of Trigeminal Neuralgia

*John M. Tew, Jr., **Jeffrey T. Keller, and **David S. Williams

*Mayfield Neurological Institute, Cincinnati, Ohio 45219, and **Christ Hospital Research Institute, Cincinnati, Ohio 45219*

The practice of surgery of the trigeminal nerve has been established for centuries. According to Krause (18), peripheral section of a branch of the trigeminal nerve was first proposed by Schlichtung in 1748. Subsequently, few advances were made until Hartley (9) and Krause (16) proposed intracranial section of peripheral branches of the trigeminal nerve. The following year, Krause (17) advocated resection of the gasserian ganglion. Horsley (11) reported that division of the sensory root might be effective, since regeneration would probably not occur after preganglionic section of the nerve. Spiller and Frazier (23) reported the first successful performance of retrogasserian rhizotomy and presented anatomical evidence that regeneration after root section was unlikely.

Following these early reports, many refinements have been made. These include: preservation of the motor root, subtotal resection of the root, and a progressive lowering of the mortality rate. Despite these refinements, due to the occurrence of continuing complications and incomplete relief of pain, other procedures such as the posterior fossa approach to the trigeminal nerve (3), percutaneous injection (6), and decompressive techniques (5,12,25) have been recommended. For many years, percutaneous techniques (7,15) were favored in most European centers. Yet these approaches failed to gain universal appeal because of undesirable side effects and an unduly high incidence of pain recurrence.

The major complications of percutaneous techniques have been largely a result of the uncontrollable spread of injected chemicals such as alcohol or phenol, or the injury of major vessels by thermal coagulation rather than a result of the injury of important structures by a penetrating electrode or needle.

As introduced by Kirschner (14), the percutaneous approach to the gasserian ganglion employed none of the attributes of functional surgery other than placement of the needle with the aid of radiographic control. Nevertheless, the speed and simplicity of the method led to widespread popularity in Europe. Unfortunately, many complications were reported (2,10,29,30). Several deaths were attributed to carotid artery injury and meningitis. Although Thiry (28) continued to use much the same crude technique as Kirschner, he was able virtually to eliminate the serious complications by reducing the intensity of the electrocautery. Schürman (21) accomplished further improvement in results by controlled partial coagulation under neuroleptic-analgesia. Sweet (24) advanced the hypothesis that the differential sensitivity of the pain fibers to heat could be exploited to achieve lasting pain control. Experimental studies by Letcher (19) and Frigyesi (4) have confirmed the validity of Sweet's premise (24). Blockade of conduction in A delta and C fibers by a temperature level less than that required to abolish transmission in A alpha fibers explains the frequent clinical preservation of touch perception in patients with superimposed analgesia.

The reproducibility of clinical results, the lowered morbidity, and the relative absence of surgical stress have led to widespread acceptance of this functional approach as the treatment of choice for trigeminal neuralgia when a destructive surgical procedure is considered.

The success of the thermocoagulation technique is most directly related to the adoption of the concepts of functional surgery or applied neuroanatomy and physiology to surgery of the trigeminal nerve. While considerable changes have occurred in our technique during the past 9 years, the following principles have proven of great value:

1. *Short-term anesthesia:* Reversible anesthesia is induced by the ultra-short-acting barbiturate, methohexital (Brevital®), administered by intravenous injection.

2. *Radiographic localization:* Precise placement of the electrode tip in the vicinity of the posterior root under radiographic control (cineradiography) according to three-dimensional external and internal landmarks.

3. *Physiologic localization:* Isolated electrical stimulation at 50 to 75 CPS, 100 to 400 mV, and a square-wave pulse of 1-msec duration localizes the electrode

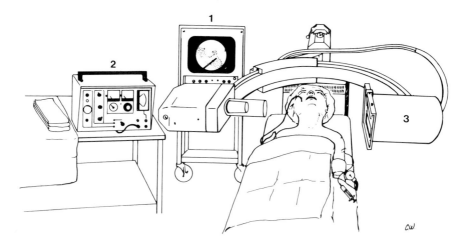

FIG. 1. The operative arrangement used for stereotactic rhizotomy of the trigeminal nerve. **1.** Image intensifier. **2.** Radiofrequency generator. **3.** C-arm cineradiographic unit.

tip in the posterior rootlets. Stimulation of paroxysms of tic-like pain provides accurate localization.

4. *Controlled lesion production with temperature monitoring.*

5. *Physiologic testing:* Rapid reversibility of the anesthetic agent permits testing of cutaneous sensation for pain and touch perception in an alert, co-operative patient. Repetitive lesioning can be conducted until the desired result is achieved.

TECHNIQUE: PERCUTANEOUS TRIGEMINAL RHIZOTOMY

The procedure is conducted in the radiography suite (Fig. 1). After the patient has been anesthetized with an intravenous injection of 30 to 50 mg of methohexital, a hollow 19-gauge needle with a terminus bare for 5, 7½, or 10 mm is selected. The electrode is placed in a stereotactic fashion by freehand manipulation although a guiding apparatus may be used if deemed helpful. Three external landmarks are placed on the skin of the face (Fig. 2). The anterior approach,

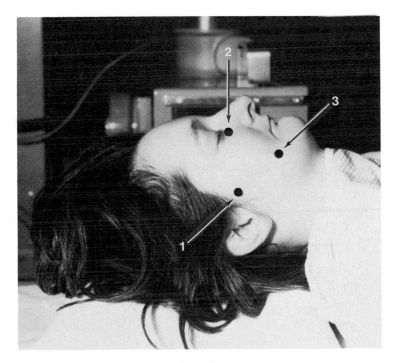

FIG. 2. Anatomic landmarks for electrode placement. **1.** A point 3 cm anterior to external auditory meatus. **2.** Medial pupillary point. **3.** Electrode entry site (3 cm lateral to oral commissure).

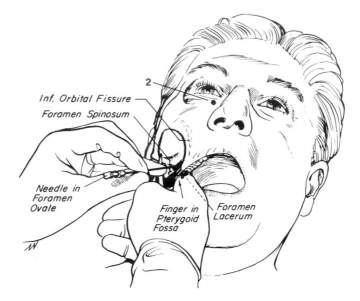

FIG. 3. Illustration demonstrating needle placement according to the technique of Härtel. (**2.** Medial pupillary line.)

as advocated by Härtel, is utilized (8), (Fig. 3). The needle is aimed toward the intersection of planes extended from: (a) a point 5 cm anterior to the external auditory meatus, and, (b) a point marking the medial aspect of the pupil. Further reliability of placement is provided by cineradiographic monitoring. In the lateral view, the needle is directed toward a point 5 to 10 mm below the floor of the sella turcica (Fig. 4). Entrance of the needle into the foramen ovale is signaled by a wince and a brief contraction of the masseter muscle, indicating contact with the mandibular sensory and motor fibers. The stylet is withdrawn to elicit the flow of cerebrospinal fluid (CSF) and to exclude penetration of the carotid artery. The needle is then advanced until the tip reaches the vicinity of the clival line (Fig. 4).

The results of anatomical studies performed in our laboratory (27) have been confirmed by physiologic stimulation and clinical observations. These findings have greatly increased the safety and ease in which this procedure can be performed. The more important of these observations follow.

Definition of Internal Landmarks

The mapping of the relationship of the trigeminal rootlets to the profile of the clivus (Fig. 5) and the distance from the foramen ovale to the retrogasserian fibers is such that with consistent reliability the rootlets of the third, second, and first divisions can be successively stimulated, by the use of a small electrode tip (5 mm), as the electrode is advanced in calibrated steps. The maxillary

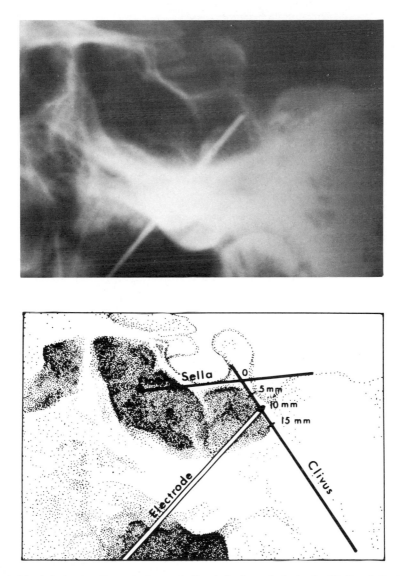

FIG. 4. (Top): Lateral radiograph demonstrating trajectory of electrode. **(Bottom):** Illustration demonstrating ideal electrode trajectory (5–10 mm below the floor of sella turcica).

rootlets can be most frequently isolated with the tip of the electrode projected at the clival line. Cisternal fluid can be aspirated in nearly all circumstances except when prior surgical exploration or alcohol injection has been performed. The relationship of the rootlets to the clival line is important, since cisternal injection studies have indicated that the subarachnoid space may be reflected

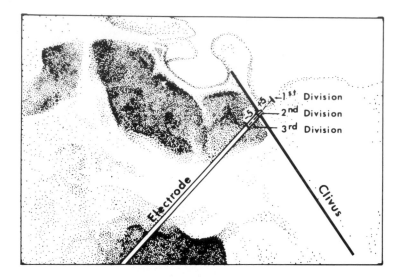

FIG. 5. Composite illustration demonstrating the relationship of the trigeminal rootlets to the profile of the clivus. With the electrode tip at −5 mm, the third division is stimulated: at 0, the second division; and at +5 mm deep to the clivus, the first division fibers are stimulated.

off the peripheral nerve. Therefore, aspiration of CSF does not invariably indicate that the needle tip has reached the retrogasserian fibers.

Definition of Neurovascular Relations

The relationship of the carotid artery to the mandibular nerve, trigeminal ganglion, and retrogasserian fibers is demonstrated in Fig. 6. The carotid artery is vulnerable to injury at three sites: (a) At the foramen lacerum, posterolateral deviation of the needle may penetrate its cartilaginous covering. (b) Immediately upon entrance into the cranial cavity (middle fossa), the carotid artery lies directly behind the mandibular nerve. The carotid canal is devoid of bony covering in 80% of cases studied anatomically. An inferior deviation of the penetrating electrode may therefore pierce the nerve and the carotid artery at the same site. Such an occurrence probably took place in the case reported by Rish (20). (c) The artery may be penetrated within the cavernous sinus if the electrode is directed too far cephalad along the clival line. Carotid cavernous fistula development has been reported (P. Williams, *personal communication*). Attention to the trajectory of the electrode has eliminated vascular complications from our experience.

Relationship of the Cranial Nerves (III, IV, and VI) to the Trigeminal Rootlets

Penetration of the foramen ovale by the proper trajectory and avoidance of excessive penetration (5 mm beyond the profile of the clivis) have eliminated

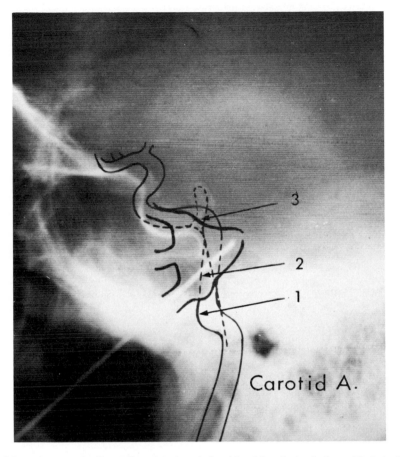

FIG. 6. A lateral composite illustration of 1. the relationship of the electrode tip and its trajectory to the mandibular nerve; 2. the carotid artery in Meckel's cave; and 3. The cavenous carotid.

ocular nerve complications in the last 200 cases. The abducens, the most frequently injured nerve, can be avoided if the electrode trajectory is maintained between the 5- to 10-mm planes and the electrode does not penetrate more than 10 mm deep into the clival line. Oculomotor and trochlear palsies rarely occur unless the needle penetrates the cavernous sinus (Fig. 7).

RESULTS: FUNCTIONAL RHIZOTOMY FOR TRIGEMINAL NEURALGIA

At the time of this report, over 500 patients have been operated upon for typical trigeminal neuralgia by the percutaneous rhizotomy approach. A thorough follow-up evaluation extending over a period of 1 to 8 years has been completed for 400 of these patients (Table 1).

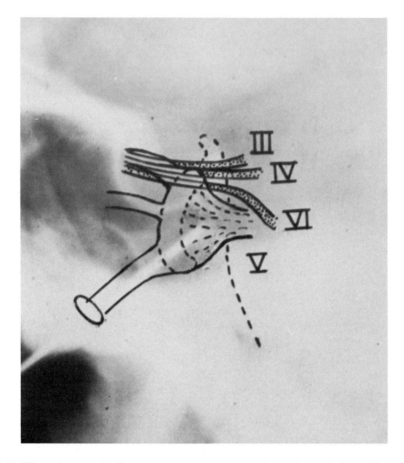

FIG. 7. A lateral composite illustration of the relationship of the electrode tip and its trajectory to the mandibular nerve, ganglion, clivus, posterior rootlets, and ocular nerves. III, IV, V, and VI = cranial nerves.

The average age was 63 years, and 60% of patients were female. In 60% of patients, pain was located on the right, and the second and third divisions of the trigeminal nerve were commonly involved. Isolated pain in the first or third division was less frequent than the second division. It is notable that 21% of patients had a significant degree of pain in the first division although pain was isolated to the first division in only 2% of patients.

The disease had been present for an average of 8 years and was characterized by increasingly severe episodes of paroxysmal pain and shortening periods of remission. Many patients had been treated by surgical methods, usually nerve avulsion or alcohol injection (32%), while 11% had a prior intracranial procedure, usually subtotal rhizotomy. Nearly all patients had been treated with either diphenylhydantoin (Dilantin®) or carbamazepine (Tegretol®), as well

TABLE 1. *Characteristics of 400 patients selected for electro-coagulation treatment*

Average age	63 years
Sex	60% female
Side of coagulation	
Right	60%
Left	39%
Bilateral	1%
Division of trigeminal nerve involved	
V-1	2%
V-2	20%
V-3	17%
V-1, V-2	14%
V-2, V-3	42%
V-1, V-2, V-3	5%

as other forms of medical and physical remedies. While diphenylhydantoin was effective in over 50% of patients, the effect was seldom lasting or satisfactory. Carbamazepine was considered more effective; 92% of patients reported significant relief of a lasting nature, but the efficacy was limited by the tendency of most patients to develop increasing side effects to the drug as higher dosage was required.

A response to follow-up was obtained for all 400 patients; however, many of the patients were not recalled for personal examination because of advanced age, disability, distance from the examining clinic, death, or for other reasons. All were contacted by questionnaire or phone, however, and a family member was contacted if the patient had died. At the time of evaluation, 93% of patients reported excellent to good results from the procedure. The remaining patients obtained only fair results (6%) because of undesirable side effects or recurrence of pain. Four patients (1%) reported that they had never received satisfactory relief of the pain at any time following the coagulation procedure.

SIDE EFFECTS

Sensory Deficit

Troublesome numbness and paresthesias resulting from the sensory deficit proved to be the most consistent adverse side effect of the procedure. Commonly, an intermittent crawling, burning, or itching sensation was described. Most patients readily adjusted to the sensory deficit, and the paresthesias usually diminished with time. In the more active and mentally alert patients, few disturbances of sensation were reported. Older patients are more prone to this complication. Constant, severe dysesthesias in an anesthetic or analgesic zone (anesthesia dolorosa) rarely occurred in these patients. One patient reported a severe burning pain which lessened considerably after several months. Forty-five patients reported a significant problem with paresthesias and 11 additional patients complained of other symptoms related to the sensory deprivation. Five patients reported a troublesome aching pain in the jaw region.

Five patients developed persistent excoriation of the skin about the face, nostril, or scalp. Many of these patients were observed to traumatize the skin by frequent scratching or manipulation. These patients were aged and demented to a major degree. This development could be controlled in most cases by the nocturnal application of mittens.

Eye Complications

Eye complications occurred in 8% of patients. Eight patients (2%) developed neurolytic keratitis. Thirty percent of this group had corneal analgesia, indicating that preservation of touch perception in the absence of pain perception does not necessarily protect against corneal ulceration. The corneal lesion was reversible in each of the patients in response to early ophthalmologic treatment. Application of a soft contact lens, meticulous eye care, and occasional tarsorrhaphy prevented permanent visual loss. Intermittent blurring of vision was a complaint in 12 patients (4%). Sixty percent of these patients had preservation of touch perception on the cornea but the corneal reflex was markedly diminished. Again, this finding suggests that preservation of touch perception on the cornea does not necessarily protect against keratitis and visual clouding. Our experience indicates that persons with some sensory preservation on the cornea adjust more rapidly to the deficit and rarely develop ulceration. Although patients with corneal anesthesia seldom develop keratitis in the late postoperative period, meticulous instruction of the patient and relatives concerning all features of eye care is mandatory. Careful adherence to this practice has probably prevented the serious eye complications sometimes seen following this procedure. Seventy patients in this group had neuralgia involving or limited to the ophthalmic division. Seventy-two percent of these patients achieved pain relief without developing a major corneal sensory deficit; only 6% of the total group developed neurolytic keratitis.

Transient diplopia occurred in 7 patients (2%), all of whom were undergoing treatment for neuralgia involving the ophthalmic division. In 5, the double vision could be explained by an abducens nerve palsy and in 2 patients the cause was trochlear palsy. The deficit was transient in all patients; the most persistent disturbance lasted for 4 months while in all others it disappeared in a few weeks.

The incidence of unwanted loss of corneal sensation and paresis of ocular nerves has been greatly reduced in recent years by performing electrocoagulation with the patient alert and cooperating in the evaluation during the final stage of production of the lesion.

Motor Paresis

Paresis of the muscles innervated by the motor root of the trigeminal occurred in 22% of patients. In most instances, the deficit was partial and transient. Weakness of masseter, temporalis, and pterygoid muscles causes a mild degree of disability owing to jaw deviation and loss of chewing power. Trismus was a more troublesome problem but could be avoided or eliminated by being careful not to strain the muscles and frequent jaw exercises.

Difficulties in hearing related to inconstant roaring and a popping sound was reported by some patients. These symptoms are attributable to paresis of the small muscles about the eustachian tube (tensor veli palatine) and tympanic membrane (tensor tympani).

Many patients reported difficulty with mastication who did not have any motor paresis. They related their difficulty to sensory loss in the mouth; however, the majority of patients did not find this to be significant, since they had been accustomed to chewing on the nonpainful side for many years.

Herpes Simplex

The lesions of herpes simplex were noted in 3% of patients. Since most of our patients were not examined more than 48 hours postoperatively, this figure is undoubtedly low.

RECURRENCE OF TRIGEMINAL NEURALGIA

The follow-up period varied from 1 to 8 years. Thirty-seven (9%) patients developed recurrent pain of sufficient severity to require repetition of the surgical prodecure. Thirteen patients (3%) had some recurrent pain but adequate control could be achieved by medical therapy. Six patients (2%) had a minor recurrence of pain but required no additional medical or surgical treatment.

Recurrence of pain following percutaneous rhizotomy of the trigeminal nerve occurred more frequently during the early years of our experience. During this period, we sought to make lesions of a minimal nature to limit the degree of sensory deficit. It was determined that the recurrence rate was high in patients with minimal sensory deficit, as had been recorded in other procedures. Subsequently, we advised patients to have lesions which would induce analgesia in the zones of pain and hypalgesia in the adjacent painful zones. The result has been a significant reduction in recurrence of pain, but, as expected, more patients have complained of troublesome numbness and paresthesias.

DISCUSSION

Trigeminal neuralgia is a common disorder that continues to stimulate controversy concerning the basic etiology and best mode of treatment. Although medical therapy is the primary method of control, it is seldom effective in eliminating the progressive recurrence of the advancing symptoms. Surgical treatment has been largely destructive in nature until the recent reports of Jannetta (13) proposed that permanent relief of pain can be obtained by vascular decompression of the trigeminal rootlets. This hypothesis provides an attractive alternative to all destructive procedures; however, the magnitude of the posterior fossa procedure limits its applicability in many aged patients having a reduced cardiovascular reserve. The major appeal of the percutaneous approach to treatment of facial pain has been its simplicity and the relative absence of serious complications. With the application of the principles of functional surgery to the well-established techniques, it is now possible to demonstrate that the procedure of stereotactic radiofrequency rhizotomy of the trigeminal nerve (22,26) is the surgical procedure of choice after medical therapy has been exhausted. The advantages of controlled thermal elimination of pain perception in a restricted zone of the face has, in our experience, been associated with a low recurrence rate (9%) and insignificant lasting side effects other than disagreeable numbness or paresthesias (12%). If recurrence of pain occurs in a patient who possesses satisfactory reserve to permit posterior fossa exploration, or if the individual abhors the thought of partial sensory deprivation, the procedure advocated by Jannetta can be wisely applied; however, the current tabulation of results of Jannetta (13) and Apfelbaum (1) do not indicate that one can expect a significant improvement in the recurrence rate or avoidance of complications, as compared to our series of cases performed by the electrocoagulation technique. Nevertheless, it is agreed that there is a compelling rationale for seeking to relieve the pain of trigeminal neuralgia and eliminating the need for sensory deprivation. Further experience and careful study will ultimately determine the precise role of these equally attractive concepts.

SUMMARY

During the last 9 years, we have been involved in a continuing clinical experience that has directed our efforts toward the development of a functional method of controlling the pain of trigeminal neuralgia. Through a process of technical evolution, the principles outlined in this chapter have been developed. The application of these principles of functional surgery to the treatment of trigeminal neuralgia has been highly effective in eliminating the early serious complications attendant to thermocoagulation.

REFERENCES

1. Apfelbaum, R. I. (1977): A comparison of percutaneous trigeminal neuralgia and microvascular decompression of the trigeminal nerve for the treatment of tic douloureux. *Neurosurg.,* 1:16–21.
2. Bauer, K. H. (1944): Die electrokoagulation des ganglion gasseri. *Chirurgia,* 16:1–5.
3. Dandy, W. E. (1929): An operation for the cure of tic douloureux: Partial section of the sensory root at the pons. *Arch. Surg.,* 18:687–734.

4. Frigyesi, T. L., Siegfried, J., and Brozzi, G. (1975): The selective vulnerability of evoked potentials in the trigeminal sensory root to graded thermocoagulation. *Exp. Neurol.,* 49:11–21.
5. Gardner, W. S. (1962): Concerning the mechanisms of trigeminal neuralgia and hemifacial spasm. *J. Neurol.,* 19:947–758.
6. Harris, W. (1921): Alcohol injection of the gasserian ganglion for trigeminal neuralgia. *Lancet,* 1:218–221.
7. Harris, W. (1940): An analysis of 1433 cases of paroxysmal trigeminal neuralgia (trigeminaltic) and the end results of gasserian alcohol injection. *Brain,* 63:209–224.
8. Härtel, F. (1914): Ueber die intracranielle injektionsbehandlung der trigeminusneuralgie. *Med. Klin.,* 10:582–584.
9. Hartley, F. (1892): Intracranial neurectomy of the second and third divisions of the fifth nerve. *New York J. Med.,* 55:317–319.
10. Hensell, V. (1957): Ist die electrokoagulation des ganglion gasseri auch heute noch berechitigt? *Chirurgia,* 28:544–548.
11. Horsley, V. (1891): Remarks on the various surgical procedures devised for relief or cure of trigeminal neuralgia. *Br. Med. J.,* 2:1139.
12. Jannetta, P. J. (1976): Microsurgical approach to the trigeminal nerve for tic douloureux. *Prog. Neurol. Surg.,* 7:180–200.
13. Jannetta, P. J. (1977): Treatment of trigeminal neuralgia by suboccipital and transtentorial cranial operations. In: *Clinical Neurosurgery,* edited by E. Keener, pp. 538–549. Waverly Press, Baltimore, Maryland.
14. Kirschner, M. (1932): Electrocoagulation des ganglion gasseri. *Zentralbl. Chir.,* 47:2841–2843.
15. Kirschner, M. (1942): Zur behandlung der trigeminusneuralgie. *Med. Wehnschr. (Munich),* 89:235–239.
16. Krause, F. (1892): Resection des trigeminus innerhalb der schadelhohle. *Arch. Klin. Chir.,* 41:821–832.
17. Krause, F. (1893): Entfernung des ganglion gasseri und des central daron gelegnen trigemenusstrammes. *Deutsche Med. Wehnschr.,* 19:341.
18. Krause, F. (1896): *Die Neuralgie des Trigeminus.* F. C. W. Vogel, Leipzig, 250 pp.
19. Letcher, F. S., and Goldring, S. (1968): The effect of radiofrequency current and heat on peripheral nerve action potential in the cat. *J. Neurosurg.,* 29:42–47.
20. Rish, B. L. (1965): Cerebrovascular accident after percutaneous rf thermocoagulation of the trigeminal ganglion. *J. Neurosurg.,* 44:376–377.
21. Schürman, M., and Butz, M. (1972): Temporal retrogasserian resection of trigeminal root versus controlled elective percutaneous electrocoagulation of the ganglion of Gasser in the treatment of trigeminal neuralgia: Report on a series of 531 cases. *Acta Neurochir. (Wien),* 26:33–53.
22. Siegfried, J. (1977): 500 percutaneous thermocoagulations of gasserian ganglion for trigeminal pain. *Surg. Neurol.,* 8:126–131.
23. Spiller, W. G., and Frazier, C. R. (1901): The division of the sensory root of the trigeminus for the relief of tic douloureux. *Univ. Penn. Med. Bull.,* 14:341.
24. Sweet, W. H. (1976): In: *Current Controversies in Neurosurgery,* edited by T. P. Morley, p. 853. Saunders, Philadelphia.
25. Taarnhoj, P. (1954): Decompression of the trigeminal root. *J. Neurosurg.,* 11:299–305.
26. Tew, J. M., and Keller, J. T. (1977): Controversy in the management of trigeminal neuralgia: The treatment of trigeminal neuralgia by percutaneous radiofrequency technique. In: *Clinical Neurosurgery,* edited by E. Keener, pp. 557–578. Waverly Press, Baltimore, Maryland.
27. Tew, J. M., Keller, J. T., and Williams, D. S.: Application of stereotaxic principles to the treatment of trigeminal neuralgia. *J. Appl. Neurophysiol. (in press).*
28. Thiry, M. S. (1962): Experience personnelle basee sur 225 cas de nevralgie essentielle du trijumeau traites par electrocoagulation stereotaxique du ganglion de Gasser entre 1950 et 1960. *Neurochirurgie,* 8:86–92.
29. Tonnis, W., and Kreissel, H. (1951): Die bedeutung einer sog faltigen differentialdiagnose fur die chirurgische behandlung der trigeminusneuralgie. *Deutsche Med. Wehnschr.,* 76:1202–1205.
30. Zenker, R. (1939): Die behandlung der trigeminus neuralgie unter besonderer Berücksichigung der grundlagen, der ausfuhrung and der ergebnisse der punktion und elektrokoagulation des ganglion gasseri nach Kirschner. *Ergeb. Chir. Orthop.,* 31:1–82.

Functional Neurosurgery, edited by T. Rasmussen
and R. Marino. Raven Press, New York © 1979.

Functional Neurosurgery of Neuroendocrine Disorders

J. Hardy

*Department of Surgery, University of Montreal and Service of Neurosurgery,
Hôpital Notre-Dame, Montreal, Quebec, Canada H2L 1M4*

The pituitary gland has for a long time been considered the master organ of the endocrine system on the basis of the many trophic hormonal secretions that control the peripheral organs: thyroid, breast, adrenals, and gonads. Its close anatomical connection with the median eminence of the hypothalamus consists of two parts: a direct neural connection through the infundibular process and neural lobe, and an indirect vascular connection through the blood vessels of the portal system. These pathways form the anatomical basis for neuroendocrine control of the pituitary gland by the central nervous system. Although the electrical impulse from the hypothalamic hypophyseal bundle was previously studied in lower animals (29,31,43,52), direct recording from the human neurohypophysis was first described in 1965 by Hardy (11,13), who postulated that this particular electrical activity of the neurohypophysis was coincident with the mechanism of transportation of the neurosecretory material from the hypothalamic neurons (12) (Fig. 1). The concept that electrical activity from specialized neurons exerting a direct action on the endocrine system is the basis for the modern specialized discipline of neuroendocrinology.

Recent data from anatomical, histological, biochemical, and clinical sources suggest that the brain is also a target organ under the influence of hormones. Although the hypothalamus plays an important role in the regulation of endocrine functions, it is not only an autonomous primary regulatory center but merely a functional relay circuit that is influenced by two major sources: It receives and transmits impulses from other regions of the brain relaying them to the pituitary by neurohumoral and nervous transmission. It also receives direct hormonal influence from upgoing flows of the pituitary and relays them to other specific cerebral structures.

Of the many hypothalamic regulatory substances so far postulated, only three have been isolated, structurally determined, and their physiological activity demonstrated: thyrotropin releasing hormone (TRH) (5,9,49); luteinizing hormone-releasing hormone (LH-RH) (50); and growth hormone releasing inhibiting hormone (GH-RIH or somatostatin) (6). The chemical nature of the others is still unknown.

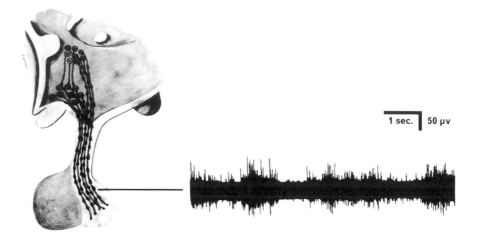

FIG. 1. Microelectrode recording of electrical activity from human neurohypophysis during transsphenoidal hypophysectomy. (From refs. 11–13.)

On anatomical grounds, our findings (17) of a selective distribution of oversecreting pituitary microadenoma in human subjects have yielded to the confirmation of a topographical distribution of nuclei or pools of cells secreting the various hormones of the pituitary (Fig. 2). Histochemical studies and immunofluorescent methods have further confirmed the same localization of these pools of cells in normal pituitary gland (33,41,42). Therefore, the adenohypophysis can no longer be viewed as a unique simple endocrine organ, but it appears to be an aggregate or a complex of several specialized glands, each one made of a specific cell type independent of the others. Furthermore, electron-micro-

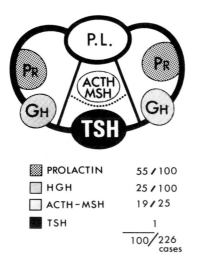

▨ PROLACTIN	55 / 100
▨ HGH	25 / 100
☐ ACTH–MSH	19 / 25
■ TSH	1
	100/226 cases

FIG. 2. Topographical distribution of hypersectomy pituitary microadenomas (lesion smaller than 10 mm in diameter). (J. Hardy, *unpublished data.*)

scopic studies have now clearly defined the structural characteristic of each cell type and its secretory granules (1,46–48). Morphological and immunofluorescent methods indicate that each adenohypophyseal hormone is produced by a distinct and separate cell type, with two exceptions, however, which remain to be clarified. Some gonadotropic cells secrete both LH and FSH, and most ACTH-secreting cells also secrete MSH or beta-lipotrophin hormone. So far, there are seven well-known pituitary hormones secreted by the adenohypophysis: TSH, ACTH, GH, LH, FSH, PRL, and MSH or β-LPH. Each of these hormones has a direct and specific activity on target organs of the body, except for LPH, the function of which has not been entirely clarified.

The classical description of the blood supply of the hypothalamic pituitary complex must be revised. After the original work of Xuereb et al. (55), the importance of the blood supply to the pituitary gland by the superior hypophyseal artery was emphasized; however, our recent studies (32) have shown that the main arterial supply to the pituitary gland is coming from the inferior hypophyseal arteries (collateral of the internal carotid artery) and that the distal branches provide the main blood supply to the posterior neural lobe, the posterior part of the pituitary stalk, and the median eminence of the hypothalamus. Other recent studies by Page and Bergland (36,37) revealed that the main venous drainage of the anterior pituitary is an upgoing circulatory supply toward the median eminence of the hypothalamus. These recent data on a new arrangement of the vascular supply between the hypothalamus and pituitary would further emphasize the concept of a mutual control between these two structures and the dependence of the hypothalamus on the secretions of the anterior lobe of the pituitary. This mutual control between hypothalamus and pituitary is divided in two parts: first, the classical downgoing flow of neurosecretory material and hypophysiotropic hormones from the median eminence to control the secretion of the anterior pituitary gland, and second, the finding of an upgoing arterial and venous supply of the anterior pituitary toward the median eminence of the hypothalamus suggests that the anterior pituitary hormones are also providing direct control of the hypothalamic functions as well as other cerebral structures (2).

From the clinical point of view, there is an increasing amount of data confirming that hormones have a direct effect on the development and activities of the central nervous system (35).

It is well known that hypothyroidism in children is associated with a high incidence of mental dificiency, suggesting that the thyroid hormone plays an important role in brain development during fetal life. Prolonged untreated myxedema can produce dementia associated with brain damage. At the opposite, severe hyperthyroidism and thyroid crisis are sometimes accompanied by acute organic psychotic disorders.

ACTH excessive secretion seen in Cushing's disease is often associated with severe mental disorders resembling the clinical picture of acute paranoid schizophrenia, even associated with electroencephalographic changes of all epileptiform nature. We have observed a case in whom the electroencephalogram returned to normal after pituitary tumor ablation.

Gonadal steroid hormone effects upon the central nervous system are now well established. Steroid anesthesia is widely used in clinical practice. More interesting are the recent observations that oversecretion of prolactin hormone in a patient harboring a pituitary tumor is associated with sexual disorders. In the male, loss of libido, sexual impotency, and azoospermia are encountered with prolactine tumors. In the female, sterility, amenorrhea-galactorrhea, and sexual frigidity are also produced by an elevated prolactin level. In the past, these symptoms were thought to be related to hormonal insufficiency resulting from a large "chromophobe" adenoma; however, our personal experience in the treatment of microadenomas demonstrates that these symptoms are caused by oversecretion of prolactin, since they are reversible after the prolactin pituitary tumor is removed (18).

The only hormone that does not seem to influence the brain is growth hormone. For instance, the absence of growth hormone does not affect the brain development in contrast to that of most other organs. In human subjects, an excess of growth hormone secretion which produces gigantism and acromegaly is not associated with mental or behavioral disorders.

We can only summarize this briefly, but there are objective data supporting the interaction between hormonal and neural mechanism. On one hand, hormones exert a direct influence on nervous process at the basis of behavioral reactions. On the other hand, neural circuits are controlling the secretions of anterior pituitary hormones, which finally control the entire hormonal secretions of the organism.

The classical concept that the final common pathway of neuroendocrine mechanism is located in the hypothalamo-hypophyseal tract will probably be revised in the future. It may only be a link to a reflex arch, but at least, it will remain the major relay circuit between neural activity of the brain and hormone secretion. The brain and the pituitary are two important organs and are closely related on the anatomical and functional basis.

Fundamental events of the human life are assured by the hormonal secretions of the pituitary: birth, growth, sexual activity, reproduction, lactation, body comfort, and the aging process are basically the major functions of the hypophysis. Neural activities of the brain appear to have an essential role for controlling the quality of these functions in providing the basic structures for motivation, driving appetite for food, and search for emotional satisfaction as well as the integration of the environmental influence.

FUNCTIONAL HYPOPHYSECTOMY

Functional hypophysectomy is essentially the removal of the normal pituitary gland. Historically, the first hypophysectomy was performed in France in 1934 by Puech (7), in a patient with severe juvenile diabetes. Puech was going on the basis of the Houssay phenomenon on the diabetogenic role of pituitary hormones. Following the extensive works of Huggins (24), who demonstrated the hormonal dependency of certain cancers of the breast and prostate, hypophysectomy was introduced in the human subject during the 1950s (34,45). After several years of empiricism, there remain only two clinical indications for which the therapeutic value of hypophysectomy has been eventually confirmed in advanced metastatic cancer of the breast and prostate, and in the prevention of blindness in progressive diabetic retinopathy.

Despite the obvious clinical results, the pathophysiological mechanism of the effects produced by hypophysectomy in the human is not yet completely understood; however, recent progress in endocrinology and experimental biological correlations have promoted certain explanations. In a recent publication (19), we have reported complete pain sedation following hypophysectomy in 92% of patients suffering from bony metastases of breast carcinoma. Other effects have been encountered in a large proportion of patients who have experienced a sudden arrest of the rapid flare-up of generalized cancerous process, objective regression of metastases, and improvement of the general condition. The striking effect of functional hypophysectomy in relieving pain from bony metastases supports the major indications for pain relief in endocrine-dependent cancer of the breast and prostate (39). The mechanism of pain relief following pituitary ablation is still a matter of controversy. In the past, the intracranial approach requiring the surgical injury and division of the pituitary stalk would have supported a neurohumoral mechanism from the hypothalamus; however, our experience in performing microsurgical selective adenohypophysectomy by the transsphenoidal approach has confirmed the major role of anterior pituitary hormones. It would appear that the sedation of osseous pain is related to the sudden suppression of growth hormone, since it has been shown that infusion of growth hormone in hypophysectomized patients reproduces the bone pain temporarily (38). Its algogenic function is also evoked clinically in adolescents who have a rapid growth and suffer from vertebral pain, the so-called "growth pain" and also, in acromegalic patients with severe arthrosic pains; these pains are suppressed immediately following the removal of the growth hormone oversecreting adenoma (21).

On the other hand, recent literature tends to emphasize the role of prolactin. It is known (30) that serum prolactin levels can be suppressed by L-DOPA, giving satisfactory pain relief for a short period of time during the action of the L-DOPA; however, both growth hormone and prolactin have a short half-life of approximately 30 minutes. This should be correlated with the fact that patients are usually relieved immediately following surgical total pituitary ablation. Finally, the recent discovery of morphine-like substances (called enkephalin and endomorphin) from the pituitary gland may contribute to the understanding of the mechanism of pain relief (25).

On the long-term effects of hypophysectomy in cancer, it is most probable that the objective results are dependent on the complete suppression of gonadotropins and even more so of prolactin, since the action of these hormones in the experimental production of breast cancer in mice has been demonstrated (53).

Similarly, the growth hormone responsible for skeletal growth until adulthood could be involved in the process of cellular growth in young neoplastic tissues. In diabetes mellitus accompanied with retinopathy, improvement of visual function associated with retinal changes following hypophysectomy could also depend upon the suppression of the diabetic hormone, a biochemical substance closely related to the growth hormone, although not necessarily with the same molecular structure. A recent report (51) has shown that selective blockage of growth hormone cells by gamma irradiation of the pituitary is the important mechanism for ocular response in the treatment of diabetic retinopathy.

The effect on diabetes mellitus is constant: following hypophysectomy, hyperglycemia is normalized and in all cases the insulin requirement is markedly reduced, even completely suppressed in some patients. The lipotropic hormone, although not yet isolated in the human subject, can be involved as well, since the normalization of hypertriglyceridemia is observed in diabetic patients following hypophysectomy (20).

FUNCTIONAL SURGERY OF OVERSECRETING PITUITARY DISORDERS

The etiology of pituitary oversecreting disorders has always been a challenge. Because of close dependence of the pituitary from the hypothalamus, which is the "neural center" of neuroendocrine functions, the pathogenesis of hyperpituitarism was for many years attributed to hypertrophy or diffuse hyperplasia of the pituitary cells secondary to a primary hypothalamic disturbance of the so-called controlling or "releasing factors."

In this regard, the brilliant work of two major groups must be cited: that of Andrew Schally from New Orleans and that of Roger Guillemin from California, both of whom have worked with unremitting intensity for almost 2 decades to identify the chemical nature of the hypophysiotropic hormones. Their findings leave no doubt about the major role of these hypothalamic humoral substances in the physiological control of the pituitary gland secretion; however, when dealing with practical therapeutic endeavor in the treatment of diseases in human subjects, a major gap persisted for a long time. For instance, the hypothesis of diffuse hyperplasia or adenomatous formation of the whole pituitary gland was mainly supported by the fact that some patients had no radiological enlargement of the sella turcica to evidence a pituitary adenoma. In the others, when there were radiological signs of an expanding lesion in the sella, the clinical syndrome was attributed to a pituitary adenoma.

The controversy between the two etiological factors, whether primary hypothalamic disturbance or primary endogenous pituitary adenoma, has maintained a confusion for many years in the literature. This has been so to such an extent that, for example, acromegaly was divided into two groups, patients suffering from acromegaly disease without a tumor or from acromegaly with a pituitary tumor (10). From the therapeutic point of view, this confusion is even more striking in a monograph entitled "Stereotaxic Surgery of the Non Tumoral Hypophysis by Radioisotopes" (54), in which is included the treatment of Cushing's disease and acromegaly.

In patients harboring an obvious radiologically enlarged sella turcica to evidence a pituitary tumor, the therapeutic purpose was the treatment of a functional disorder associated with a tumoral process. In other patients with radiologically normal sella turcica, functional systemic disease may have been related to a possible functional disorder of the hypothalamic-pituitary axis without evidence of an organic lesion.

In the meantime, considerable progress in the field of transsphenoidal pituitary surgery with the development of microsurgical procedure (14–16) has allowed us to identify within a normal-sized pituitary gland a well-circumscribed nodule localized in a specific area of the gland (17). These early detected pituitary lesions have been termed *microadenomas* when they were smaller than 10 mm in diameter, which is the lower limit of normal dimension of the pituitary gland. With the use of magnification, good illumination, and microsurgical technique of dissection, these tiny intrapituitary lesions have been selectively removed while preserving the remaining normal secreting pituitary tissue (Fig. 3). The finding of these obvious organic lesions, although minimal in size, has kept open the controversy between functional and organic surgery.

In other fields of neurosurgery, pathological findings have often demonstrated

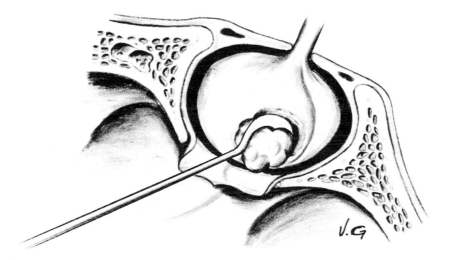

FIG. 3. Illustration of transsphenoidal microsurgical selective microadenomectomy. (From ref. 17*a*.)

an organic lesion at the basis of a functional disorder. For example, treatment of epilepsy by temporal lobe removal appeared to be a true functional surgical procedure; however, the high incidence of the finding of incisural sclerosis by Penfield and Jasper (40) and the finding of small tumors in the amygdala by Falconer (8) provide an organic basis of a pathological process at the origin of a functional disorder; however, the lesion itself is not the primary cause of neuronal overactivity. Hughlings Jackson (26) clearly stated that it is the surrounding injured or suffering nervous tissue which is delivering abnormal electrical discharges that is responsible for epilepsy. The same is true nowadays in the treatment of the so-called "idiopathic" or essential trigeminal neuralgia, facial hemispasm, and other dysfunction of the cranial nerves in which an organic cause has been found with microsurgical exploration (3,4,27,28,44). Thus, the boundary between functional and organic surgery is rather arbitrary.

In the field of pituitary surgery, there is an obvious overlapping between functional and organic disease. Oversecreting pituitary disorders appear to serve as the best example for reunification of both disciplines. On the one hand, the major endocrine disturbance producing systemic disorders is a result of an oversecretion of hormones (ACTH, prolactin, growth hormone). The final aim of treatment is the normalization of the oversecretion by any means; however, in our experience, this oversecretion has always been produced by a localized pool of cells that have also acquired a functional disorder of their own reproductive function, resulting in the growing of a neoplastic benign lesion. Both secretion and cellular multiplication are functions of pituitary cells. Since the oversecreting disorder is caused by a functional tumor, surgical treatment is, therefore, a functional therapeutic approach.

Moreover, these technical developments in microsurgery have permitted such refinements that it is now possible clearly to distinguish between contiguous tissues which are otherwise histologically different (16). This has opened the field of histological functional microsurgery. As the result of considerable acquired experience, new therapeutic concepts in oversecreting pituitary disorders and better knowledge about their pathophysiology have been brought about. The most interesting progress in the past several years was obtained in the treatment of acromegaly-gigantism, Cushing's disease, and galactorrhea-amenorrhea syndrome. Detailed reports on these subjects are published separately elsewhere (17,18,21–23).

The functional approach to the treatment of neuroendocrine disorders has led to new concepts about the etiology of oversecreting pituitary disorders. In the past, the hypothesis that oversecreting pituitary lesions originate from a primary hypothalamic disturbance of the releasing factors resulting in hyperplasia of pituitary cells and eventually to a tumor formation has been supported for a long time on the basis of nonautonomous behavior of pituitary hormone secretion in oversecreting tumors. On the contrary, our experience with the selective adenomectomy has led us to propose the alternative hypothesis that a feed-back mechanism from primary elevated pituitary hormones is modulating the hypothalamic factors controlling the various patterns of normal secretions of the pituitary. After total selective removal of an oversecreting adenoma, a complete clinical and biological cure can be obtained in acromegaly, Cushing's disease, and galactorrhea-amenorrhea syndromes. The final evidence is the restoration of normal diurnal variations of growth hormone, ACTH, and prolactin now and thereafter under the normal physiological control of hypothalamic hormones.

In conclusion, there is so far no evidence in humans to support the hypothesis of primary hypothalamic disturbance at the origin of pituitary oversecreting tumors. Our original hypothesis postulated 10 years ago (43) that the oversecreting pituitary diseases are due to a primary pituitary adenoma or microadenoma has been confimed. In the treatment of hyperpituitarism, the ideal goal of restoring a state of eupituitarism can now be obtained by transsphenoidal microsurgery.

REFERENCES

1. Baker, B. L. (1974): Endocrinology. In: *Handbook of Physiology*, edited by R. O. Greep and E. B. Astwood p. 45. American Physiological Society. Williams & Wilkins, Baltimore, Maryland.
2. Bergland, R. M., Davis, S. L., and Page, R. B. (1977): Pituitary secretes to brain: Experiments in sheep. *Lancet*, 2:276–278.
3. Bertrand, R. A., Molina, P., and Hardy, J. (1977): Surgical Treatment of Hemi-Facial Spasm. *Facial Nerve Surgery*, edited by V. Fisch, pp. 512–520. Kugler Medical Publications, Amsterdam.
4. Bertrand, R. A., Molina, P., and Hardy, J. (1977): Vestibular syndrome and vascular anomaly in the cerebello-pontine angle. *Acta Otolaryngol. (Stockh.)*, 83:187–194.
5. Blackwell, R. E., and Guillemin, R. (1973): Hypothalamic control of adenohypophysial secretions. *Ann. Rev. Physiol.*, 35:357.
6. Brazeau, P., et al. (1973): Hypothalamic polypeptide that inhibits the secretion of immunoreactive pituitary growth hormone. *Science*, 179:77.
7. Chabanier, H., Puech, P., Lobo-Onell, C., and Lelu, E. (1936): Hypophyse et diabète. *Presse Méd.*, 44:986–989.
8. Falconer, M. A., and Cavanagh, J. B. (1959): Clinico-pathological considerations of temporal lobe epilepsy due to small focal lesions. *Brain*, 82:483–504.
9. Guillemin, R., Burgus, R., and Vale, W. (1971): The hypothalamic hypophysiotropic thyrotropin releasing factor. *Vitam. Horm.*, 29:1.
10. Guiot, G., Oproiu, A., Hertzog, E., and Fredy, D. (1969): Adénomes Hypophysaires. *Encyclopédie Médicochirurgicale*, Paris. 5:17–40.
11. Hardy, J. (1965): Electrophysiology of the Human Hypophysis. *Can. Med. Assoc. J.*, 92:866–867.
12. Hardy, J. (1966): Activité Electrique de la Neuro-hypophyse Humaine. *Union Med. Can.*, 95:586–592.
13. Hardy, J. (1966): Microelectrode recording of electrical activity in the human hypophysis. *Can. Med. Assos. J.*, 94:665.
14. Hardy, J. (1969): Microsurgery of the Hypophysis: Subnasal transsphenoidal approach with television magnification and televised radiofluoroscopic control. In: *Microneurosurgery*, edited by R. W. Rand, pp. 87–103. C. V. Mosby.
15. Hardy, J. (1969): Trans-nasal, transsphenoidal approach to the pituitary gland. In: *Microsurgery as Applied to Neurosurgery*, edited by M. G. Yasargil, pp. 180–194. Thieme Varlag Co., Germany.
16. Hardy, J. (1969): Transsphenoidal microsurgery of the normal and pathological pituitary. In: Clinical Neurosurgery, Vol. 16, pp. 185–217. Waverly Press, Baltimore, Maryland.
17. Hardy, J. (1973): Transsphenoidal surgery of hypersecreting pituitary tumors. In: *Diagnosis and Treatment of Pituitary Tumors*. Proceedings of a Conference held in Bethesda, Maryland. *Excerpta Med.*, pp. 179–194.

17a. Hardy, J. (1975): *Transsphenoidal Operation on the Pituitary.* Codman & Shurtleff, Inc., Signature series.
18. Hardy, J. Beauregard, H., and Robert, F. (1978): Prolactin-secreting pituitary adenomas: Transsphenoidal microsurgical treatment. In: Progress in Prolactin Physiology and Pathology, edited by C. Robin and M. Harter, pp. 361–370. Elsevier/North Holland, Amsterdam.
19. Hardy, J. Grisoli, F., Leclercq, T. A., and Somma, M. (1975): Le Traitement du Cancer du Sein Métastatique par l'Hypophysectomie Transsphénoïdale: Expérience de 160 cas. *Union Med. Can.,* 104:1557–1562.
20. Hardy, J., Panisset, A., Marchildon, A., and Lanthier, A. (1969): Microsurgical selective anterior pituitary ablation for diabetic retinopathy. *Can. Med. Assos. J.,* 100:785–792.
21. Hardy, J., Robert, F., Somma, M., and Vezina, J. L. (1973): Acromégalie-Gigantisme: Traitement chirurgical par exérèse transsphénoïdale de l'adénome hypophysaire. *Neurochirurgie,* 19 (Suppl. 2):184.
22. Hardy, J., Somma, M., and Vezina, J. L. (1976): Treatment of Acromegaly: Radiation or surgery? In: *Current Controversies in Neurosurgery,* edited by J. P. Morley, pp. 377–391. W. B. Saunders, Co., Philadelphia, Pennsylvania.
23. Hardy, J., and Vezina, J. L. (1976): Transsphenoidal neurosurgery of intracranial neoplasm. *Adv. Neurol.,* 15:261–274.
24. Huggins, C. (1942): Effect of orchidectomy and irradiation on cancer of the prostate. *Ann. Surg.,* 115:1192–1200.
25. Hughes, J., Smith, T. W., and Kosterlitz, H. W., et al. (1975): Identification of two related pentapeptides from the brain with potent opiate agonist activity. *Nature,* 258:577.
26. Jackson, J. H. (1931): *Selected Writings of John Hughlings Jackson,* Vol. 1. On Epilepsy and Epileptiform Convulsions, edited by J. Taylor. Hodder & Stoughton, London. 500 pp.
27. Jannetta, P. J. (1970): *Microsurgical Exploration and Decompression of the Facial Nerve in Hemifacial Spasm: Current Topics in Surgical Research,* Vol. 2, pp. 217–220. Academic Press, New York.
28. Jannetta, P. J., and Rand, R. W. (1967): Arterial compression of the trigeminal nerve in patients with trigeminal neuralgia. *J. Neurosurg.* (suppl.), 26:159–162.
29. Kandel, E. R. (1964): Electrical properties of hypothalamic neuroendocrine cells. *J. Gen. Physiol.,* 47:691–717.
30. Kleinberg, E. L., Noel, G. S., and Frantz, S. G. (1971): Chlorpromazine stimulation and levodopa suppression of plasma prolactin in man. *J. Clin. Endocrinol. Metab.,* 33:873.
31. Koisumi, K., Ishikawa, T., and McBrooks, C. (1964): Control of activity of neurons in the supra-optic nucleus. *J. Neurophysiol.,* 27:878–892.
32. Leclercq, T. A., Grisoli, F., and Hardy, J. (1974): Blood Supply of the Human Pituitary. Presentation at the Congress of Neurological Surgeons, Vancouver, British Columbia, Canada.
33. Leznoff, A., Fishman, J., Talbot, M., et al. (1962): Localization of ACTH in the human pituitary. *J. Clin. Invest.,* 41:1720–1724.
34. Luft, R., and Olivecrona, H. (1953): Experiences with hypophysectomy in man. *J. Neurosurg.,* 10:301–316.
35. Martin, J. B. Reichlin, S., and Brown, G. M. (1977): Effects of Hormones on the Brain. In: *Clinical Neuroendocrinology,* Vol. 14, pp. 275–303. Waverly Press, Baltimore, Maryland.
36. Page, R. B., and Bergland, R. M. (1977): The Neurohypophyseal capillary bed: Anatomy and arterial supply. *Am. J. Anat.,* 148:345–358.
37. Page, R. B., and Bergland, R. M. (1977): *Pituitary Vasculature,* pp. 9–17. Academic Press, New York.
38. Pearson, O. H., and Ray, B. S. (1958): Physiological effects of adrenalectomy and hypophysectomy. In: *Endocrine Aspects of Breast Cancer,* pp. 90–94. Livingston, Edinburg, Scotland.
39. Pearson, O. H., and Ray, B. S. (1959): Results of hypophysectomy in the treatment of metastatic mammary carcinoma. *Cancer,* 12:85–92.
40. Penfield, W., and Jasper, H. (1954): Temporal lobe and incisural sclerosis. In: *Epilepsy and the Functional Anatomy of the Human Brain,* p. 333. Little, Brown and Company, Boston.
41. Phifer, R. F., Orth, D. N., and Spicer, S. S. (1974): Specific demonstration of the human hypophyseal adrenocorticomelanotropic (ACTH/MSH) cell. *J. Clin. Endocrinol. Metab.,* 39:684–692.
42. Phifer, R. F., Spicer, S. S., and Orth, D. N. (1970): Specific demonstration of the human hypophyseal cells which produce adrenocorticotrophic hormone. *J. Clin. Endocrinol. Metab.,* 31:347–361.

43. Potter, D. D., and Lowenstein, W. R. (1955): Electrical activity of neurosecretory cells. *Am. J. Physiol.,* 183:652.
44. Provost, J., and Hardy, J. (1970): Microchirurgie du Trijumeau: Anatomie Fonctionnelle. *Neurochirurgie,* 16:459.
45. Ray, B. S., and Pearson, O. H. (1956): Hypophysectomy in the treatment of advanced cancer of the breast. *Ann. Surg.,* 144:394–403.
46. Robert, F. (1973): L'adénome hypophysaire dans l'acromégalie gigantisme. *Neurochirurgie,* 19(Suppl. 2):117–162.
47. Robert, F., and Hardy, J. (1975): Prolactin-secreting adenomas: A light and electron microscopical study. *Arch. Pathol.,* 99:625–633.
48. Robert, F., Pelletier, G., and Hardy, J. (1977): Pituitary adenomas in Cushing's disease: A histologic, ultrastructural and immunocytochemical study, *Arch. Pathol. Lab. Med.,* 102:448–455.
49. Schally, A. V., Arimura, A., and Kastin, A. J. (1973): Hypothalamic regulatory hormones. *Science,* 169–341.
50. Schally, A. V., Arimura, A., Kastin, A. J., Matsuo, H., Redding, T., Nair, R. M. G., and Debeljuk, L. (1971): Gonadotrophin releasing hormone: One polypeptide regulates secretion of luteinizing and follicle-stimulation hormones. *Science,* 173:1036–1038.
51. Schaub, C., Szikla, G., Drouin, P., Bluet-Pajot, M. T., Mejean, L., Debry, G., and Talairach, J. (1977): Interstitial gamma irradiation by ^{198}Au of the pituitary in diabetic retinopathy. *J. Neurosurg.,* 46:703–716.
52. Siggs, E. B., and Shapiro, T. D. (1961): Evoked and spontaneous potentials in the pituitary gland. *Physiologist,* 4:110.
53. Smithline, F., Sherman, L., and Kolodny, H. D. (1975): Prolactin and breast carcinoma: Medical progress. *N. Engl. J. Med.,* 784–792.
54. Talairach, J., Sedan, R., et al. (1966): La Chirurgie Stéréo-taxique de l'Hypophyse non Tumorale par les Radio-isotopes. *Neurochirurgie,* 2:302.
55. Xuereb, G. P., Prichard, M. M. L., and Daniel, P. M. (1954): Arterial supply and venous drainage of human hypophysis cerebri. *Q. J. Exp. Physiol.,* 39:199.

Functional Neurosurgery, edited by T. Rasmussen
and R. Marino. Raven Press, New York © 1979.

Advances in Psychiatric Surgery

H. Thomas Ballantine, Jr., and Ida E. Giriunas

*Department of Surgery (Neurosurgery), Harvard Medical School, and the Neurosurgical
Service, Massachusetts General Hospital, Boston, Massachusetts 02114*

The history of the development and progress of psychiatric surgery is fascinating but also, at times, disheartening. Since the first paper on the subject by
Egas Moniz in 1936 (13), the treatment of psychiatrically disabled persons by
neurosurgical intervention has been the subject of high praise at one time and
of bitter criticism at another. For example, in 1949 Moniz received a Nobel
Prize for his introduction of prefrontal leukotomy. Twenty-four years later,
the legislature of the state of Oregon, bowing to pressure from political extremists,
passed "psychosurgical legislation" so restrictive that psychiatrists and neurosurgeons in Oregon have virtually abandoned modern psychiatric surgery.

Recent scientific and (in the United States) sociopolitical developments have,
however, provided guidelines for the practice and use of psychiatric surgery
which have attracted the attention of thoughtful psychiatrists, psychologists,
and neurosurgeons. It would seem appropriate at this time, therefore, to reflect
upon the past, present, and future of this specialized form of functional neurosurgery.

THE EVOLUTION OF PSYCHIATRIC SURGERY

The development of neurosurgical procedures for the treatment of psychiatric
patients can be roughly separated into four overlapping stages since the first
publication on the subject by Moniz and Lima:

1. Radical frontal leukotomy
2. Restricted frontal leukotomy, including orbital undercutting
3. Cingulectomy
4. Stereotactic procedures, including:
   a. Inferomedial leukotomy
   b. Subcaudate tractotomy
   c. Cingulotomy
   d. Amygdalotomy
   e. Thalamotomy
   f. Hypothalamotomy
   g. Multitarget procedures (amygdalotomy, cingulotomy, zona innominata)

Departures from the original radical operation of Moniz and Lima have been the result of a continuing search for a safer, more effective, and simpler procedure. It should be remembered, however, that these radical leukotomies were not without success.

A little-known but most important evaluation of this type of surgery for psychiatric illness was initiated in 1950 by Jenkins and Holsopple in six U.S. Veterans Administration Hospitals (1). The clinical material of the authors consisted of 373 patients, all but 12 of whom had been diagnosed as schizophrenic. The patients were divided into two groups, consisting of 185 patients who were controls and 188 patients who were subjected to the following operations:

1. Radical frontal leukotomy (140 patients)
2. Bimedial frontal leukotomy (26 patients)
3. Orbital gyrus undercutting (13 patients)
4. Transorbital leukotomy (9 patients)

Four years after their operations, 17.8% of the 140 patients with the standard radical operation had been discharged from the hospital in contrast to 9.7% of the controls. Of the 26 patients who had undergone the bimedial operation, 23% had been discharged.

The treatment of the affective psychoses was even more successful. In general, it had been shown that at least 60% of patients suffering from disabling disorders of affect were improved by this procedure. Unfortunately, however, the operation caused neurological and psychiatric complications and carried a small but distressing mortality rate. As a result, this operation has been abandoned.

The original operation of Moniz transected the central core of white matter just anterior to the anterior horns of both lateral ventricles. This approach was modified by Freeman and Watts, who sectioned the inferior portions of both frontal lobes about the level of the tragus. These procedures were "blind" in that the surgeon could not see the tissue being transected. Lyerly (11) subsequently transected the same fibers under direct vision. Later Poppen (14) devised a technique of bimedial leukotomy from a superior frontal approach.

In 1948, Scoville (16) further restricted the frontal lobe operation by interrupting under direct vision only the fibers in the orbital gyri, which he calls "orbital undercutting." At about the same time Geoffrey Knight (9), in England, began to use this surgical approach.

Knight concluded from his experience that the maximum effect of orbital undercutting was produced when the path of transection included the last 2 cm of the subcaudate region of the orbital gyrus. He began in 1960, therefore, to place radioactive yttrium seeds in this tissue under stereotactic control.

In 1947, the distinguished Yale physiologist, John Fulton, suggested the operation of cingulectomy, and about a year later Sir Hugh Cairns at Oxford and Professor Jacques LeBeau undertook the procedure. The results in 52 patients operated upon by Cairns were reported in 1961 by Lewin (10). Twenty-one of 26 patients suffering from intractable affective illnesses demonstrated "significant improvement" 1 to 11 years after the operation, which consisted of removing by suction, under direct vision, the anterior 4 cm of both cingulate gyri. This rather formidable surgical exercise has been largely replaced by the stereotactic approach.

Anterior stereotactic cingulotomy was introduced in 1962 by Foltz and White (8), whose report led me to use this technique at the Massachusetts General Hospital in 1962 for the alleviation of intractable psychiatric illness and pain. Our first 5 years of experience was recorded in 1967 (2), and I am much indebted to my colleague Raul Marino for his invaluable assistance in the preparation of that report.

In 1968, Brown and Lighthill recorded their experiences with stereotactic "anterior selective cingulotomy" (6). As early as 1949, Spiegel and Wycis reported the results of stereotactic thalamotomy for the treatment of psychiatric illness (20). Since that date, there have been many publications dealing with the effects of amygdalotomy, thalamotomy, and hypothalamotomy on a variety of psychiatric disorders. Most of these operations have been performed on patients whose uncontrollable violence was a major symptom of their psychiatric illness. More recently, combined operations have been performed by Richardson in London (12) and M. Hunter Brown in California (7).

In this brief and incomplete review, I have attempted to emphasize the progress of psychiatric surgery from its relatively crude beginnings to a point today where all surgeons use precise, limited, operative approaches and most of them perform their procedures under stereotactic control.

SELECTION OF PATIENTS

The selection of patients for psychiatric surgery is still a matter of some debate because of the lack of uniformity in diagnostic classification. For example, disorders diagnosed by American psychiatrists as "paranoid schizophrenia" or "schizoaffective" illness might well be classified as examples of severe manic-depressive psychosis by their British colleagues.

It is generally agreed, however, that individuals disabled by disorders of affect such as depression, anxiety, anorexia nervosa, obsessive-compulsive neurosis, and phobias are most likely to benefit by psychiatric surgery, whereas patients suffering from pure cognitive disorders of early onset, long duration, and diagnosed as "schizophrenic" are not. There are, however, patients with combinations of disorders of affect and cognition; therefore, if an individual is disabled by a psychiatric illness in which emotional suffering is a major symptom that has not responded to vigorous nonoperative treatment, psychiatric surgery should be seriously considered.

THE RESULTS OF MODERN SURGICAL PROCEDURES

The only "open" operations currently performed with any frequency are bimedial leukotomy and orbital undercutting. Most psychiatric surgery today is of the "closed" stereotactic type, usually subcaudate tractotomy, anterior cingulotomy, or "multiple-target" procedures. Bimedial leukotomy under direct vision can be expected to produce significant improvement in 70 to 85% of patients suffering from disorders of affect. This procedure does, however, carry a significant risk of psychiatric complications. Post and Schurr (15) have reported, for example, that in a series of 64 patients, there were side effects which were felt to be undesirable by the patients and their relatives in 21% of the cases and to be serious in 8%. This complication rate has led these authors to turn more often to stereotactic procedures.

Orbital undercutting, originally performed by both Scoville and Knight about 30 years ago, is probably the first clear departure from frontal leukotomy. In 1975, Scoville (16) presented the results of this procedure in 109 patients. Seventy-six percent of the patients had "good to excellent outcomes"; 15 of 17 patients (88%) with depression and 30 of 36 (83%) with obsessive-compulsive neurosis achieved excellent to good postoperative states. Complications included a 4% mortality rate; 13% of the survivors had one or more seizures; and "there were two blood clots and one minor 'stroke' which subsided in a matter of days. . . ." "Temporary mental changes of apathy and lethargy occurred and lasted for one to three months. Irritability and hostility lasted for one month, and certain patients experienced a transitory stage of over-talkativeness."

Stereotactic subcaudate tractotomy as a substitute for orbital undercutting was initiated by Knight in 1960. One of the stimuli that prompted this change was the report by Sykes and Tredgold (18) that, in Knight's hands, orbital undercutting carried a 16% risk of postoperative epilepsy, a 5% risk of undesirable personality change, and a 1.5% mortality rate.

According to Knight (9), his stereotactic procedure aims to create, by the insertion of radioactive yttrium, small bilateral lesions at a "site of convergence . . . which will exert widespread effects on connexions of the agranular cortex and projections to the substantia innominata." The coordinates for the center of this target are given by his co-workers, Bartlett and Bridges, as a point 15 mm lateral to the midline, 5 mm rostral to the anterior limit of the third ventricle, and 11 mm superior to the orbital plate (4).

In 1972, Knight (9) reported a series of 580 cases of subcaudate tractotomy. There was one death resulting from a placement error, and the incidence of postoperative epilepsy was less than 1%. A review by Strom-Olsen and Carlisle (17) of 210 of the patients in this series showed that there were no adverse effects on personality in 86%, an insignificant adverse change in 11.4%, and moderate change in 2.6%. There were no adverse effects that were disabling. Over 70% of patients with depression showed satisfactory postoperative improvement, and only one of the 210 patients was classified as "worse" postoperatively. By 1975, the series had been enlarged to include over 700 patients.

At this point, I should like to consider stereotactic anterior cingulotomy, which has not only stood the test of time but has been evaluated by a number of clinical investigators. The most comprehensive review of this operation occurred in 1972 at a Symposium on Cingulotomy held in Philadelphia, the proceedings of which were, unfortunately, never published. Nevertheless, according to my records of the meeting, seven participants reported a total of 683 stereotactic cingulotomies. Complications numbered three: one death and two incidences of hemiplegia. There was no mention of postoperative psychiatric deterioration. Satisfactory improvement was reported in 70 to 90% of patients suffering from diabling disorders of affect. Symptoms most often favorably affected were those of depression and anxiety, obsessive-compulsive neurosis, and anorexia nervosa. In general, the techniques are those described by Ballantine (2): The cingulate bundle is interrupted bilaterally at loci ranging from 1 to 4 cm posterior to the anterior tips of the lateral ventricles.

Our own experience at the Massachusetts General Hospital was most recently reported in detail at the Fourth World Congress of Psychiatric Surgery in 1975 and published in 1977 (3). We found that 75% of 154 patients with disabling affective disorders showed satisfactory improvement after bilateral stereotactic anterior cingulotomy. There were no serious surgical, neurological, or psychiatric complications.

COMBINED PROCEDURES

Cox and Brown reported in 1975 [with publication in 1977 (7)] the results in 66 patients of "six target limbic surgery," i.e., placing bilateral lesions in the cingulum, amygdala, and zona innominata. These operations were performed in California by Hunter Brown, and the patients were evaluated by A. W. Cox, Associate Professor of Psychiatry, Tulane University School of Medicine.

The series consisted of 32 schizophrenic patients and 19 "violent-aggressive" individuals who had multitarget surgery as the initial procedure. In 15 other patients in whom cingulotomy had failed, additional lesions were placed in the amygdala and zona innominata. Statistically significant improvement was noted in all three groups, although it was somewhat less impressive in the 19 violent-aggressive patients.

A recent publication by Mitchell-Heggs, Kelly, and Richardson (12) records their experiences with multitarget lesions in the cingulum, lower medial quadrants of the frontal lobes, and (occasionally) in the genu of the corpus callosum. They report an overall improvement in 76% of their patients. Most striking is their statement that favorable results were obtained in 89% of patients suffering from obsessional neurosis and in over 80% of "the small number of schizophrenics treated."

THE SOCIOPOLITICAL PROBLEMS OF PSYCHIATRIC SURGERY

Since its first introduction as a form of therapy, psychiatric surgery has been under scrutiny and criticism from the scientific and medical communities, but it is only in the last 10 years that the general public and the politicians in the United States and elsewhere have become involved in attempting to assess the effectiveness and appropriateness of these operations.

It has been alleged (despite the evidence presented earlier in this chapter) that reliable information on cost/benefit and outcomes from psychiatric surgery is substantially lacking. Moreover, it has been proposed that surgery for psychiatric illness could easily be used as a form of "social control" of minority groups and for other political purposes. So great has been the influence of certain radical, vocal, and misguided groups that in one American state (Oregon) and one country (Japan) it has become all but impossible to perform these operations.

In response to the public concern in America over psychiatric surgery and certain other medical research and therapeutic endeavors, the United States Congress created in 1974 a National Commission for the Protection of Human Subjects of Biomedical and Behavioral Research. On May 23, 1977, the report of the Commission concerning the "Use of Psychosurgery in Practice and Research: Report and Recommendations for Public Comment" was published in the United States Federal Register. In summary, the Commission recommended that "psychosurgery be used only to meet the health needs of individual patients and then only under strict limitations and controls, with added safeguards when the patient is a prisoner, a minor, or in a mental institution."

The recommendations were based primarily upon three investigations which were independent of one another and were performed by investigators not associated with the practice of psychiatric surgery.

At Boston University, a team headed by two neuropsychologists, Allan F. Mirsky and Maressa H. Orzack, evaluated 27 patients subjected to the following operations: orbital undercutting in eight patients, bilateral cingulate lesions in seven patients (sometimes in association with additional lesions placed in the amygdala and/or substantia innominata), ultrasonic prefrontal lesions (10 patients), and anterior prefrontal leukotomy (2 patients).

Mirsky and Orzack reported that 78% of the 27 patients studied were significantly improved and that depression was the symptom most favorably affected. There were two cases that were considered worse postoperatively. Although difficult to assess with precision because of the retrospective nature of the study, they concluded that there was no evidence of significant cognitive deficit attributable to the surgery. They did find a cognitive loss (lowered performance of the Wisconsin Card Sorting task) in those patients who were greatly improved by surgery, and speculated that this "loss" permitted the patients to "function in a more effective and less troubled way." Finally, those patients with favorable outcomes postoperatively had significantly higher scores on psychological testing than did a group of eight controls.

The Commission also provided for expansion of an ongoing study at Massachusetts Institute of Technology by two neuropsychologists, Professor Hans-Lukas Teuber and Suzanne Corkin, with the collaboration of a neurologist, Thomas Twitchell.

This group studied 34 patients operated upon by me at the Massachusetts General Hospital during the period 1962 to 1976: 18 of these had both preoperative and postoperative evaluation. A brief review of their findings is included in the Proceedings of the Fourth World Congress of Psychiatric Surgery (19).

Repeated analyses of data accumulated on these 34 patients failed to disclose any obvious "costs" of intervention. There were no new neurological deficits, no lasting effects on performance of 24 behavioral tasks. The patients were capable of appropriate depths in their feelings of pleasure and sadness, and patients operated upon for pain were still sensitive to new forms of noxious stimuli.

The benefits observed were significant therapeutic improvement in 80% of patients suffering from pain and depression, 75% of patients with depressive mood disorders, and 50% of patients with schizophrenic disorders. Significant improvements were found in the full scale verbal and performance I.Q. ratings; improvement in frontal lobe function (Wisconsin Card Sorting Test) in patients 40 years of age or younger (unchanged in patients over 40); and, finally a slight gain in employment status, postoperatively.

Also observed was a phenomenon reported by many others that pain patients obtained almost immediate relief postoperatively, whereas patients with depression or schizophrenia required several weeks or months and, in some cases, repeat operations to obtain relief.

Finally, the Commission contracted with Elliot Valenstein, a Professor of Psychology at the University of Michigan, to survey the recent literature on "psychosurgery." This survey revealed that 85% of patients afflicted with disorders of affect were reported as significantly improved following frontal lobe or cingulate surgery but that patients with "schizophrenia" had a lower success rate. He was critical of the scientific merit of most of these reports and expressed some skepticism concerning the reported lack of side-effects of psychiatric surgery. Nevertheless, he did state that "it is unlikely that many neurosurgeons would rate their results as excellent on the basis of elimination of troublesome behavior without considering other aspects of the patients' overall adjustment. It would take overt deceit, not self-deception to assign a rating of "excellent" to a patient who spends the days sitting passively and unresponsively at home even if no longer a burden to anyone."

These reports were the foundation for the Commission's statement that psychosurgery should be used to meet the health needs of an individual patient. The report also stated that "These studies appear to rebut any presumption that all forms of psychosurgery are unsafe and ineffective. . . . Because of this finding . . . the Commission has not recommended a ban on psychosurgery."

The Commission opined, nevertheless, that "The safety and efficacy of specific psychosurgical procedures for the treatment of particular disorders, however, have not been demonstrated to the degree that would permit such procedures to be considered 'accepted' practice." For this reason, and because of the possibility that psychosurgery might be misused, the Commission recommended for the present that psychosurgical procedures be performed only after review (such as generally precedes the conduct of research) by an IRB [Institutional Review Board] whose composition and procedures for review of psychosurgery have been approved by the Department of Health, Education, and Welfare.

Another important recommendation was that "The Secretary of the Department of HEW is encouraged to conduct and support studies to evaluate the safety of specific psychosurgical procedures and the efficacy of such procedures in relieving specific psychiatric symptoms and disorders. . . ."

THE FUTURE OF PSYCHIATRIC SURGERY

The report of the National Commission, cited above, should restore this type of functional neurosurgery to its previous state of respectability. At the same time, however, all workers in this field have been given added responsibilities; among them are the following:

1. To assess all patients carefully both before and after operation.
2. To describe the operative approach in such detail that it can be performed by other surgeons.
3. To follow patients postoperatively in order to evaluate the long-term results of such surgery.
4. To record in the scientific literature the results of surgical intervention.
5. To choose patients for operation in a manner that will allay any remaining doubts on the part of the public regarding the ethical issues of this form of treatment.

In the realm of clinical research, many questions remain to be answered, as, for example:

1. Is there a specificity of anatomical interruption that can be applied to a specific psychiatric disorder?
2. Are multiple lesions more effective for the treatment of certain psychiatric disorders?
3. What is the underlying reason for the therapeutic benefit of psychiatric surgery?

This third question is probably the most important, and it offers certain exciting opportunities to advance our understanding of psychiatric illness. Teuber, in his report to the Commission, made the following comment: "In attempting a physiologic interpretation of the beneficial effects of psychiatric surgery, one can only speculate that the therapeutic effects that were seen in this group, particularly in cases of persistent pain (whenever in excess of placebo effects), might be due to the induction of some change in chemically-specific pathways, possibly at some remove from the area directly approached."

In this regard, Bridges et al. (5) have recently reported a most important study. Their synopsis follows:

Tryptophan and 5-hydroxyindoleacetic acid (precursor and metabolite respectively of 5-hydroxy-tryptamine) were determined in ventricular CSF of psychiatric patients undergoing stereotactic subcaudate tractotomy. Tyrosine and homovanillic acid (precursor and metabolite respectively of dopamine) were also determined. Results suggest an association between affective state and the above precursor amino acids with lower concentrations in primary depression and higher ones when anxiety or agitation predominate. This leads to lower 5-hydroxyin-doleacetic acid concentrations in depression and higher concentrations in anxiety and agitation.

We have, with the collaboration of our colleagues at Massachusetts Institute of Technology, embarked on a similar attempt to determine whether there is a defect in serotonin metabolism in psychiatric patients. This effort is designed to lay the groundwork for testing the hypotheses that the major affective psychoses are, in fact, precipitated by neurotransmitter abnormalities; and that the beneficial effects of psychiatric surgery are a result of chemical changes induced by anatomical interruption.

Should these hypotheses be shown to be correct, our understanding of the nature of a group of psychiatric disorders that are responsible for major disability and premature death would be immensely enhanced.

SUMMARY

Surgery for psychiatric illness has been performed since 1935 for the alleviation of the torture of intractable, disabling psychiatric illness. The surgical approaches have progressed from radical and crude interventions to the placement of precise lesions at small sites usually within the limbic system; psychiatric and neurological complications are now rare. The risks and benefits of certain of these operations, particularly cingulotomy, subcaudate tractotomy, and bimedial leukotomy are sufficiently well known so that they no longer require their classification as "experimental" or "innovative."

Nevertheless, a substantial number of patients (15–30%) with disabling disorders of affect are not improved by psychiatric surgery. Moreover, we do not have a clear understanding of the reasons for our successes and failures.

We are still working our way through the darkness of ignorance, but careful evaluation by clinicians and neuroscientists of the effects of psychiatric surgery must inevitably lead to a better understanding of the nature of psychiatric illness and thus to better methods of treatment. Surgery for psychiatric illness stands at the threshold of an exciting era through which the advancement of knowledge and the alleviation of suffering can proceed together for the benefit of all mankind.

REFERENCES

1. Ball, J., Klett, G. J., and Gresock, C. J. (1959): The Veterans Administration study of prefrontal lobotomy. *J. Clin. Exp. Psychopathol. Q. Rev. Psychiatr. Neurol.*, 20:205–217.
2. Ballantine, H. T., Jr., Cassidy, W. L., Flanagan, N. B., and Marino, R., Jr. (1967): Stereotaxic anterior cingulotomy for neuropsychiatric illness and intractable pain. *J. Neurosurg.*, 26:488–495.

3. Ballantine, H. T., Jr., Levy, B. S., Dagi, T., and Giriunas, I. B. (1977): Cingulotomy for psychiatric illness: Report of 13 years experience. In: *Neurosurgical Treatment in Psychiatry, Pain, and Epilepsy,* edited by W. H. Sweet, S. Obrador, and J. G. Martin-Rodriguez, pp. 387–398. University Park Press, Maryland.
4. Bartlett, J. R., and Bridges, P. K. (1977): The extended subcaudate tractotomy lesion. In: *Neurosurgical Treatment in Psychiatry, Pain, and Epilepsy,* edited by W. H. Sweet, S. Obrador, and J. G. Martin-Rodriguez, pp. 387–398. University Park Press, Maryland.
5. Bridges, P. K., Bartlett, J. R., Sepping, P., Kantamaneni, B. D., and Curzon, G. (1976): Precursors and metabolites of 5-hydroxytryptamine and dopamine in the ventricular cerebrospinal fluid of psychiatric patients. *Psychol. Med.,* 6:399–405.
6. Brown, M. H., and Lighthill, J. A. (1968): Selective anterior cingulotomy: A psychosurgical evaluation. *J. Neurosurg.,* 29:513–519.
7. Cox, A. W., and Brown, M. H. (1977): Results of multi-target limbic surgery in the treatment of schizophrenia and aggressive states. In: *Neurosurgical Treatment in Psychiatry, Pain, and Epilepsy,* edited by W. H. Sweet, S. Obrador, and J. G. Martin-Rodriguez, pp. 469–479. University Park Press, Baltimore.
8. Foltz, E. L., and White, L. E. (1962): Pain "relief" by frontal cingulumotomy. *J. Neurosurg.,* 19:89–100.
9. Knight, G. (1972): Psychosurgery today. *Proc. R. Soc. Med.* 65:1099–1108.
10. Lewin, W. (1961): Observation on selective leucotomy. *J. Neurol. Neurosurg. Psychiatry,* 24:37–44.
11. Lyerly, J. G. (1939): Transection of the deep association fibers of the prefrontal lobes in certain mental disorders. *South. Surgeon,* 8:426–434.
12. Mitchell-Heggs, N., Kelly, D., and Richardson, A. (1976): Stereotactic limbic leucotomy: A follow-up at 16 months. *Br. J. Psychiatry,* 128:226–240.
13. Moniz, E. (1936): Essai d'un traitement chirurgical de certaines psychoses. *Bull. Acad. Med.,* 115:385–392.
14. Poppen, J. L. (1948): Technic of prefrontal lobotomy. *J. Neurosurg.,* 5:514–520.
15. Post, F., and Schurr, P. H. (1977): Changes in the pattern of diagnosis of patients subjected to psychosurgical procedures, with comments on their use in the treatment of self-mutilation and anorexia nervosa. In: *Neurosurgical Treatment in Psychiatry, Pain, and Epilepsy,* edited by W. H. Sweet, S. Obrador, and J. G. Martin-Rodriguez, pp. 261–266. University Park Press, Baltimore, Maryland.
16. Scoville, W. B., and Bettis, D. B. (1977): Results of orbital undercutting today: A personal series. In: *Neurosurgical Treatment in Psychiatry, Pain, and Epilepsy,* edited by W. H. Sweet, S. Obrador, and J. G. Martin-Rodriguez, pp. 189–202. University Park Press, Baltimore, Maryland.
17. Strom-Olsen, R., and Carlisle, S. (1971): Bi-frontal stereotactic tractotomy. *Br. J. Psychiatry,* 118:141–154.
18. Sykes, M. K., and Tredgold, R. F. (1964): Restricted orbital undercutting: A study of its effects on 350 patients over ten years 1951–1960. *Br. J. Psychiatry,* 110:609–640.
19. Teuber, H.-L., Corkin, S. H., and Twitchell, T. E. (1977): Study of cingulotomy in man: A summary. In: *Neurosurgical Treatment in Psychiatry, Pain, and Epilepsy,* edited by W. H. Sweet, S. Obrador, and J. G. Martin-Rodriguez, pp. 355–362. University Park Press, Baltimore, Maryland.
20. Wycis, H. T. (1972): The role of stereotaxic surgery in the compulsive state. In: *Psychosurgery,* edited by E. Hitchcock, L. Laitinen, and K. Vaernet, pp. 115–116. Charles C Thomas, Springfield, Illinois.

Functional Neurosurgery, edited by T. Rasmussen
and R. Marino. Raven Press, New York © 1979.

Psychological Assessment of Neurosurgical Patients

Laughlin B. Taylor

*Montreal Neurological Institute and Hospital, 3801 University Street,
Montreal, Quebec H3A 2B4, Canada*

For more than 20 years, the psychology laboratory at the Montreal Neurological Institute has played an essential role in the assessment of patients being considered for elective neurosurgery. During this time, we have been preoccupied with the examination of patients with intractable epilepsy; however, we have also examined patients with Parkinson's disease, dystonia, and other movement disorders, as well as an increasing number of patients with vascular anomalies or deficiencies of blood supply to the brain. By working closely with our neurosurgeons, we have been able to identify a number of psychological measures that have not only furthered our knowledge of brain function, but in addition have been of help to the surgeons in four principal ways:

1. Understanding the cerebral organization of the patient, particularly with regard to the complementary specialization of language and spatial skills of the dominant and nondominant cerebral hemispheres, respectively.
2. Diagnosis of the area of epileptic lesion and other areas of the brain where there is evidence of dysfunction or interference with function.
3. Identifying the risks of surgery to essential psychological functions such as speech, memory, and other less well-defined functions that are necessary for effective daily life.
4. Prognosis as to the success of the surgery in relieving symptoms associated with the disease process, and the patient's reactions to his postoperative status, where age, intelligence, variations of cognitive skills, emotional factors, and family and community relationships are all important.

Inevitably, in the application of our findings, it is the individual patient who concerns us. For each individual, the characteristic mild psychological deficits that are usually evident before surgery may be grossly apparent or not present and they may be exaggerated or relieved by surgery, but before we can look at such individual cases we must first briefly review our accumulated data on the psychological measures we have found useful in detecting anomalies of brain function [a more detailed review is available in Milner (21)]. At the same time, we shall have the opportunity to illustrate how we are able to explore the contributions made by discrete areas of the brain to functional systems.

GENERAL INTELLIGENCE

All our patients have their intelligence assessed before and after surgery, using the Wechsler intelligence scales. The principal reason for giving these tests is to obtain a reference point for the interpretation of other test data. Frequently, however, the general level of intelligence reflects the extent of damage to the brain, and the pattern of subtest scores serves as a useful indicator of specific psychological deficits or of diffuse pathological processes. Differences between the Verbal and Performance I.Q. ratings can be associated with damage to the dominant or nondominant cerebral hemisphere (14,15,28), but the effects of culture, education, and perhaps sex differences, as well as the representation of aspects of the same intellectual factor in both hemispheres, can complicate their interpretation. Nevertheless, these differences are important and are frequently the first clues to alert us to the possibility of atypical representation of speech.

The mean level of intelligence of our patients is in the high average range. Postoperative testing 2 weeks after a discrete cortical removal or thalamotomy usually shows a slight decline of the intelligence rating, but in follow-up testing there is a recovery from this loss, and for all our groups of epileptic patients, regardless of the side or site of lesion, the follow-up Full Scale I.Q. rating is higher than it was before surgery (21). The removal of the interfering epileptogenic process is, therefore, clearly beneficial as Narabayashi (Chapter 16, *this volume*) has also reported. Although there are many factors that can affect this recovery in individual cases, sometimes resulting in dramatic increases of intelligence levels, the one general exception to this finding is the slow recovery made by patients over the age of 40, particularly in the first postoperative year, if surgery in the posterior temporal area of the dominant hemisphere has resulted in an exacerbation of language and verbal memory deficits.

TEMPORAL LOBES

The functional specialization of the two cerebral hemispheres is apparent in the memory deficits found with lesions in the temporal lobes. Damage to the dominant, left, temporal lobe results in verbal memory deficits, whereas damage to the right temporal lobe results in impairment of nonverbal memories. This is true regardless of the modality of presentation or the method of testing (recall or recognition), except for occasional tasks that readily can be solved by either hemisphere.

We have used the stories (Logical Memory) and paired words (Associate Learning) of the Wechsler Memory Scales as measures of immediate and delayed recalls of verbal memory, and have found the delayed recall condition particularly sensitive to the function of the left temporal lobe (15). As can be seen in Fig. 1, the mean number of items recalled by the left temporal lobe group in the delay condition is lower than that of any other group at each testing time: before surgery, when the score is diagnostically low; in the immediate postopera-

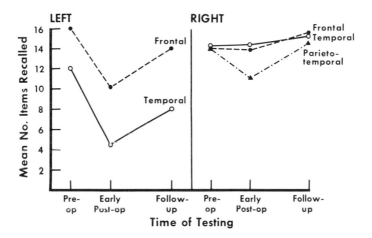

FIG. 1. Mean preoperative, early postoperative, and long-term follow-up scores for delayed recall of verbal material for 48 patients who had cortical excisions for the relief of epilepsy.

tive period; and in long-term follow-up 5 or more years later. Characteristically, measures of such specific psychological functions of discrete areas of the brain, as opposed to the measures of general intelligence already mentioned, result in a curve of performance as portrayed in Fig. 1, commencing with a significantly low score before surgery, dropping to a still lower score as a consequence of the immediate effects of surgery, and then recovering in follow-up to an intermediate score which represents a residual defect. This slight increase of deficit is exchanged in most instances for the relief or significant lessening of epileptic seizures in over two-thirds of our patients, as reported by Rasmussen (Chapter 17, *this volume*).

To test the nonverbal memory function of the right temporal lobe, we have used the simple designs of the Wechsler Memory Scale, but as we find them limited in diagnostic usefulness, we have adopted the Rey Complex Figure for our assessment before surgery and an alternate form (30) for postoperative testing. A printed copy of one of these geometric figures is placed before a patient with instructions to "Copy this drawing as well as you can—Make sure you do not leave out anything." Exposure of the figure for copying is limited to 5 minutes. Then 45 minutes later the patient is asked to reproduce as much of the figure as he can remember. Although these designs do not differentiate between right and left temporal lobe function before surgery as well as our verbal memory tasks do, partly because of unfamiliarity with the nonverbal task, nevertheless right temporal lobe patients perform significantly worse than left temporal lobe patients on the recall of such designs before surgery, and on the copy and recall after surgery, both in the immediate postoperative period and in long-term follow-up. Again the follow-up results point to a residual defect, in this instance of a nonverbal memory defect for right temporal lobe patients.

Patients with left temporal lobe lesions usually produce a copy of the design that closely approximates the original, and a good delayed recall before and after surgery. Representative drawings of a left temporal lobe patient are illustrated in Fig. 2, where only a few slight copying errors are evident and the recalls contain about 70% of the detailed spatial arrangement of the design. In contrast, the drawings of a right temporal lobe patient in Fig. 3 show many copying errors and delayed memory for less than half of the designs both before and after surgery. It should be noted that while the left temporal lobe patient was producing good drawings, he recalled very few verbal items in postoperative testing, whereas while the right temporal lobe patient was efficiently recalling verbal items, he was unable to copy or recall accurately the geometric figures. These results illustrate the double dissociation between verbal and nonverbal memory and the function of the left and right temporal lobes, respectively.

Although we measure various perceptual skills that are associated with the function of the temporal lobes (perception of verbal material such as dichotically presented digits with the left temporal lobe and nonverbal material such as melodies and faces with the right), we continue to emphasize memory testing not only because the temporal lobes as a whole are involved in the consolidation of memories (6), but also because of the risk of a global amnesic syndrome developing as the consequence of a unilateral temporal removal that includes hippocampal structures when mesial temporal areas of the opposite hemisphere are damaged as well (23). In our routine assessments, the vulnerability of mesial temporal function is best revealed to us by studying the rate of learning of recurring digit and block pattern sequences, as was done by Corsi (22). If the

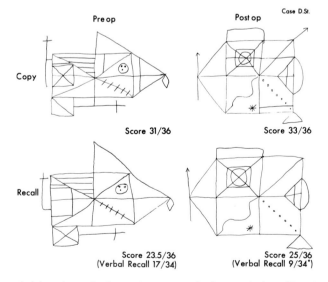

FIG. 2. Copy and delayed recall of complex geometric figures, before (Rey figure, **left**) and after (Taylor figure, **right**) left temporal lobectomy. (*), significantly low score.

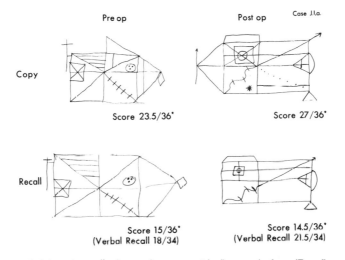

FIG. 3. Copy and delayed recall of complex geometric figures, before (Rey figure, **left**) and after (Taylor figure, **right**) right temporal lobectomy. (*), significantly low score.

memory systems of both temporal lobes are found to be defective, we do sodium amobarbital (Amytal) tests for memory (20) as a final check on whether or not mesial temporal tissue can be included in the proposed surgery.

Finally, we are also aware that our assessment of temporal lobe patients is subtly influenced by our clinical impressions of how they react when we meet and work with them. Recent studies of Bryan Kolb, in our laboratory, on the defective perception of facial expressions and production of facial movements by frontal lobe patients, as opposed to right temporal lobe patients' reduced capacity to recognize faces (19), have encouraged us to begin quantifying these impressions to help in the understanding of observed behavioral differences between patient groups.

FRONTAL LOBES

Inappropriate responses frequently differentiate frontal lobe patients from other patient groups. These responses seem to be related to a lack of inhibition as well as an inefficient assimilation of information included in test instructions, rather than difficulty with the test per se. Numerous trials are therefore required to learn tasks such as stylus mazes, both tactual (2) and visual (18), as the performance of frontal lobe patients is marred by rule infractions. On tasks such as the Rey Complex Figure, the variant performance often takes the form of unusual intrusions and distortions of details, more for right than left frontal lobe patients, presumably because of the spatial nature of the test. For standard tests of intelligence and memory not demanding sustained or original learning, frontal lobectomy results in little or no change of test scores unless the damage is extensive and bilateral, as is occasionally seen after trauma or with large midline tumors.

Quality of response is also a distinguishing feature of the inefficient performance by frontal lobe patients of the Wisconsin Card Sorting Test (9) which, since the first report of Milner (16), we have come to rely on as one of our principal means of determining frontal lobe dysfunction. Again, frontal lobe patients seem unable to make adequate use of the information with which they are provided throughout the test. Instead, they continue using the first strategy they happen to adopt in sorting, even after being informed that their responses are incorrect. As a result, they make many perseverative errors and generally achieve less than half of the six possible sorting categories (color, form, and number, each sorted twice). Although this task can be performed by an average 7-year-old child, very bright frontal lobe patients persist in making perseverative responses, sometimes even after having described the possible categories. This test is sensitive to function in dorsolateral areas of both frontal lobes, but more to the left than the right, as some patients with lesions in the right dorsolateral frontal area can perform the task and in follow-up testing there tends to be recovery of ability to do the test after right-sided surgery, but not after left.

Patients with lesions confined to more inferior parts of the frontal lobes are generally proficient at sorting tasks, but they have difficulty with fluency tasks. For the left hemisphere, this translates as a lack of spontaneous speech or inability to generate language, which is very noticeable in left inferior frontal patients. To detect this lack of verbal fluency we use the Chicago Word Fluency Test (32), which requires the subject to write as many different words beginning with S as possible in 5 minutes, and as many four-letter words beginning with C in 4 minutes. The results for frontal lobe patients are the same whether they respond orally (1), or in writing (17). Because of the verbal nature of this test, it is most sensitive to left frontal lobe function; however, right frontal lobe patients also display limited word fluency relative to other patient groups (26). In addition, frontal lobe patients produce words that other patient groups and normal control subjects reject as being socially unacceptable. Jones-Gotman and Milner's report of an analogous fluency task involving the production of meaningless designs, on which frontal lobe patients score poorly (right worse than left), further suggests that a general factor of fluency is associated with the function of the inferior parts of the frontal lobes (10).

CENTRAL AREA

A sizable percentage of our patients have removals of epileptogenic tissue from the central (Rolandic) area. Before surgery, somatosensory testing on the hands of these patients yields contralateral deficits if the area of damage includes the postcentral gyrus, or if there is interference in the central area from neighboring epileptic tissue. If part of the postcentral gyrus is excised, the sensory deficits become more severe and bilateral deficits are more likely to be evident, particularly if both the hand and face areas have been removed (4). Follow-up testing generally results in the expected partial recovery of function, but deficits persist if the excision has invaded the postcentral gyrus. Severe deficits are found in only those patients where the surgery has necessitated the invasion of the contralateral hand area (3).

Although the surgeon is reluctant to invade the central area, in particular the hand or foot regions, over the years we have accumulated a small group of patients who have had a surgical removal including part or all of the lower central, face, area. As somatosensory function on the face is of interest in these patients, we have modified measures of two-point discrimination, point localization, and pressure sensitivity to meet the particular needs of testing on the face. A preliminary look at our data suggests that, unlike the hand, and in keeping with the known diffuse sensory representation of the face (27), long-lasting sensory deficits on the face are seldom seen even with complete removal of both the precentral and postcentral gyri of the lower central area shown by stimulation at the time of surgery to represent the face.

Another finding with these face area patients is that certain aspects of their language are impaired. For example, they achieve an even lower score on the word fluency test than do our frontal lobe patients (31). They also are unable to make effective use of the phonetic elements of language. When asked before surgery to discriminate phonemes embedded in nonsense words (29), face area patients correctly identify less than half of the 108 sounds they have heard, whereas other patient groups score significantly higher on the task (Table 1). After surgery, the typical curve for specific skills is again seen, with the scores for face area patients falling still lower and then recovering to a level that represents a residual deficit. These same patients are also poor spellers, occasionally writing words that are unrecognizable.

Data collected on two recent face area patients (Fig. 4), one with a left hemisphere lesion and the other with a right, serve to illustrate these findings. Before surgery, the left hemisphere patient, a 13-year-old male, who subsequently had a total removal of the precentral and postcentral face area, had only a mild contralateral 2-point deficit, whereas the right hemisphere patient, a 23-year-

TABLE 1. *Mean number of correct discriminations of 108 phonemes embedded in nonsense words*

Patient group	Time of testing		
	Preoperative	Postoperative	Follow-up
Temporal			
Left	77.4	70.8	77.1
Right	71.5	78.3	77.4
Frontal			
Left	62.9	62.3	67.8
Right	65.1	70.0	68.2
Central			
Left	45.6	30.6	37.4
Right	68.5	73.9	65.1

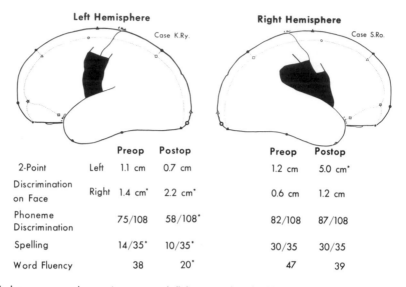

			Preop	Postop		Preop	Postop
2-Point		Left	1.1 cm	0.7 cm		1.2 cm	5.0 cm*
Discrimination on Face		Right	1.4 cm*	2.2 cm*		0.6 cm	1.2 cm
Phoneme Discrimination			75/108	58/108*		82/108	87/108
Spelling			14/35*	10/35*		30/35	30/35
Word Fluency			38	20*		47	39

FIG. 4. Language and somatosensory deficits associated with lesions of the lower central (face) area. (*), significant deficit.

old male who later had all of the postcentral face area removed as well as the parietal opercular area behind the face area and most of the precentral face area, had a high threshold on the contralateral side of the face, but not a deficit. Early postoperative testing after face area removals yielded expected deficits, but even with removal of the entire left face area the young boy developed only a moderate contralateral deficit, which is not likely to be significant in follow-up testing. In contrast, the older right hemisphere patient exhibited a severe contralateral deficit after removal of most of the face area and tissue posterior to it, but we expect that in follow-up testing this deficit, although still evident, will be slight. In general, then, we see only mild, transitory, sensory deficits on the face even after total removal of the central face area, but deficits do tend to be more persistent and severe if the surgical removal extends into the central hand area or behind the face area in the parietal lobe.

On the phoneme discrimination and word fluency tasks, the left face area boy had normal scores before surgery, but his spelling was poor. In early postoperative testing, however, he had significantly low scores on all these language tests, although he was not dysphasic. The right face area patient, conversely, had no deficits on any of these language tests in either preoperative or postoperative testing.

PARIETAL AND OCCIPITAL LOBES

Of more than 1,000 patients we have seen who have had unilateral brain surgery, less than 20 have had either a pure occipital or parietal lobectomy.

This low frequency is partly accounted for by the reduced tendency for tissue in these areas to become epileptiform and the smallness of the occipital lobe. Many left parietal lobe patients are also eliminated from our series because the posterior speech area continues to be present in this lobe, making the risk of possible speech loss too great for these patients to be considered for elective surgery. Early injury to either parietal lobe results in a reorganization of function (unlike our findings for temporal lobe patients), with the right hemisphere assuming at least some major language function if the left posterior speech area is damaged, whereas with damage to the right parietal lobe the left hemisphere may subsume spatial function. Data from these patients with atypical cerebral organization cannot, of course, be included in our regular analyses. In time we shall be able to comment more fully on such patients and on the function of the right parietal lobe.

CEREBRAL ORGANIZATION

Cerebral organization does not become a matter of primary concern to us for the majority of our patients, as most of them are right-handed, and our diagnosis of the side of lesion usually agrees with the clinical impression gained from the seizure pattern and EEG and radiological findings. For all non-right-handed patients, however, we automatically do intracarotid sodium amobarbital tests for speech (33) because of the high incidence of atypical speech representation in these patients (Chapter 17, *this volume*). We also do amobarbital tests on all those patients where our impression of the side of lesion differs from other clinical findings: i.e. if the site of lesion is diagnosed by other laboratories as being in the right hemisphere and we find that the patient is experiencing verbal difficulties, or conversely, the lesion is thought to be on the left and we do not find any verbal deficits, there is then the possibility of atypical organization of speech, which the surgeon needs to have verified before surgery. This is not possible in all instances, particularly in children under about the age of 12 years.

A variety of language tests give us details of the patient's perception, comprehension, expression, and organization of speech. One of these, the Dichotic Digits Test, is of particular value to us, as Kimura (12) has shown a relationship between the perception of digits presented simultaneously to the two ears and the cerebral representation of speech. For most right-handed normal subjects, and patients known to have speech in the left hemisphere as shown by amobarbital tests, digits presented to the right ear are perceived more accurately than those presented to the left. [A converse, left-ear effect is found for nonverbal material such as melodies (13) and environmental sounds (7)]. Although this test is not reliable (8), nevertheless the absence of the right-ear effect is sometimes our only indication of atypical speech representation, and so if it is absent we arrange for amobarbital speech tests.

As we now use catheters rather than needles to do these tests, a 3 cm³ angiogram can be performed, which provides us with the likely distribution of the drug when we later inject 3 cm³ of 175 mg of 10% sodium amobarbital. Both sides of the brain are tested for speech and memory, one side on each of two different days, as interpretation is often not possible without the results from both sides, particularly if speech is represented bilaterally.

1976 PATIENT SAMPLE

During 1976, our psychology laboratory investigated 83 patients who had unilateral cortical excisions for the relief of epilepsy (Table 2). Of these patients, 43 were male and 40 female, and they ranged in age from 6 to 64 years with a mean age of 24 years and a mean level of general intelligence in the high average range. There were slightly more excisions in the left hemisphere than in the right, a general finding with our patient sample over the years. Most of the patients had temporal lobectomies, but 16 (20%) had frontal lobectomies. Only 3 patients had removals confined to the parietal or occipital lobes and 3 others had removals mainly of the face area. As would be expected, surgery involving more than one lobe of the brain was more prevalent in the right hemisphere than in the left, and the two hemicortisectomies performed were of the right, nondominant, hemisphere.

Thirty-nine, or 47%, of the patients, were referred for sodium amobarbital testing, 25 for verification of speech representation, and 14 to establish memory capacity. Speech representation in relation to handedness is shown for these patients in Table 3, without taking into account whether damage to the left cerebral hemisphere was early or late. Generally, the findings parallel those presented by Rasmussen (Chapter 17, *this volume*) as most right-handers were found to have speech represented in the left hemisphere, whereas less than half of the non-right-handers had speech only in the left hemisphere. Although there were instances of right hemisphere and bilateral speech representation for both handedness groups, these atypical patterns were almost 3 times as

TABLE 2. *Site of cortical excision in 83 epileptic patients studied in 1976*

	Number of patients	
Cortical removal	Left hemisphere	Right hemisphere
Temporal	26	19
Frontal	8	8
Parietal	2	—
Occipital	1	—
Central (face area)	2	1
Frontotemporal	4	8
Frontoparietal	1	—
Temporo-occipital	—	1
Hemicortisectomy	—	2
Total	44	39

TABLE 3. *Speech lateralization as related to handedness in 39 patients tested with intracarotid amobarbital*

| Handedness | N | Speech representation | | |
		Left	Bilateral	Right
Right	30	24 (80%)	4 (13%)	2 (7%)
Left or mixed	9	4 (45%)	3 (33%)	2 (22%)

frequent for the non-right-handers; however, fully 20% of the right-handed sample had speech either all in the right hemisphere or bilaterally represented, emphasizing that even for right-handers left hemisphere dominance for speech cannot be taken for granted. There was a higher representation of bilateral speech in both the right-handed and non-right-handed patients of the past year than in our previously reported sample, probably because of the increasing complexity of seizure problems that are being considered for surgery now as opposed to a few years ago, but also because experience has subtly altered our criteria for the classification of speech.

Although the amobarbital procedure for memory is usually reserved for temporal lobe patients, in 1976 one frontal lobe tumor patient had his memory function checked because he was experiencing generalized memory difficulties. In Table 4, the results of amobarbital memory testing with the remaining 13 patients, all of whom had temporal lobe epilepsy and were exhibiting some generalized memory defects before surgery, illustrate findings we have come to expect from these tests. Memory disturbance is frequently seen with injection of the cerebral hemisphere contralateral to the lesion, as it was in 9 of these patients, thus confirming the inability of the damaged hemisphere to process memory material efficiently when it is left to function on its own, that is, while the undamaged hemisphere is affected by the drug. In contrast, there is usually no disturbance of memory with injection of the hemisphere ipsilateral to a unilateral lesion. As can be seen, however, one of the left temporal lobe patients did have disturbance of memory from both the ipsilateral and contralateral injections, thus

TABLE 4. *Incidence of memory disturbance for 13 temporal lobe patients after intracarotid amobarbital tests for memory*

| Site of lesion | N | Site of injection | |
		Ipsilateral to lesion	Contralateral to lesion
Left temporal	6	1/6	4/6
Right temporal	7	0/7	5/7

rating her as a high-risk patient for the development of an amnesic state if the surgical removal involved mesial areas of either temporal lobe. Memory function was judged not to be at risk for the remaining 12 patients, even though they displayed general memory deficits on our psychological testing before surgery. On the basis of EEG and radiological studies, in addition to the psychological evidence, these patients probably have bitemporal lobe damage, but not sufficient damage in the hemisphere contralateral to the lesion to develop a global amnesia after unilateral mesial temporal lobe surgery.

CASE STUDIES OF COMPLEX SEIZURE PROBLEMS

Since many of our patients have been thoroughly investigated elsewhere, they are known to be good candidates for focal epileptic surgery before we see them. Others, who are referred primarily because of the desperate nature of their seizure disorders, require extensive study before a decision can be made concerning the advisability of surgery. Presentation of the psychological protocols for two such patients, who have had surgery within the past year, will illustrate the part psychological tests play in the preoperative examination of these complex cases, and what the immediate effects of surgery are on essential psychological functions.

Case Histories

Patient M. Kr: A 20-year-old, right-handed, married woman with two children had a series of convulsions at age 2 years and was then seizure-free until age 13, when she began having frequent seizures with an aura of upper abdominal discomfort followed by automatisms, rigidity, and occasional falling and urinary incontinence. There was no memory for events after the aura in these episodes. In 1974, she was admitted for possible surgery but, as EEG studies yielded no definite lateralization of epileptic activity, she was sent home for a further trial of medication. Two years later she was readmitted, as she had become unable to manage her home, and spent most of her day in bed. Bitemporal abnormality continued to be seen on her EEGs, so multiple electrodes were implanted bilaterally in the hippocampus and amygdala. During prolonged recording, sharp waves predominated on the right side and a seizure was recorded which started in the right temporal lobe. Results of a pneumoencephalogram were ambiguous but could be interpreted as suggesting atrophy in the right temporal lobe.

The psychological test results of this woman are listed in Fig. 5. Before surgery, she was of average intelligence, but with a Verbal I.Q. significantly lower than the Performance I.Q. rating. This discrepancy, together with slight naming difficulties and the inefficient perception of dichotically presented digits, is consistent with impaired function in the dominant, left hemisphere. Specific dysfunction of the left temporal lobe was pointed to by poor delayed recall of stories and paired words, but damage in the right temporal lobe was also suggested by the inadequate memory of nonverbal material in the form of the Rey Complex Figure. Because of this memory difficulty for both verbal and nonverbal material, a sodium amobarbital test for memory was requested. Injection of the left hemisphere resulted in a significant impairment of memory, consistent with the suspected inability of the right hippocampal system to process memory material adequately on its own. There was no impairment of memory function with injection of the right hemisphere, indicating that surgery involving the right temporal lobe could safely invade mesial structures.

A right temporal lobectomy, extending 7.2 cm along the base and 5.0 cm along the Sylvian fissure, and including the amygdala and hippocampus, was carried out by Dr. Olivier. Pathological analysis revealed a developmental anomaly in the form of a hamartoma in the hippocampus.

	Case M.Kr.	
Handedness- Right (23/90)		
	Preop.	Postop.
Full Scale I.Q.	98	108
Verbal I.Q.	92*	104
Performance I.Q.	105	110
Delayed Verbal Recall	10.0/34*	15.0/34
Delayed Nonverbal Recall	13.5/36'	16.0/36*
Wisconsin Card Sorting	3.5 categories	6 categories
Word Fluency	36	37
Object Naming	17/26*	17/26*
Spelling	31/35	30/35
Dichotic Digits	157/192*	164/192*

FIG. 5. Psychological test results before and after right temporal lobectomy. (*), significantly low score.

Postoperative psychological test results suggested a general lessening of interference with function, particularly in the left hemisphere, as the Verbal I.Q. and verbal memory scores increased significantly after surgery and the six categories of the card sorting test were quickly achieved. Evidence of some dysfunction in the dominant hemisphere remained, however, as the perception of dichotically presented digits and naming tasks were still performed at below expected levels. Continuing difficulty with the recall of a complex geometric figure reflected the known damage in the right temporal lobe. The daily function of this woman was markedly improved in the early postoperative period. Six months after her discharge from the hospital she wrote, "It seems as if my husband, two daughters and I are enjoying a little heaven here on earth. As each day ends I'm very grateful that the operation was a success. I have now been seizure-free for 6 months and very optimistic that possibly I may be for the rest of my life, as long as I take my medicine."

Patient E. Sa: A 32-year-old man, a patient of Dr. Rasmussen's, developed seizures at the age of 22 years, 1 week after a head trauma. Since that time, the seizures have remained the same, occurring two or three times a day and beginning with an aura of a strange feeling in the head followed by automatisms for which he is amnesic. As he works with heavy machinery and on occasion has been belligerent when restrained during the course of a seizure, his company gave him a leave of absence, telling him that if his seizure problem had not improved within 6 months he would be without a job. On admission to the hospital, independent foci over both temporal regions were recorded on EEGs, whereas radiological examinations showed only mild ventricular dilation without evidence of significant focal atrophy. It was decided to monitor seizure activity with a computor and bilateral temporal, chronically implanted, depth electrodes directed at both limbic and neocortical structures. EEG recordings then revealed electrographic seizures originating in the hippocampal region. Three typical clinical seizures were recorded, all of which started in the right temporal lobe.

Psychological test results for this patient are shown in Fig. 6. He was found to be of average intelligence, but he had difficulty copying and recalling nonverbal geometric figures, pointing to dysfunction of the nondominant temporal lobe. In addition, his word fluency score was very low and, although he is completely right-handed and comes from a right-handed family, his perception of dichotic digits was better for those digits presented to the left ear than to the right, consistent with at least some speech representation in the right hemisphere. The right-sided sodium amobarbital test produced speech arrest for 30 sec and both naming and serial

Case E.Sa.		
Handedness - Right (18/90)		
	Preop.	Postop.
Full Scale I.Q.	98	89
Verbal I.Q.	101	90
Performance I.Q.	96	88
Delayed Verbal Recall	15/34	6/34*
Delayed Nonverbal Recall	12.5/36*	4/36*
Wisconsin Card Sorting	4.4 categories	4.1 categories
Word Fluency	15*	14*
Object Naming	23/26	15/26*
Spelling	29/35	16/35*
Dichotic Digits: Left	91/96	70/96
Right	81/96	75/96
Total	172/192	145*/192

FIG. 6. Psychological test results before and after right, dominant, temporal lobectomy. (*), significantly low score.

speech errors. There was no disturbance of speech with injection of the left hemisphere. This man would seem, therefore, to be one of those rare individuals of right-handed stock whose speech naturally developed in the right hemisphere, as we have no evidence of damage occurring early enough in the left hemisphere to force the development of speech on the right. Rather, we have evidence of trauma in adult life resulting in a lesion of the right temporal lobe which, as would be expected, has not resulted in any rearrangement of speech representation. It is noteworthy that the only clues of this right hemisphere dominance for speech came from the left-ear effect on the dichotic digits test and the limited word fluency. There was no significant interference with memory function from either injection.

An anterior right temporal lobectomy was then carried out, including the pes and about 1 cm of the hippocampus. Gross abnormality was found to be unusually well localized to the hippocampal region.

Postoperative recovery of this patient was much slower than usual (probably owing to the occurrence of a major convulsion during the operation), and was reflected in an uncharacteristic general decrease of all intelligence ratings (Fig. 6) when testing was done 2 weeks after surgery. Interference with language function was evident on most verbal tests, and verbal memory scores were particularly low as a consequence of the invasion of hippocampal structures of the dominant temporal lobe. The hippocampal removal may also have resulted in the drop of the nonverbal memory score, but on the basis of the amobarbital memory testing this should prove transient. The sharp decrease in the perception of digits presented to the left (contralateral) ear on the dichotic task is a customary finding after removal of the dominant temporal lobe (11). There was little change in the performance of tests sensitive to frontal lobe function. It is expected that in follow-up testing in a year's time, a general recovery will be evident on all tests but particularly on nonverbal tests. At that time, there should no longer be any interference with language function, and only minimal accentuation of memory deficits.

OTHER PHENOMENA

Generally, the findings discussed above are common to a wide range of patients, including those undergoing psychiatric surgery (5) and stereotactic surgery for

Parkinson's disease (24,25), and also to children. There are, however, many aspects of human behavior that we are not measuring, either because they are phenomena we do not as yet understand or of which we are unaware. One such phenomenon of spatial displacement has been seen by us in 3 male Parkinsonian patients of Dr. Bertrand's, all of whom had a right-sided thalamotomy. After surgery, the men were oriented as to person and time, but thought they were in a hospital other than ours. One patient became quite disturbed, as his displacement became involved with an elaborate delusional system. In another patient, the displacement was not uncovered for more than a week, as the only clue to his disorientation was in his effusive greeting of the doctors as they made rounds each morning, and his comments on the extraordinary care he was receiving. Finally it was discovered that he thought the rounds party was traveling 100 miles to his home hospital each morning. These spatial displacements have lasted up to 10 days, and then have cleared without explanation. Such phenomena deserve our close attention, as they are obviously important for our understanding of human function, and they illustrate the need for comprehensive base-line studies whenever possible before elective surgery.

REFERENCES

1. Benton, A. L. (1968): Differential behavioral effects in frontal lobe disease. *Neuropsychologia,* 6:53–60.
2. Corkin, S. (1965): Tactually-guided maze learning in man: Effects of unilateral excisions and bilateral hippocampal lesions. *Neuropsychologia,* 3:339–351.
3. Corkin, S., Milner, B., and Rasmussen, T. (1970): Somatosensory thresholds: Contrasting effects of postcentral gyrus and posterior parietal-lobe excisions. *Arch. Neurol.,* 22:41–58.
4. Corkin, S., Milner, B., and Taylor, L. (1973): Bilateral sensory loss after unilateral cerebral lesion in man. *Trans. Am. Neurol. Assoc.,* 98:118–122.
5. Corkin, S., Teuber, H.-L., and Twitchell, T. E. (1977): A study of cingulotomy in man: A summary. In: *Neurosurgical Treatment in Psychiatry, Pain, and Epilepsy,* edited by W. H. Sweet. University Park Press, Baltimore, Maryland.
6. Corsi, P. M. (1972): *Human Memory and the Medial Temporal Region of the Brain.* Unpublished Ph.D. thesis, McGill University.
7. Curry, F. (1967): A comparison of left-handed and right-handed subjects on verbal and non-verbal dichotic listening tasks. *Cortex,* 3:343–352.
8. Goodglass, H. (1967): Binaural digit presentation and early lateral brain damage. *Cortex,* 3:295–306.
9. Grant, D. A., and Berg, G. A. (1948): A behavioral analysis of degree of reinforcement and ease of shifting to new responses in a Weigl-type card-sorting problem. *J. Exp. Psychol.,* 38:404–411.
10. Jones-Gotman, M., and Milner, B. (1977): Design fluency: The invention of nonsense drawings after focal cortical lesions. *Neuropsychologia,* 15:653–674.
11. Kimura, D. (1961): Some effects of temporal-lobe damage on auditory perception. *Can. J. Psychol.,* 15:156–165.
12. Kimura, D. (1961): Cerebral dominance and the perception of verbal stimuli. *Can J. Psychol.,* 15:165–171.
13. Kimura, D. (1964): Left-right differences in the perception of melodies. *Q. J. Exp. Psychol.,* 16:355–358.
14. Meyer, V., and Jones, H. G. (1957): Patterns of cognitive test performance as functions of the lateral localization of cerebral abnormalities in the temporal lobe. *J. Ment. Sci.,* 103:758–772.

15. Milner, B. (1958): Psychological defects produced by temporal-lobe excision. *Res. Publ. Assoc. Nerv. Ment. Dis.,* 36:244–257.
16. Milner, B. (1963): Effects of different brain lesions on card sorting. *Arch. Neurol.,* 9:90–100.
17. Milner, B. (1964): Some effects of frontal lobectomy in man. In: *The Frontal Granular Cortex and Behavior,* edited by J. M. Warren and K. Akert. McGraw-Hill, New York.
18. Milner, B. (1965): Visually-guided maze learning in man: Effects of bilateral hippocampal, bilateral frontal, and unilateral cerebral lesion. *Neuropsychologia,* 3:317–338.
19. Milner, B. (1968): Visual recognition and recall after right temporal-lobe excision in man. *Neuropsychologia,* 6:191–209.
20. Milner, B. (1972): Disorders of learning and memory after temporal-lobe lesions in man. *Clin. Neurosurg.,* 19:421–446.
21. Milner, B. (1975): Psychological aspects of focal epilepsy and its neurosurgical management. In: *Advances in Neurology,* Vol. 8, edited by D. P. Purpura, J. K. Penry, and R. D. Walter. Raven Press, New York.
22. Milner, B. (1978): Clues to the cerebral organization of memory. In: *Cerebral Correlates of Conscious Experience* (INSERM 6), edited by M. Jouvet. Elsevier North-Holland, Amsterdam, Holland.
23. Milner, B., and Penfield, W. (1955): The effect of hippocampal lesions on recent memory. *Trans. Am. Neurol. Assoc.,* 80:42–48.
24. Perret, E., Kohenof, M., and Siegfried, J. (1969): Influences de lesions thalamiques unilatérales sur les fonctions intellectuelles, mnésiques et d'apprentissage de malades Parkinsoniens. *Neuropsychologia,* 7:79–88.
25. Proctor, F., Riklan, M., Cooper, I. S., and Teuber, H.-L. (1963): Somatosensory status of parkinsonian patients before and after chemothalamectomy. *Neurology,* 13:906–912.
26. Ramier, A.-M., and Hécaen, H. (1970): Rôle respectif des atteintes frontales et de la latéralisation lesionnelle dans les déficits de la "fluence verbale." *Rev. Neurol.,* 123:17–22.
27. Rasmussen, T., and Penfield, W. (1947): Further studies of the sensory and motor cerebral cortex of man. *Fed. Proc.,* 6:452–460.
28. Reitan, R. M. (1955): Certain differential effects of left and right cerebral lesions in human adults. *J. Comp. Physiol. Psychol.,* 48:474–477.
29. Stitt, C., and Huntington, D. (1969): Some relationships among articulation, auditory abilities, and certain other variables. *J. Speech Hear. Res.,* 12:576–593.
30. Taylor, L. B. (1969): Localisation of cerebral lesions by psychological testing. *Clin. Neurosurg.,* 16:269–287.
31. Taylor, L., Milner, B., and Darwin, C. J. (1975): Verbal disabilities associated with lesions of the left face area. *(Manuscript in preparation).* Summarized in The 17th International Symposium of Neuropsychology, Ettlinger, G., Teuber, H.-L. and Milner, B. *Neuropsychologia,* 13:125–133.
32. Thurstone, L. L., and Thurstone, T. G. (1943): *The Chicago Tests of Primary Mental Abilities.* Science Research Associates, Chicago, Illinois.
33. Wada, J., and Rasmussen, T. (1960): Intracarotid injection of sodium Amytal for the lateralization of cerebral speech dominance: Experimental and clinical observations. *J. Neurosurg.,* 17:266–282.

Functional Neurosurgery, edited by T. Rasmussen
and R. Marino. Raven Press, New York © 1979.

Depth Recordings and Stimulation of the Human Brain: A Twenty Year Experience

*Blaine S. Nashold, Jr., **William P. Wilson,
and *Elizabeth Boone

*Department of Surgery Division of Neurosurgery, and the **Department of Psychiatry,
Duke University Medical Center, Durham, North Carolina 27710*

We must approach the brain of a man as Sherrington approached the nervous
system of other mammals. We must identify individual reflex mechanisms
wherever possible and yet strive to understand how these mechanisms are
integrated into a functional whole. This is the underlying problem of
neurophysiology.

— Wilder Penfield

The introduction of chronic depth electrodes into the human brain for diagnosis is not new. In the early 1950s, several investigators began to develop the
surgical technique for electrode implantation and electroencephalographie (EEG)
recording of subcortical activity in patients undergoing psychosurgery. These
investigators hoped that the electrical activity of the deeper brain structures
could be used as an electrophysiologic guide to psychosurgery. The hope of
these investigators was not fulfilled in relation to psychosurgery but it did encour-
age the use of depth electrode recordings and stimulation in other neurological
disorders. In 1953, Bickford, Dodge, and Sim-Jacobsen, at the Mayo Clinic,
reported to the American EEG Society preliminary studies (20,21) using depth
electrodes, and since then the technique has had worldwide use.

The initial interest of investigators was the recording of electrical activity
from the brain. Where the stereotactic technique was used deep electrodes could
be introduced safely and accurately into specific subcortical brain areas. These
depth electrodes were used for monitoring electrical activity, and specific physiological responses were elicited by electrical stimulation. The results of stimulation
and EEG recording with depth electrodes made possible more precise localization
of therapeutic stereotactic lesions. Heath, in the 1950s (4), used depth electrode
stimulation as a modality of treatment in certain psychiatric disorders, and
more recently deep brain stimulation has been used to treat intractable pain.

During the past 20 years, we have employed depth electrode studies for diagnostic purposes in neurological diseases such as epilepsy, involuntary movements,
and intractable pain. EEG recordings and electrical stimulation were carried
out in order to evaluate physiological responses and to make subsequent therapeutic lesions more effective.

A summary of our clinical observations over a 20-year period is reported here. Readers interested in more specific details can refer to the original papers listed in the references.

It should be emphasized that the clinical observations in man were carried out within the strictest ethical controls and with the full consent of the patient and, in most instances, a member of his family. Clinical protocols were approved in advance by the Duke Medical Center committee on "Human Experimentation." The purpose of electrode implantation was always considered as an adjunct to diagnosis related to a specific treatment to relieve the individual patient.

Stereotactic localization of a target area in the brain always has an inherent element of error, owing in part to the variation in the human brain structures plus certain variables of the surgical technique. Detailed stereotactic atlases of the deep brain structures are available and strict stereotactic techniques were employed by us. Improved localization of therapeutic lesion in the brain must depend on anatomical, physiological, behavioral, and electrographic data. A certain element of experimentation using these advanced techniques is always present not only because of the complexity of the disease process itself, but also the lack of detailed information of normal brain function in man. The ultimate goal for the use of depth electrodes was to improve the localization of the subsequent therapeutic lesion that would relieve the patients' symptoms, and to reduce the morbidity and mortality rates of the stereotactic surgical operation. The surgical mortality rate of stereotactic neurosurgical operations and depth electrode implantation is less than 1%, with a morbidity rate ranging from 4 to 8%.

METHODS

Stereotactic Technique of Electrode Implantation

Depth electrode implantation was carried out using the standard stereotactic neurosurgical technique. The instruments for electrode implantation included the Bertrand, Todd-Wells, and Reichert-Mundinger stereotactic instruments.

The depth electrodes were originally designed and manufactured by Schryver. They were multicontact electrodes made up of Teflon coated stainless steel (wire diameter 0.002 inches, Quad-coated Teflon 0.0035) (Fig. 1).[1] The electrodes can be made in 10 different configurations, depending on their specific application within brain structures (Table 1).

The depth electrodes were introduced through a burr hole placed in the appropriate location on the skull, anchored by silk sutures to the scalp, and protected in a special net head dressing. Postoperative skull roentgenograms were made to check the electrode position and to note any change in position. Postoperative complications were nil, and no hemorrhage, infection, or neurological deficit

---

[1] These same electrodes are commercially available from Rhodes Medical Instruments, Woodland Hills, California.

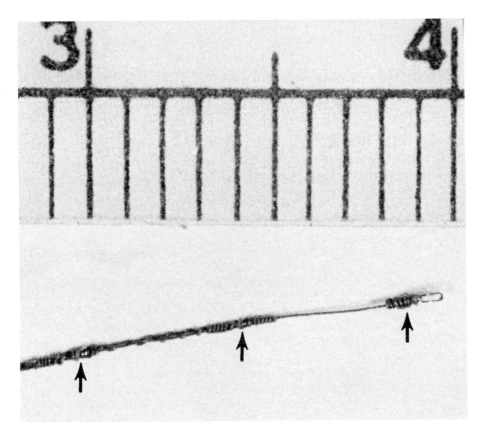

FIG. 1. Schryver electrode.

TABLE 1. *Depth electrodes*

Type	Contact spacing center to center (mm)	No. of contacts	Length of contact winding (mm)	Average approximate area of each contact (sq. mm)
EX-19	5	6	0.5	0.628
EX-20	10	6	0.5	0.628
EX-29	5	3	0.5	0.628
EX-51	10	6	1.0	1.256
EX-55	5	6	1.0	1.256
EX-60	5	3	1.0	1.256
EX-61	2	6	1.0	1.256
EX-63	5	6	3.0	3.769
EX-88	10	3	3.0	
EX-89	10	3	6.0	

Wire is 0.0035 inch quad Teflon coated.

was noted. The electrodes were left in the brain for periods up to 6 months, depending on the nature of the patient's disease and the information collected (Fig. 2).

EEG Recording Sessions

EEG recordings from the electrodes were usually delayed for several days to allow time for stabilization of the electrical impedance. Measurements of impedance that were made the first day reveal high electrical resistance (over 100,000 ohms), and the electrical recordings tended to be unstable with artifacts. The average electrical resistance of the Schryver electrodes described in this chapter range from 50,000 to 70,000 ohms. Weekly measurements showed that the impedance remains stable for months. If the electrical resistance of a particular electrode began to rise, the EEG recording was usually discontinued.

Stimulation Sessions

Stimulations were carried out after preliminary EEG recordings (7 days). The patient was in a quiet room where he was comfortable and able to communicate freely with the observers. Stimulation sessions usually lasted from 30 min to 1 hr, and only rarely were they carried on for longer periods. The patient always had the option of discontinuing the stimulation. Physiological responses were monitored by the appropriate recordings on a polygraph or movie film. Written and voice records were kept, and several observers attended each stimulation session.

The stimulation parameters employed varied from low to high frequencies with both unidirectional and bidirectional square waves (Grass stimulator and isolation unit). A current of 2 mA was never exceeded. Bipolar stimulation was carried out between adjacent contacts or closely adjacent contacts on the same electrode. Each electrode was systematically explored and the physiological responses noted were rechecked at later sessions.

OCULAR RESPONSES FROM DEEP BRAIN STIMULATION IN CONSCIOUS MAN

Spiegel and Wycis (24) were the first to record eye movements in conscious patients during stereotactic operations. In 1967, we recorded preliminary observations of ocular reactions resulting from brain stimulation in the conscious human with chronic implanted electrodes (5,6,9–11,13). Stimulation was done in a variety of subcortical areas (thalamus, mesencephalon) as well as in the dentate nucleus of the cerebellum. The ocular reactions resulting from thalamic and midbrain stimulation included pupillary changes, conjugate eye deviations, lid retractions, along with head and neck movements. The subject was usually

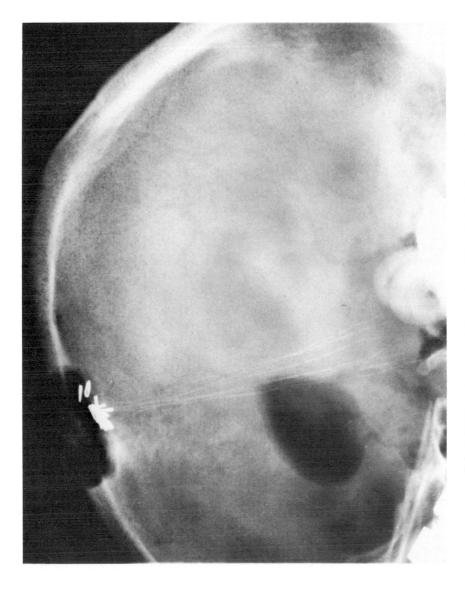

FIG. 2. Roentgenogram of skull of patient with multiple depth electrodes.

aware of his ocular movements and could detect their onset before they were observed.

Medial rectus and upper eye movements resulted from stimulation at several brain sites. One such site was near the midline just ventral to the third nerve nucleus where low-intensity and low-frequency stimulations resulted in rhythmical contractions of the ipsilateral upper lid at the same rate as the stimulus frequency. By increasing the stimulation frequency, tonic lid contractions of both lids occurred from an area 5 mm lateral to this point. Ipsilateral abduction of the eye occurred near the ventral border of the red nucleus. Further laterally and ventrally, ipsilateral abduction was produced from the vicinity of the subthalamic nucleus adjacent to the substantia nigra, while ipsilateral eyelid elevation and abduction of the eyes occurred at both medial and lateral sites. The infranuclear neural connections responsible for these eye reactions appear to pass in close anatomical apposition in the ventral mesencephalon.

Conjugate eye movements occurred at multiple sites in the thalamus, subthalamus, and mesencephalon. The deviation was always contralateral and the direction of the contralateral gaze was either up, down, or oblique in direction, depending on the area stimulated. Stimulation of the thalamus produced contralateral gaze from the regions of the medial pulvinar, central medianum, and the central thalamic gray (nonspecific midline nuclei). Stimulation of the zona incerta, fields of Florel H1, H2, and the prerubral area resulted in both horizontal and oblique upward conjugate gaze. In the rostral mesencephalon, the sites for horizontal and conjugate gaze deviation were situated in the regions of the central tegmentum and the periaqueductal gray. There was a dorsoventral orientation for these conjugate responses with the contralateral oblique upward gaze sites situated more dorsal than the sites to horizontal gaze. Upward eye movements were produced more dorsally near the posterior commissura, while downward gaze sites were more caudal. Pure vertical conjugate vertical movements were produced by stimulation within 2 mm of the midline of the rostral mesencephalon at the level of the posterior commissura. In addition to the vertical movements, there was slight divergence, closure of the eyelids, and bilateral pupillary constriction. Upward gaze resulted from stimulation of sites ventral to the aqueduct near the border of the red nucleus, and in this location both eyelids opened as the eye deviated vertically but without pupillary change. Downward gaze was also elicited from the ventral mesencephalon at sites between the red nucleus and substantia nigra; however, no ocular responses were elicited from the center of the red nucleus; although from this location complex motor reactions were noted with increased contralateral muscle tone plus extension of the head.

Ocular convergence resulted from stimulation ventral to the periaqueductal gray near the third nerve nucleus and slightly more dorsal and mesial. Head and neck movements were noted as well but not always associated with full eye deviations. Stimulation in the region of the anterior limb of the internal capsule adjacent to the anterior thalamus resulted in contralateral head rotation with minimal eye deviation. Head extension elicited from the red nucleus was not associated with full eye ocular deviation. The horizontal oblique and vertical conjugate gazes from the subthalamic and midbrain stem were as a rule associated with appropriate change in the posture of the head and neck. An exception to this was conjugate lateral gaze elicited from the superior collicular region associated with a visual hallucination without head rotation. The ocular movements always preceded the head rotation and the total oculocephalic response simulated the normal voluntary action observed with spontaneous turning of the eyes and head. A visual hallucination (phosphene) seen by the patient in his contralateral visual field resulted during stimulation in the region of the superior colliculus. The electrode was situated approximately 5 mm from the midsagittal plane just beneath the surface of the left superior colliculus. Eye deviation occurred to the right without head movement. The patient reported "bright lights in the eyes," "something flashed in front of me" (phosphene), indicating that the visual hallucination seemed to be localized to the right visual field in the direction of the eye movement. The sensation of "lights" also occurred when he closed both eyes and did not seem to be distorting his vision. The phosphenes produced by stimulation of the vicinity of the superior colliculus appear similar to those reported by Brindley and others from stimulating the primary visual cortex in man.

Somatosensory and visual hallucinations were reported by some patients during the ocular moments. One sensation described was that of a vague unpleasant feeling localized within the eyes, and the oral and nasal cavities. This was elicited from regions in the rostral periaqueductal region as well as from the pulvinar and parafascicular thalamic areas.

Closure of both eyes without ocular deviation also occurred at collicular levels when the stimulation was near the mesial mesencephalon and the region of the periaqueductal gray. These ocular responses were also associated with an unpleasant feeling referred to the central region of the face, eyes, nose, and mouth. Similar feelings were noted by the patients when the midline thalamic nuclei were stimulated. Horizontal nystagmus was produced during stimulation of the central tegmental region, dorsal to the red nucleus, and it also occurred from the same sites as the mesencephalon tegmentum, from which contralateral horizontal deviation occurred.

Electrical stimulations were also carried out in the depths of the cerebellum in the region of the dentate nucleus and in the midline cerebellum nuclei prior to the placement of stereotactic therapeutic lesions for relief of spasticity and abnormal involuntary movements (12). Ocular reactions produced by stimulation of the perimedian nuclear regions of the cerebellum (dentate nucleus) resulted in pupillary dilatation, an ipsilateral eye movement up and outward, and a contralateral eye movement down and in (skew deviation). Ipsilateral conjugate gaze, bilateral eye closure, and contralateral nystagmus resulted from dentate stimulation. Similar ocular responses have been reported by Fisher in patients with acute deep cerebellar hemorrhage (1).

Stereotactic therapeutic lesions placed within the dentate nucleus resulted in transient ocular disturbances such as pupillary dilatation, with sluggish light reflexes and unequal pupils (12). Transient contralateral head and horizontal eye deviation, loss of vertical gaze, absence of "Doll's head" and optic kinetic nystagmus, and subjective sensations of dizziness were seen after dentate lesions but they cleared within days. The same lesion produced reduction of flexor tone in the ipsilateral extremities plus a reduction of the patient's involuntary movements.

The results of ocular deviations and visual sensations produced in man by deep brain stimulation closely corresponded to observations made in the higher primates; however, in our patients, it was not possible to confirm anatomically the precise localizations of the electrode contacts.

THE USE OF IMPLANTED DEPTH ELECTRODES IN EPILEPSY

Surface electrodes placed on the cerebral cortex and depth electrodes have been used extensively in patients with temporal lobe epilepsy, centrencephalic seizures, and reflex epilepsy. EEG recordings have also been made in patients with central pain (thalamic syndrome) and involuntary movement disorders (2,8,14,16,18).

In 1973, a group of five patients with bitemporal epilepsy were evaluated by implantation of depth electrodes into both hippocampi and amygdalae (8). The epilepsy in these patients had been proven intractable after many years of drug treatment. The scalp EEGs in these patients had revealed repeated bilateral epileptic discharges usually independent and with shifting lateralization.

The depth electrodes were introduced stereotactically via frontal bur holes into the mesial temporal regions (hippocampus and amygdala). Extensive depth electrode recordings were made, and the temporal lobe was stimulated to evaluate behavioral changes associated with epileptic afterdischarge.

In all patients, bilateral slow waves, spike, spike and wave, or repetitive spikes were noted in the amygdalae and hippocampi. These were nearly always bilaterally asynchronous, but they were frequently synchronous between the amygdala and hippocampus on one side. The hippocampus appeared more active electrographically than did the amygdala. There was usually less low-voltage, fast activity on the side interpreted as having the greatest electrographic abnormality, especially apparent during sleep activation. A few spontaneous and pentylenetetrazol(Metrazol ®)-activated seizures were recorded, sometimes with a clear focus of onset but usually without it. In every case, in addition to recording from subcortical electrodes, scalp and nasopharyngeal electrodes were used for simultaneous recording. Although persistent and repetitive abnormal discharges were being recorded from the subcortical structures, only rarely did spike or spike-wave activity occur in a scalp or nasopharyngeal recording of diagnostic degree. When surface or nasopharyngeal electrodes recorded subcortical activity, it was even observed in some patients to be contralateral to abnormalities being recorded in the amygdalae and hippocampi.

Afterdischarges were obtained frequently from both amygdalae and hippocampi. At times, these were associated with clinical phenomena related to the seizure pattern; at other times, they were unrelated. An afterdischarge caused by stimulation in the amygdala always spread to the ipsilateral hippocampus and occasionally to the opposite side. An afterdischarge from stimulation of the hippocampus usually, but not always, spread from the hippocampus to the amygdala. Afterdischarges were obtained from the side opposite the presumed focus. No significant differences in the parameters of stimulation were noted. As in spontaneous activity, afterdischarges clearly recorded by the depth electrodes were most frequently unaccompanied by significant scalp or nasopharyngeal electrode abnormalities.

Behavioral Results of Stimulation

In three patients, clinical seizures were activated by depth stimulation, and in each case the clinical activation and EEG focus were localized to the amygdaloid nucleus. Although the clinical seizure could be activated by stimulation of the amygdaloid region in these three patients, the physiological effects produced by electrical activation were often far more complex than the patient's own spontaneous seizures. Stimulation of the amygdaloid nuclear region, irrespective of whether it was the site of the clinical focus, always resulted in a greater variety of physiological and behavioral responses than stimulation of the hippocampus.

Amygdaloid stimulation resulted in motor, sensory, autonomic, and emotional changes which at times were quite complex. Only motor and epigastric sensations were noted from hippocampus activation. In one patient, both hippocampi were stimulated simultaneously, resulting in bilateral motor behavior, salivation, respiratory changes, and a marked postictal confusion. The poststimulation confusion was reminiscent of the mental changes noted in those few patients with bilateral temporal lobe lobectomies.

Except when a clinical focus was activated, the presence of clinical foci in the mesial temporal lobe structure did not appear to influence the kinds of responses that occurred during stimulation.

The general impression from stimulation was that the physiological effects may not only represent the local activation of the mesial temporal region but also activation of distant brain structures. No instance of aggressive behavior was associated with stimulation, and only one patient had a history of aggressive acts.

Stereotactic therapeutic lesions using an HF probe were made in three patients with combined unilateral amygdaloid-hippocampal lesion, while two patients had either a single hippocampal or amygdaloid lesion. Four patients showed a marked reduction of seizure intensity and frequency following combined amygdaloid-hipppocampal lesions but required low maintenance of anticonvulsant medication. One patient had no change in seizure frequency, but the intensity of the seizure subsided, with reduction in his aggressive behavior, which had been a problem preoperatively.

Reflex Epilepsy: Observations in Two Children with Implanted Electrodes in the Brainstem and Thalamus

Afferent stimuli under certain conditions may evoke an epileptic seizure designated as reflex epilepsy. These afferent stimuli appear to exert a facilitating influence upon the epileptic focus. Penfield favored the cortex as the site for this reflex facilitation (19) while Gastaut believed that the brainstem reticular formation was the site for the myoclonus activated by sensory stimulation (3). Depth electrode studies were carried out in two children who suffered from intense myoclonic seizures activated by simply touching the shoulder (18). These children were totally incapacitated from normal life because the seizures could not be controlled by medication.

It was reasoned that if the afferent stimulus could be blocked from reaching the cortex or thalamus, better control of the seizures might occur. Chronic electrodes were implanted in the sensory thalamus, ascending sensory pathways of the dorsolateral midbrain, and the fields of Forel. Extensive scalp and depth electrode recordings were made during afferent stimulation by simply tapping the child on the affected shoulder. In one patient, a 7-year-old female, myoclonic seizures were triggered by touching the left shoulder. Scalp EEGs revealed bilateral epileptic abnormalities, more in the right cortex than the left. A tap on the patient's left shoulder activated spike, and spike and wave in the right Rolandic region. The depth electrode recordings from the thalamus and brainstem revealed major subcortical epileptic discharges occurring from the left midbrain at the collicular level from the region of the dorsolateral tegmentum. The midbrain discharges followed the cortical discharges by 100 mscc. In the right brain, occasional discharges were noted in the prerubral region and the ventral thalamus. These also followed the cortical discharges. There was no correlation between the cortical and subcortical epileptic discharges. Immediately following the implantation of the depth electrodes, the seizures could no longer be elicited by touching the shoulders. The electrodes were simply withdrawn after several months and no further reflex seizures have occurred for 7 years. The patient may experience occasional spontaneous myoclonic seizures, but these have never been associated with a cutaneously evoked seizure caused by tapping the shoulder.

The second child was a 9-year-old female, who also suffered from severe reflex epilepsy activated mainly by touching the region of the left shoulder, or leg, as well as by loud sounds and startle. Medication was of no value, and the child was showing rapid signs of mental deterioration. Thalamic and midbrain electrodes were implanted, and preoperative scalp EEGs revealed lateralized slow sharp waves as well as bilateral cortical epileptic abnormalities. Bilateral cortical epileptic abnormalities were noted more frequently in the right central region as well as bilateral paroxysmal bursts of slow activity in the delta and theta frequency. Independent epileptic spikes were recorded in the pulvinar. Tactile stimulation of the left shoulder (site of reflex seizure) evoked bilateral cortical and subcortical diffuse abnormalities. Stimulation of the right shoulder evoked fewer cortical responses and diffuse subcortical discharges. A stereotactic lesion made to interrupt the spinoreticular pathways in the mesencephalon as well as the spinothalamic pathway resulted in no improvement in the child's reflex epilepsy. Postlesion examination of the child revealed no evidence of sensory deficit following the stereotactic lesions.

THE SLEEP RHYTHMS OF THE SUBCORTICAL NUCLEI OBSERVED IN MAN

A group of five patients were evaluated with studies of EEG sleep rhythm (25). Three had been admitted for evaluation of intractable central pain, one for epilepsy, and one for a severe dystonic syndrome. Briefly, it was observed that unique electrical activity was observed in the dorsal tegmentum which was specific for rapid eye movement (REM) sleep. In the C(2), D(3), and E(4) stages of sleep, the tegmental rhythms had a progressively wider range of rhythm than other subcortical areas. Sigma rhythms were seen only in the thalamus and were recorded primarily from the nucleus dorsalis medialis and the nucleus ventralis anterior.

Evoked photic responses were recorded in man from the thalamus and the midbrain (26). These included areas of the tegmentum, tectum, and ventral medial thalamus-medial pulvinar. Subcortical areas from which these evoked responses were obtained were contiguous. In addition, a variety of sensory, motor, and autonomic responses were obtained when these areas were stimulated.

EVALUATION OF CENTRAL PAIN SYNDROMES WITH DEPTH ELECTRODES

In 1966, Wilson and I reported a woman with a central pain syndrome following a vascular insult to the left thalamus and midbrain (15). She suffered from severe paroxysmal right facial pain, not unlike that described in trigeminal neuralgia, and was not relieved by a unilateral frontal lobotomy, peripheral neurectomy, or retrogasserian neurotomy. Following the experience of Spiegel and Wycis (23), a stereotactic mesencephalotomy was planned to relieve her pain, but in order to improve the localization of the stereotactic lesion, depth electrodes were implanted in the left midbrain and thalamus. To our surprise, spontaneous epileptic activity was recorded from the left dorsolateral mesencephalon at the level of the superior colliculus during her paroxysms of spontaneous facial pain.

Electrical stimulation of the same midbrain region reproduced her pain exactly, and subcortical epileptic afterdischarges were recorded from the same electrodes. A stereotactic lesion of the dorsolateral mesencephalon relieved her pain for 3 years, then she died of cardiac failure.

Three more patients with central pain were studied using depth electrodes, and we concluded that under some conditions central pain seemed to originate from spontaneous or stereotactically induced lesions of the dorsolateral portion of the midbrain, probably involving the spinothalamic or quintothalamic pathways. Electrical stimulation of these regions would activate the spontaneous pain, whereas a medially placed stereotactic midbrain lesion in the spinoreticular pathways would reduce it. Spontaneous or electrically evoked epileptic activity such as spikes and spike afterdischarges were recorded following stimulation of the dorsal midbrain, pretectum, and pulvinar in these three patients with central pain syndrome; however, spontaneous epileptic phenomena, as noted in the first woman, were not always associated with the patient's spontaneous pains. We have postulated that central pain may be an epileptic phenomenon.

THE MIDBRAIN AND PAIN

In 1969, Wilson and I reported on patients with intractable pain syndromes in which chronic stimulation was carried out in the rostral mesencephalon prior to the placement of a stereotactic lesion aimed at the spinothalamic, quinto-thalamic, and reticulospinal pathways, which lie in a close apposition adjacent to the periaqueductal gray at the level of the superior colliculus (17). Our observations of the patient's response to stimulation of this complex neural area led us to propose that the rostral mesencephalon was an important area for the integration of pain and its emotional components and that certain intractable pain suffering syndromes were in fact caused by pathophysiological changes of the mesencephalon. Further, we suggested that in the mesencephalon there was represented a lower level of conscious awareness to painful experience. Recent observations in awake animals, in which the median raphae nuclei have been stimulated with modification of the animal's response to pain, along with the new biochemical data suggesting that the endorphin may function as a neurotransmitter in the pain pathways, seem to support our concept that the mesencephalon and the central gray area represent important regions for the neural and biochemical basis of painful experiences in both animal and man.

Originally, Spiegel and Wycis reported a variety of sensory experiences when acutely stimulating patients undergoing stereotactic operations (23). Their patients reported a vague, unpleasant feeling usually localized to the central regions of the body. Stimulation was in or near the central gray of the rostral mesencephalon. Later, we extended these studies using chronic implanted electrodes in the midbrain prior to the placement of a therapeutic stereotactic lesion to relieve the patient's intractable pain. Our patients experience a variety of complex sensory, autonomical, and emotional responses, dependent on the location of the electrode within the dorsal midbrain, as well as the kind of electrical parameters used in the stimulation. Our observations revealed a topographic organization for sensation and emotion in the dorsolateral tegmentum. Based on our experience with electrical stimulation, the dorsolateral mesencephalon was divided into two distinct zones: a medial one extending from the lateral edge of the aqueduct to 5 mm laterally, and an area which included the periaqueductal gray and the surrounding tegmentum. A second more lateral zone lies between 5 and 12 mm from the midsagittal plane and includes the quintothalamic tract, lateral tegmentum, and lateral spinothalamic tract. The electrical stimulations of the mesencephalon were carried out when the patients were alert and cooperative. They described feelings such as "numbness," "electric shock," and "burning pain," and they quantitated the response such as "weak," "strong," "tense," "unpleasant," or "fearful." These patients were able to localize the site of evoked sensation accurately within a localized area of their bodies. They described the sensations as either superficial, i.e., situated in the skin, or deep in the bones or the abdominal and/or thoracic cavities. The quality of sensation varied at different sites of stimulation. Stimulating the region of the lateral spinothalamic tract produced rather "bright," "sharp," more "painful" feelings, while those sensations evoked nearer the medial lemniscus were described as less intense and as "numbness" or "tingling." High-frequency stimulation in both of these regions was often described as "painful." Stimulations in the more lateral zone were always referred to the contralateral side of the body, while those stimulations of the central gray were less exactly localized. Central gray stimulation was usually unpleasant, and the patient referred it to the head, neck, chest, or abdomen. A sensation of abnormal taste in the mouth was experienced by one patient. Another had a sensation around the heart without any change in the heart rate, while one woman complained of periumbilical and bladder sensations and a desire to void during central gray stimulation. The most striking findings were the strong emotional reactions experienced by the patient when stimulation occurred at the edge or nearby the central gray. Feelings of fear and death were often expressed. Autonomic activation consisted of contralateral piloerection, sweating, increase in the pulse and respiratory rate, blushing over the entire face and neck bilaterally, and, in some cases, epileptic afterdischarges were recorded from the electrode spontaneously as well as a poststimulus effect. These originated from the medial zone near the periaqueductal gray. These complex sensory reactions produced by stimulating the mesial midbrain area were reminiscent of the spontaneous reactions seen in some patients undergoing an intense painful experience or in those patients who were suffering from prolonged chronic pain. A small therapeutic lesion confined to the mesial mesencephalon did not result in analgesia but produced marked calming of the patient and relieved his suffering and pain. This was particularly striking in those patients suffering from the intractable pain of carcinoma of the head and neck (7).

It appears that the role of the mesencephalon in the genesis of certain types of spontaneous pain has taken on greater significance. Evidence in man and animals suggests that the dorsal rostromesencephalon is important for the integration of painful and emotional experiences, and restricted stereotactic lesions in this region, although not producing analgesia, do reduce the pain and suffering. It is to be hoped that the biochemical studies of this region of the brain will further advance our understanding of pain physiology and that pharmacological treatment can be devised to relieve the patient without resorting to neurosurgically placed lesions in the central nervous system.

REFERENCES

1. Fisher, C. M. (1965): Acute hypertensive cerebellar hemorrhage: Diagnosis and surgical treatment. *J. Nerv. Ment. Dis.,* 140:38–57.
2. Flanigin, H. F., Nashold, B. S., Jr., Wilson, W. P., and Nebes, R. (1976): Stimulation of the temporal lobe and thalamus in man and its relationship to memory and behavior. In: *Brain Stimulation Reward,* edited by A. Wauquier and E. T. Rolls, pp. 521–526. North Holland Publishing Co., The Netherlands.
3. Gastaut, H., and Pellegrin, J. (1947): L'epilepsie myoclonique. *France Med.* No. 4, April.
4. Heath, R. G., Peacock, S. M., Jr., Monroe, R. R., and Miller, W. H., Jr. (1954): *Studies in Schizophrenia.* Harvard University Press, Cambridge, Mass.
5. Nashold, B. S., Jr. (1970): Ocular reactions from brain stimulation in conscious man. *Neuro-Ophthalmology,* 5:92–103.
6. Nashold, B. S., Jr. (1970): Phosphenes and horizontal gaze produced by electrical stimulation of the midbrain in conscious man. *Arch. Ophthalmol.,* 84:433–435.
7. Nashold, B. S., Jr. (1972): Extensive cephalic and oral pain relieved by midbrain tractotomy. *Confin. Neurol.,* 34:382–388.
8. Nashold, B. S., Jr., Flanigin, H., Jr., Wilson, W. P., and Stewart, B. (1973): Stereotactic evaluation of bitemporal epilepsy with electrodes and lesions. *Confin. Neurol.,* 35:94–100.
9. Nashold, B. S., Jr., and Gills, P., Jr. (1967): Ocular signs resulting from brain stimulation and lesions in the human. *Arch. Ophthalmol.,* 77:609–618.
10. Nashold, B. S., Jr., Gills, J. P., Jr., and Wilson, W. P. (1967): Ocular signs of brain stimulation in the human. *Confin. Neurol.,* 29:169–174.
11. Nashold, B. S., Jr., and Seaber, J. H. (1972): Defect of ocular motility after stereotactic midbrain lesions in man. *Arch. Ophthalmol.,* 245–248.
12. Nashold, B. S., Jr., and Slaughter, D. G. (1969): Effects of stimulating or destroying the deep cerebellar regions in man. *J. Neurosurg.,* 31:172–186.
13. Nashold, B. S., Jr., Slaughter, D. G., and Gills, J. P., Jr. (1969): Ocular reactions in man from deep cerebellar stimulation and lesions. *Arch. Ophthalmol.,* 81:538–543.
14. Nashold, B. S., Jr., Stewart, B., and Wilson, W. P. (1972): Depth electrode studies in centrencephalic epilepsy. *Confin. Neurol.,* 34:252–263.
15. Nashold, B. S., Jr., and Wilson, W. P. (1966): Central pain: Observations in man with chronic implanted electrodes in the midbrain tegmentum. *Confin. Neurol.,* 27:30–44.
16. Nashold, B. S., Jr., and Wilson, W. P. (1966): Thalamic and mesencephalic epilepsy in the human. *Acta Conventus Neuropsychiatrici. EEG,* 25:441–450.
17. Nashold, B. S., Jr., and Wilson, W. P. (1970): Central pain and the irritable midbrain. In: *Pain and Suffering,* edited by B. L. Crue, pp. 95–118. Charles C Thomas, Springfield, Illinois.
18. Nashold, B. S., Jr., and Wilson, W. P. (1970): Reflex epilepsy: Observations in humans with implanted electrodes in brain stem and thalamus. *Activitas Nervosa Superior,* 12:181.
19. Penfield, W., and Jasper, H. (1954): *Epilepsy and the Functional Anatomy of the Human Brain.* Little, Brown, and Company, Boston.
20. Sem-Jacobsen, C. W., Petersen, M. C., Dodge, H. W., Jr., Lazarte, J. A., and Holman, C. B. (1956): Electroencephalographic rhythms from the depths of the parietal, occipital and temporal lobes in man. *Electroencephalogr. Clin. Neurophysiol.,* 8:263–278.
21. Sem-Jacobsen, C. W., Petersen, M. C., Lazarte, J. A., Dodge, H. W., and Holman, C. B. (1955): Electroencephalographic rhythms from the depths of the frontal lobe in 60 psychiatric patients. *Electroencephalogr. Clin. Neurophysiol.,* 7:193–210.

22. Spiegel, E. A. (1953): Mesencephalotomy in treatment of intractable facial pain. *Arch. Neurol. Psychiatr.,* 69:1–5.
23. Spiegel, E. A., and Wycis, H. T. (1962): *Stereoencephalotomy.* II. *Clinical and Physiological Applications.* Grune & Stratton, New York.
24. Spiegel, E. A., and Wycis, H. T. (1964): Stimulation of Forel's field during stereotactic operations in the human brain. *Electroencephalogr. Clin. Neurophysiol.,* 16:537–548.
25. Wilson, W. P., and Nashold, D. S., Jr. (1969): The sleep rhythms of subcortical nuclei: Some observations in man. *Biol. Psychiatry,* 1:289–296.
26. Wilson, W. P., and Nashold, B. S., Jr. (1973): Evoked photic responses from the human thalamus and midbrain. *Confin. Neurol.,* 35:338–345.

Functional Neurosurgery, edited by T. Rasmussen
and R. Marino. Raven Press, New York © 1979.

Stereotactic Neuroradiology and Functional Neurosurgery: Localization of Cortical Structures by Three-Dimensional Angiography

Gabor Szikla

*Service de Neurochirurgie Fonctionnelle, Centre Hospitalier Sainte-Anne, 1, rue Cabanis
75674 Paris Cedex 14, France*

The original title suggested for this chapter was Functional Neuroradiology. Obviously, there is a sort of logical inconsistency in this title, as X-ray studies, however sophisticated, will never show functions, but only the form of the brain. We therefore changed the title to "Stereotactic Neuroradiology and Functional Neurosurgery." Still, in spite of its apparently contradictory terms, the first title emphasizes a fundamental point, which is that precise three-dimensional radiologic information on brain anatomy is not only an indispensable instrumental tool for stereotactic procedures, but can constitute *a basic framework for the study of functional neuroanatomy in living man.* This might be particularly useful in the study of the pathology of specifically human higher nervous functions related to specific structures of the brain cortex, such as speech.

"By this means, every cubic millimeter in the brain can be easily identified, recorded, and referred to." This ambitious statement, quoted from the first description of Clarke and Horsley (2), characterizes the aim of the stereotactic approach to cerebral anatomy. Because of the efforts of a great number of devoted students, this precise transcription of the anatomy of the brain in three-dimensional coordinates was progressively elaborated for many species of laboratory animals, and illustrated by an ever growing number of stereotactic brain atlases.

Guided by the experience gained in animal experimentation, the stereotactic anatomy of the deep nuclear masses and fiber tracts of the human brain was established some decades later. In the field of the human brain cortex, however, to the study of which the stereotactic methods were progressively extended, the present state of our knowledge of the three-dimensional anatomy lags far behind the aim expressed by Clarke and Horsley: *in vivo* localization of the gyri and sulci in man is clearly worlds away from the ambitiously fixed goal of identification of the "cubic millimeter."

But even giving up the idea of such precision (whose usefulness might even be questioned), one is still struck by the extraordinary contrast between our knowledge of the minute details of the three-dimensional organization of the smallest subnuclei and their neuronal circuitry in experimental animals and the crudely approximate localization of even the principal morphologic elements of the brain cortex in living man.

One of the reasons contributing to such a discrepancy is undoubtedly related to the complex and variable folding pattern of the human telencephalon. On the other hand, while the concept of "target points" with three spatial coordinates may be applied—at least theoretically—to diencephalic nuclei, it is clearly inadequate to express the three-dimensional pattern of gyri and sulci representing complex and comparatively large volumes and surfaces extending over several centimeters.

Such information, however, is necessary and in fact indispensable in several fields of functional neurosurgery, the best example of which is the delimitation and removal of cortical epileptogenic areas. Similarly, stereotactic methods were introduced in the past years in other fields such as focal irradiation of small hemispheric tumors and treatment of some arteriovenous malformations. In all these fields, knowledge of the three-dimensional functional anatomy of the human brain cortex can contribute to the planning of surgical procedure or radiation therapy, to the evaluation of functional risks, and to the understanding of the consequences of the various procedures.

In spite of this obvious practical necessity, not much has to be changed today in the words of W. Penfield (7) written more than 20 years ago: clinicians and psychologists are left "stranded upon the vast shores of the cerebral cortex *with no chart and no compass to guide them.*" Though much data have been collected since this statement, our knowledge still remains fragmentary and consists for the greater part of more or less hazardous extrapolations from animal to man.

This chapter therefore illustrates the contribution of stereotactic methods, and of stereotactic angiography in particular, to a more precise knowledge of the functional anatomy of the human telencephalon and especially the brain cortex.

TECHNICAL NOTE

The application over the past 20 years of stereotactic investigation to the surgery of focal epilepsy, especially the localization of cortical epileptogenic foci by stereo-EEG, has gradually enlarged the field of stereotactic procedures—first to the temporal lobe (14) and then to the whole cerebral cortex (1). Obviously, the introduction of intracerebral electrodes as well as the interpretation of the recorded data necessitate the detailed localization of the structures investigated. The need for precision has prompted considerable anatomoradiographic research at our institution over a long period of time; this has resulted in a stereotactic system of localization of telencephalic structures (15). This system was based on the study of serial sections of the brain, oriented in sagittal, horizontal, and vertical planes with reference to the midline and to a line drawn between the anterior and posterior commissures of the third ventricle (AC-PC line) and on neuroradiologic examinations obtained by orthogonal teleradiography with the patient's head fixed in the stereotactic frame (Fig. 1).

Though several major cortical structures can be recognized on pneumoencephalograms, air studies yield only fragmentary information concerning the localization of sulci and gyri, especially on the lateral and inferior aspects of the hemispheres. This shortcoming of direct visualization led us to develop an indirect localization system based on stereotactic reference planes. We employed the relatively constant relationships existing between the commissures of the third ventricle and the principal fissures of the cortex in order to define statistically their zone of variability, with reference to the bicommissural orientation lines. The width of the distribution bands of the large sulci is on the order of 1 cm, by this method of indirect statistical localization (Fig. 2).

CORTICAL LOCALIZATION BY THREE-DIMENSIONAL ANGIOGRAPHY

The need for more precision led us to study the anatomoradiologic correlations of the cerebrovascular system, trying to develop a method for the direct identification of sulci and gyri in the individual patient by angiography. This second study of radiographic localization of cortical structures, done in the course of the past 5 years, has shown that the entire surface anatomy of the hemispheres is inscribed in the tortuous course of the cortical blood vessels and can be extracted from the angiogram by an adequate way of reading.

Our first attempt (15) to use angiography for cortical localization, trying to apply data from the current literature such as the templates of Ring (8) or of Salamon (9) to our stereotactic localization studies, however, demonstrated a disappointing variability of vascular patterns without a consistent topographic relationship to already established data on stereotactic neuroanatomy. In retrospect, this was because, like other workers, we considered the *entire course* of an arterial branch as seen on the *lateral view* only, and tried to identify *specific arteries* ("rolandic," "angular," etc.) corresponding to the generally used terminology. Actually, we only rarely found a rolandic artery whose course conformed topographically to the statistical distribution band of the central sulcus.

In our studies, however, we became progressively more aware of the frequent repetition of some details such as loops and changes in direction of arteries in the same areas on the radiographs obtained during stereotactic procedures. This prompted us to study the anatomic correlation of these "vascular landmarks"

FIG. 1. (See pages 200–201) Stereotactic neuroradiology: orthogonal 4.3 m teleradiographs are taken with the patient's head fixed in the Talairach frame. **(A):** Head and frame. *Arrows:* X-ray incidences. **(B–D):** Identical geometry of all radiographs allows for detailed three-dimensional anatomic interpretation, right-left comparison, and **(E,F)** for comparison with control study 1 year later. (From ref. 12.)

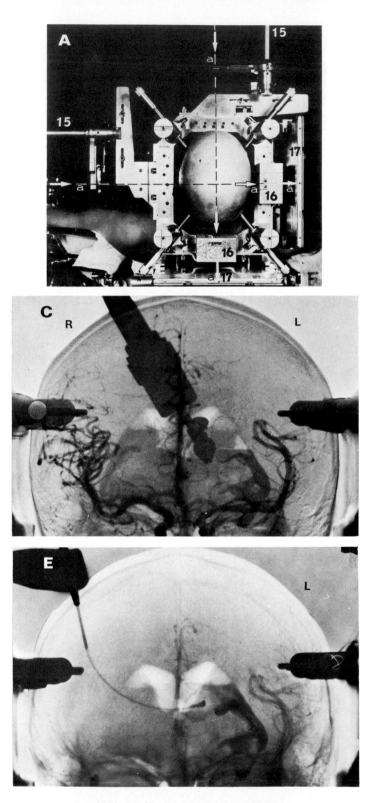

FIG. 1A-F. See legend page 199.

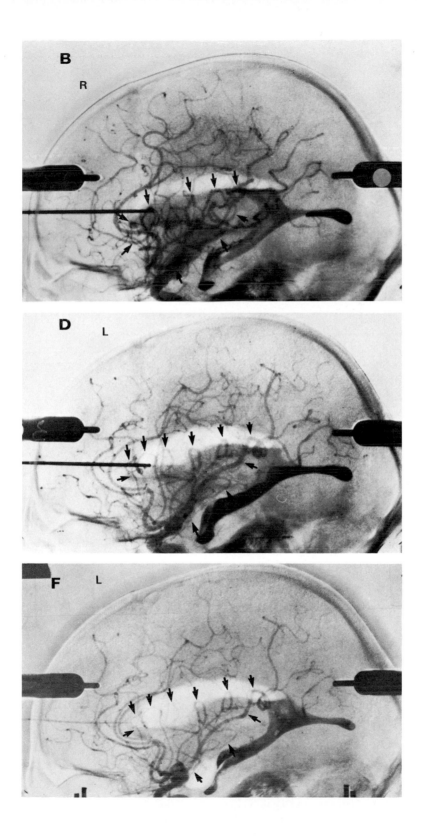

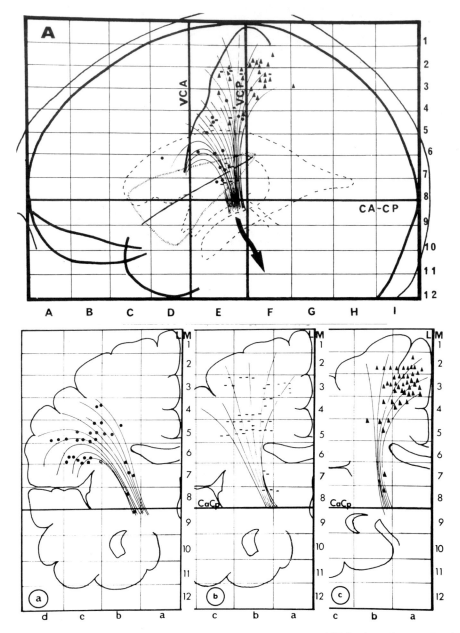

FIG. 2. Statistical localization of some cortical structures by the ACPC-oriented proportional grid. **(A):** Topography of motor points (●, face-tongue; —, upper, and ▲, lower extremity contractions elicited by intracerebral 1 cps threshold bipolar electrical stimulation in 30 surgical epilepsy cases). The upper figure shows the lateral view. The statistical projection area of the central sulcus redrawn from sagittal sections of 20 hemispheres is shaded. The lower figure shows the frontal projection. **(B):** Statistical localization of 1. inferior frontal sulcus; 2. insula; 3. sylvian fissure, surface; 4. superior temporal sulcus; 5. middle temporal sulcus; 6. central fissure; 7. parieto-occipital; and 8. calcarine sulci. (From ref. 12.)

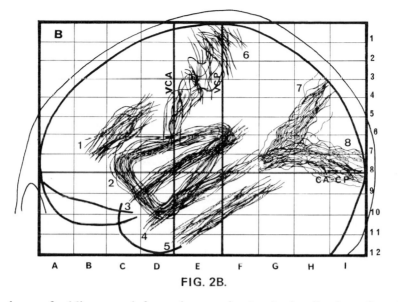

FIG. 2B.

in the hope of adding new information on the *in vivo* localization of cortical structures.

Soon it became clear that the true significance of an angiographic detail cannot be reliably established on the basis of the lateral view alone. A loop suggesting the existence of a sulcus might as well occur on the free surface of a gyrus, for instance. This led us to follow blood vessels simultaneously on both lateral and frontal projections and to use more and more stereoscopic angiograms. The latter proved especially useful and soon became the principal tool allowing for the three-dimensional, "anatomical," interpretation of the cortical angiogram (10,11,13).

The basic anatomic fact emerging from our anatomoradiological studies can be summed up briefly and is illustrated in Figs. 3–5. Between their main trunks and their terminal intraparenchymal branches, the cerebral arteries—and, to a lesser extent, the cerebral veins—adhere intimately to the cortical surface on which they run.

The cortical angiogram reflects the embryonic development of the cortex. Uneven regional growth leads to infolding of the originally smooth curved surface of the telencephalic vesicle. The sulci, as they appear, form a constant three-dimensional pattern related to local structural and eventually functional differences of the cortex (5). While in the early fifth month the vessels constitute a regular fan of straight dichotomizing branches, the progressive deepening of sulci between the developing gyri introduces a distortion in the simple original pattern (Figs. 3A and 5).

As shown by the artist's drawing (Fig. 4B), beneath the crevice visible on the cortical surface, the infolded cortex of the sulcal walls attains a great depth and has a characteristic three-dimensional pattern. It might be recalled here

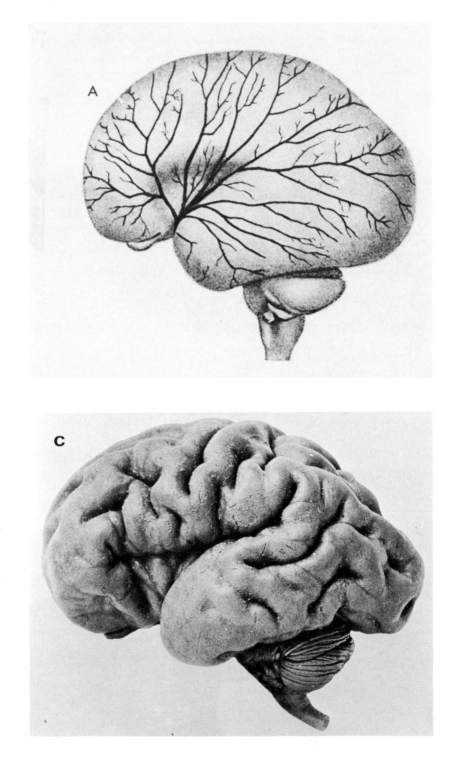

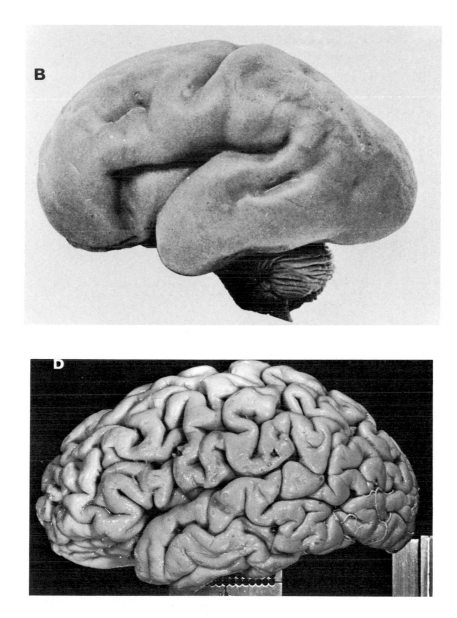

FIG. 3. Successive stages of the cortical folding process: **(A):** Early fifth, **(B):** sixth, and **(C):** seventh month embryo. (D): Adult hemisphere. (**A, B,** and **C** from Retzius, 1895; **D** from ref. 12.)

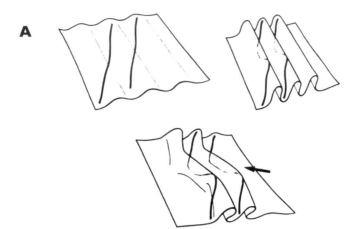

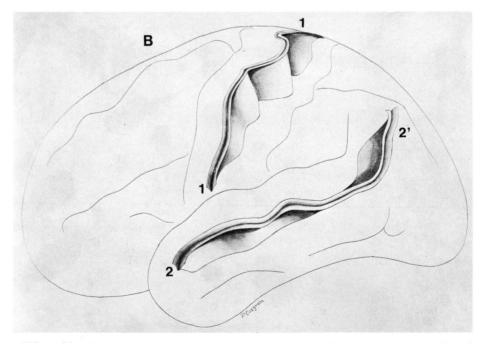

FIG. 4. Distortion of the initially regular vascular pattern (see Fig. 3A) by the formation of sulci and gyri. **(A):** Diagram of the rolandic region at three successive stages. The infolding of the inferior frontal sulcus bends the originally straight rolandic sulcus (genu inferior, *arrow*). **(B):** Depth and typical three-dimensional pattern of 1. central and 2. superior temporal sulci. **(C):** Vascular lamina of the central sulcus, composed of all arteries running on its walls. The precentral gyrus is removed, but vessels on its posterior aspect are preserved. Frontal view. (From ref. 12.)

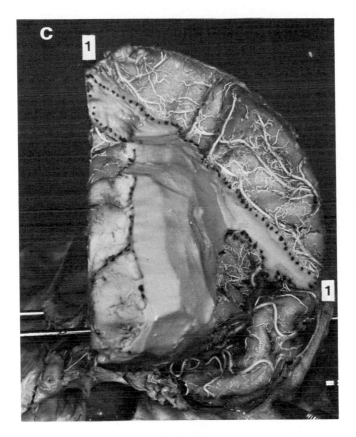

FIG. 2C.

that more than two-thirds of the cortex is buried in the depth of the sulci. Localization of these hidden surfaces by angiography must take into account their depth, form, and orientation. Generally, the courses of cortical arteries and veins do not follow a sulcus or gyrus for its entire length and as Duret (3) stated as early as 1874—"they do not have to provide branches for each of them in particular." Anatomically, after traversing the free surface of a gyrus, the arteries then enter the sulcus, descending more or less obliquely into its depth, then climb back to the surface on the opposite wall and become visible again on the neighboring gyrus.

Major sulci are crossed in this way by several arterial branches whose courses follow the invaginated deep surfaces. The initial extracerebral segments of cortical veins likewise follow the surface of the buried cortex, imprisoned between the sulcal walls. These deep segments of arteries and veins, taken together, form the composite vascular lamina, corresponding to and therefore outlining the location of the sulci. Figure 4C shows the vascular lamina in the central

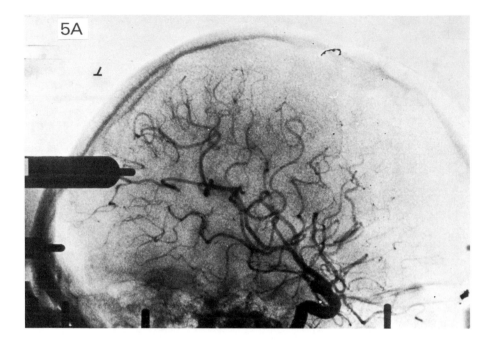

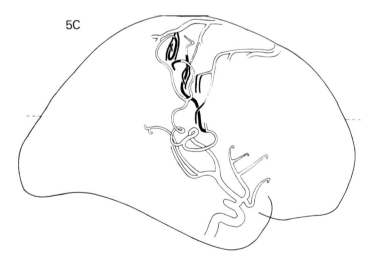

FIG. 5. Example of a sulcal pattern extracted from a three-dimensional angiogram. **(A** and **B)**: Stereoscopic angiogram of the middle cerebral artery. **(C)**: Diagram of arteries and veins in the region of central sulcus. Deep intrasulcal segments are drawn in black. **(D):** Intrasulcal segments. Arrows show points where vessels enter or leave the depth of the sulcus. **(E):** Representation of the central sulcus. [Compare with (6) in Fig. 2B.] (From ref. 12.)

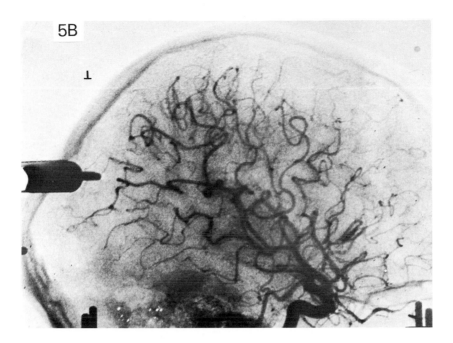

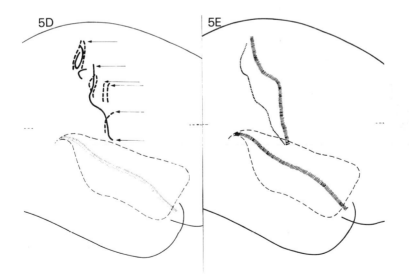

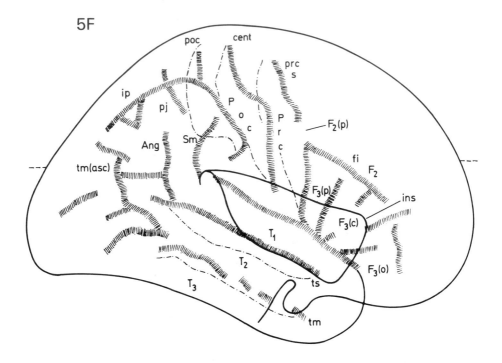

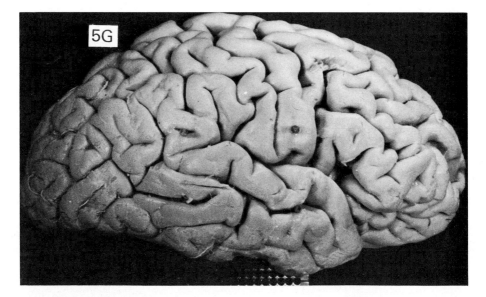

FIG. 5F and G. Example of a sulcal pattern extracted from a three-dimensional angiogram. **(F):** Surface pattern of the territory of the middle cerebral artery, extracted from the above angiogram. **(G):** Note resemblance of angiographic sulcal pattern to the lateral view of a random anatomical specimen. (From ref. 12.)

sulcus of a specimen where the arteries have been injected. Such images clearly reflect the fact that independently of the variable branching pattern of individual arteries, it is the *depth* of the vessels that provides the clue for the anatomic understanding of cortical patterns. The pia mater carrying the arteries and the initial part of the veins adheres intimately to the cortical surface, free or buried. It constitutes a vascular envelope for the brain, comparable to a tightly fitting garment, "tunica vascularis," revealing the shape of the underlying body, that is, the convexities and concavities, gyri and sulci of the cortical surface.

It is therefore the tortuosity of the cerebral vessels that reflects the anatomy of the underlying cortex, and it is by the separation of the superficial and deep segments in their course that one can extract the topographic information present in an angiogram.

For example, Fig. 5C shows the courses of some arteries and veins in the central region. The deep segments buried in the central sulcus are drawn in black. Figure 5D shows the isolated intrasulcal segments forming a mold, as it were, of the sulcus, represented in Fig. 5E.

The topographic information contained in the middle cerebral angiogram reproduced in stereoscopy on top of Fig. 5 is summarized—at least in part— in the diagram of Fig. 5F. Comparison of the surface anatomy revealed by the stereoscopic view of this clinical angiogram with the photograph of a random anatomic specimen (Fig. 5G) shows a striking similarity.

As Egas Moniz (6) wrote in an early publication: "If one is somewhat familiarized with the anatomy of the convolutions and of the more important parts of the brain, one can easily read the radio-arteriographic document *as a photograph of the morphology of the particular brain.*"

In the light of our studies we fully agree with this statement. In our everyday practice, angiography became a fundamental tool to recognize and thereby localize the different structures of the cerebral cortex *in vivo* (12). Experience has shown, however, that such detailed anatomic reading of the angiographic pictures, the mental transformation of the image of the brain vascular tree into a photograph of the brain, is probably less easily acquired than was foreseen by Moniz. The difficulty seems to be twofold: difficulty of conceiving the three-dimensional anatomy of the brain as it really is and as it appears in radiographic projections, and difficulty of considering the angiographic images in three dimensions, so as to reconstitute the anatomy of the surfaces bearing the opacified vessels. Teaching experience, however, has also shown that the necessary initial anatomic and stereoradiographic effort is usually largely compensated by the spatial view of the patient's brain given by stereoangiography.

PATHOLOGIC DEPTH PATTERNS: DISTORTION OF THE SULCAL VASCULAR PATTERN BY SPACE-OCCUPYING AND ATROPHIC LESIONS

As is well known, major sulci penetrate deeply into the brain substance, some of them approaching the ventricular wall and occasionally indenting it.

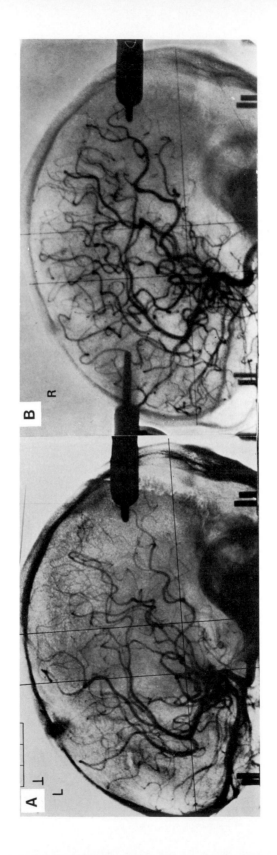

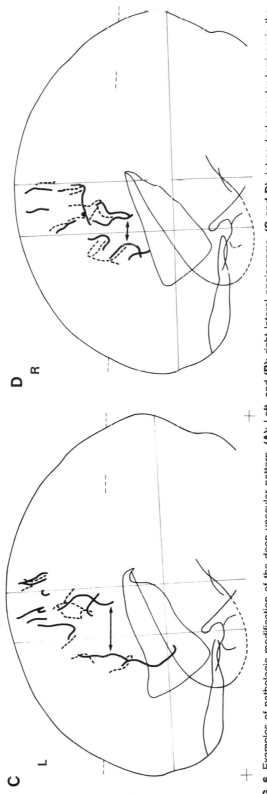

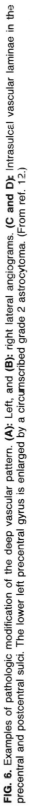

FIG. 6. Examples of pathologic modification of the deep vascular pattern. **(A):** Left, and **(B):** right lateral angiograms. **(C and D):** Intrasulcal vascular laminae in the precentral and postcentral sulci. The lower left precentral gyrus is enlarged by a circumscribed grade 2 astrocytoma. (From ref. 12.)

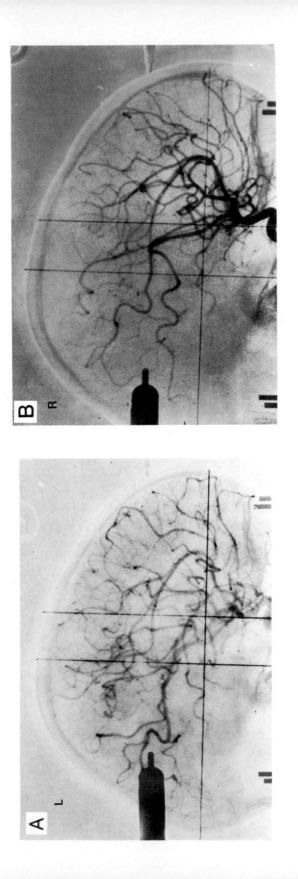

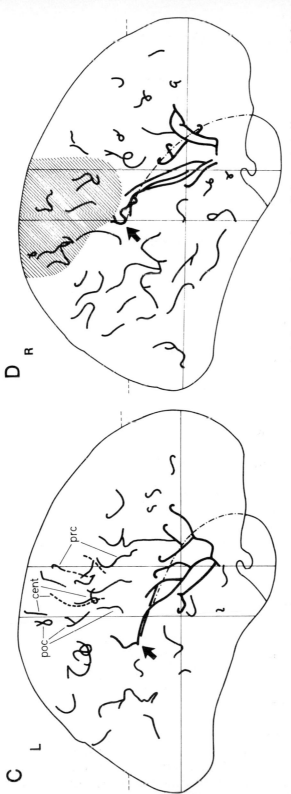

FIG. 7. (A and B): Left and right lateral angiograms. **(C and D):** A right-sided local cortical atrophy in the upper rolandic region, well demonstrated by pneumoencephalography *(shaded area)*. The deep vascular pattern, normal in the left hemisphere **(A and C)**, is shallow and irregular in the right hemisphere **(B and D)**. Sylvian fissure and insula are attracted toward the atrophic area *(arrows)*. (From ref. 12.)

They thus subdivide the volume of the hemispheres into more or less separate compartments. The pial membrane, which contains the blood vessels, penetrates into the depth of the sulci. Obviously, pathologic displacements of the brain substance will modify the pattern of the sulci and consequently the topography and general pattern of the corresponding vascular laminae. These distortions may be caused by space-occupying lesions or they can result from atrophic processes. Just as in the case of the well-known shifts of the midline blood vessels, an expanding lesion displaces the intrasulcal vascular laminae away from its center, while local atrophy draws them in toward the lesion. Such distortions may be caused either by immediate local pressure or by the attraction exerted directly by the pathologic process, but it may also appear at a distance, resulting from the displacement of neighboring brain tissue. Pathologic modifications of the cortical vascular patterns are illustrated in Figs. 6 and 7. The first four pictures (Fig. 6A–D) demonstrate angiographic changes induced by a relatively small expanding lesion without other major neuroradiologic signs.

Changes of the sulcal vascular pattern caused by space-occupying lesions may be summed up very simply: (a) Sulci overlying an expanding lesion are flattened out or disappear completely. (b) Neighboring sulci are distorted and/ or shifted away from the lesion. (c) A tumor growing in a gyrus pushes apart the sulci lying on its sides (Fig. 6A–D: superficial astrocytoma grade 2 in left lower precentral gyrus).

Figure 7A–D shows the effect of focal cortical atrophy distorting the pattern of sulci. In opposition to the mass effect of expanding lesions, the retraction of the corticomeningeal scar tissue exerts a reversed action on the brain that might be called a "negative mass effect," displacing the structures toward the lesion.

In this case, atrophy of the right superior central region was well demonstrated by pneumoencephalography (shaded in diagram). Angiographically, the vascular pattern of the right central region (Fig. 7B–D) is shallow and atypical in contrast to the normal pattern on the left (Fig. 7A–C). Moreover, upward displacement of the posterior part of the right sylvian fissure (arrow) together with the posterior cingulate and marginal sulci, appears clearly in three-dimensional angiography.

CONCLUDING REMARKS

The foregoing material was intended to illustrate that the precise three-dimensional X-ray information obtained in stereotactic projections gives a detailed definition of the anatomy of the individual brain. Stereoscopic-stereotactic angiography in particular reveals the complex surface pattern of the human brain cortex, allowing for direct visualization of sulci and gyri, normal or pathologically distorted.

The functional correlates of some elements of the gyral pattern are well known, especially with regard to the primary sensorimotor areas such as the central gyri, the lips of the calcarine sulcus, or the cortex of Heschl's transverse gyrus. While the precise localization of these areas in the brain of the individual patient can have an obvious practical utility in surgery, detailed information on brain anatomy *in vivo* might serve the purposes of further research on higher brain functions as well. By relating data recorded or elicited from the different parts of the human brain cortex to anatomically distinct structures, or by careful localization of cortical excisions and detailed analysis of their functional consequences (as will be illustrated by the presentation on removal of cortical epileptogenic areas), our knowledge of the functional anatomy of the human brain might be significantly improved.

Thus, for example, the existence of statistically significant asymmetry in the gyral patterns of the left and right cerebral hemispheres has been repeatedly reported in recent years (4,16). Stereoangiographic study of the posterior sylvian region has allowed the establishment in a quantitative way of the fact of the same asymmetry in living patients (10,13). This in turn might well provide the clue for establishing how far this morphologic asymmetry is related to hemispheric dominance and speech functions.

REFERENCES

1. Bancaud, J., Talairach, J., Bonis, A., Schaub, C., Szikla, G., Morel, P., and Bordas-Ferrer, M. (1965): *La Stéréo-Électro-Encéphalographie Dans L'épilepsie.* Masson, Paris.
2. Clarke, R. H., and Horsley, V. (1906): On a method of investigating the deep ganglia and tracts of the central nervous system (cerebellum). *Br. Med. J.,* 2.1799–1800.
3. Duret, H. (1874): Recherches anatomiques sur la circulation de l'encéphale. *Arch. Physiol. Norm. Pathol.,* Ser. 2, 1:316–353, 646–693, 919–957.
4. Geschwind, N., and Levitsky, W. (1968): Left-right asymmetries in temporal speech regions. *Science,* 161:186–187.
5. Le Gros Clark, W. E. (1947): Deformation patterns in the cerebral cortex. In: *Essays on Growth and Form presented to D'Arcy Wentworth Thompson.* Clarendon Press, Oxford, England.
6. Moniz, E., Dias, A., and Lima, A. (1928): La radio-artériographie et la topographie cranioencéphalique. *J. Radiol. (Paris),* 12:72–82.
7. Penfield, W., and Jasper, H. (1954): *Epilepsy and the Functional Anatomy of the Human Brain.* Little, Brown, and Company, Boston, Massachusetts.
8. Ring, B. A., and Waddington, M. M. (1967): Angiographic identification of the motor strip. *J. Neurosurg.,* 26:249–254.
9. Salamon, G., Gonzalès, J., Raybaud, C., and Guidicelli, G. (1971): Analyse angiographique des branches corticales de l'artère sylvienne. A propos d'un nouveau procédé de repérage angiographique. *Neurochirurgie,* 17:177–189.
10. Szikla, G., Bouvier, G., and Hori, T. (1975): Localization of brain sulci and convolutions by arteriography: A stereotactic anatomoradiological study. *Brain Res.,* 95:497–502.
11. Szikla, G., Bouvier, G., and Hori, T. (1976): Encéphalographie arterielle. Étude stéréotaxique des repères vasculaires corticaux. *Ann. Radiol.,* 19:217–222.
12. Szikla, G., Bouvier, G., Hori, T., and Petrov, V. (1977): *Angiography of the Human Brain Cortex: Atlas of Vascular Patterns and Stereotactic Cortical Localization.* Springer-Verlag, Berlin.
13. Szikla, G., Hori, T., and Bouvier, G. (1975): The third dimension in cerebral angiography: A stereotactic study on cortical localization and hemispheric asymmetry in living man. In: *Advances in Cerebral Angiography,* edited by G. Salamon. Springer-Verlag, Berlin.
14. Talairach, J., David, M., and Tournoux, P. (1958): *L'exploration Chirurgicale Stéréotaxique du Lobe Temporal dans l'épilepsie Temporale.* Masson, Paris.
15. Talairach, J., Szikla, G., Tournoux, P., Prosalentis, A., Covello, L., Bordas-Ferrer, M., Jacob, M., and Mempel, E. (1967): *Atlas D'Anatomie Stéréotaxique du Télencéphale.* (French-English edition). Masson, Paris.
16. Wada, J. A., Clarke, R., and Hamm, A. (1975): Cerebral hemispheric asymmetry in humans: Cortical speech zones in 100 adult and 100 infant brains. *Arch. Neurol.,* 32:239–246.

Functional Neurosurgery, edited by T. Rasmussen
and R. Marino. Raven Press, New York © 1979.

Stereotactic Neuroradiological Concepts Applied to Surgical Removal of Cortical Epileptogenic Areas

Jean Talairach and Gabor Szikla

*Department of Functional Neurosurgery, Université René Descartes, Hôpital Ste. Anne,
75014 Paris, France*

This presentation is intended to illustrate that the precise information obtained by stereotactic techniques can guide open surgical procedures as well as those performed with stereotactic methods.

Some basic concepts should be considered first, especially the meaning of the term *stereotaxis.* While often understood in a limited sense as being synonymous with specific procedures performed essentially at the level of the basal ganglia using specific stereotactic devices, stereotaxis is in fact a general diagnostic and therapeutic concept which has as its aim the precise three-dimensional representation of the entirety of the patient's brain. The three-dimensional representation is based on anatomical, neuroradiological, and other localizing information, the spatial integration of which allows for a more precise "anatomical" approach to the human brain and to the surgical management of localized pathological processes. Literally, stereotaxis means "orientation in space." Taken in this general sense, all surgical procedures obviously are, or at least should be, "stereotactic."

At our institution, stereotactic methods have been progressively applied over the past 25 years to deep and cortical telencephalic structures, mainly for the management of surgical epilepsies and intracranial tumors.

Excision of cortical epileptogenic areas represents a good example of the utilization of precise neuroradiological and stereoelectroencephalographic information at craniotomy.

Unquestionably, recent progress in neuroradiology has contributed greatly to the amelioration of neurosurgical techniques. Nevertheless, a certain disparity persists between the information furnished by conventional neuroradiology and that which would be most useful at the time of surgery. Despite the ever finer details detected by sophisticated neuroradiological procedures, at craniotomy the neurosurgeon still has but a rather approximate anatomical orientation on the exposed brain. This is particularly true with regard to the cortical territory that neither his vision nor the conventional radiographic documents allow him to recognize and to localize with satisfactory accuracy. In fact, inspection of the exposed cortex gives but a poor orientation to the surgeon. One might

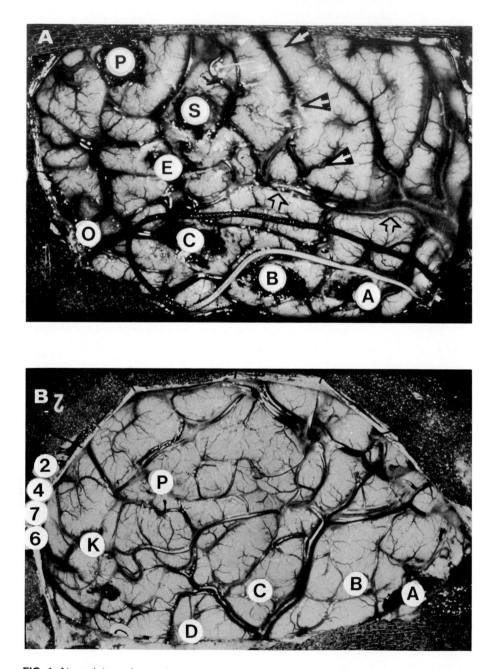

FIG. 1. At craniotomy, inspection of the exposed cortex gives only poor anatomical orientation. **(A):** Sylvian and sometimes Rolandic fissures (open and white arrows, respectively) can be recognized. **(B** and **C):** In most cases, the exposed gyri and the underlying deep (e.g., ventricular) structures can only be identified by comparison with radiographic data. Capital letters indicate electrode penetration points.

quote the words of Wilder Penfield: "The sylvian and interhemispheral fissures are the only landmarks on the brain surface which can be recognized with any degree of accuracy. Indeed, the rolandic fissure can hardly be recognized until after stimulation has identified it." (Fig. 1).

This information deficit can be filled by neuroradiology, provided studies are performed in a precise three-dimensional manner within a stereotactic framework. According to our experience, such stereotactic neuroradiological data can give to the surgeon exact orientation on the exposed cortex as well as on the topography of the underlying deep structures.

Technical details of stereotactic neuroradiological procedures and their three-dimensional interpretation have been repeatedly described (4–6) and are briefly summarized in Chapter 14 of this book. Here we will only stress the basic requirement of orthogonal biplane radiography with a common reference system in both frontal and lateral projections, allowing for three-dimensional reconstruction of all visualized structures. At craniotomy, adequate orientation of the patient's head according to radiological planes facilitates the transposition of the natural size teleradiographic data to the operative field (Fig. 2).

SURGICAL ASPECTS OF STEREO-EEG INVESTIGATION AT EPILEPSY

We cannot discuss here methods and general concepts of Stereo-EEG investigations (1,2,5) (Fig. 3). Some practical aspects relevant to surgical techniques and orientation will only be mentioned briefly.

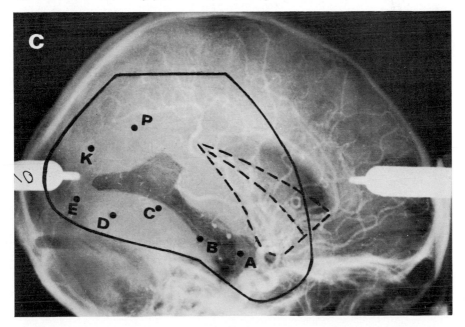

FIG 1C.

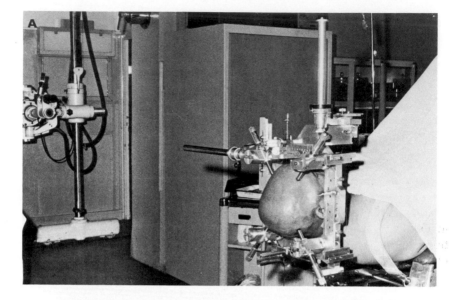

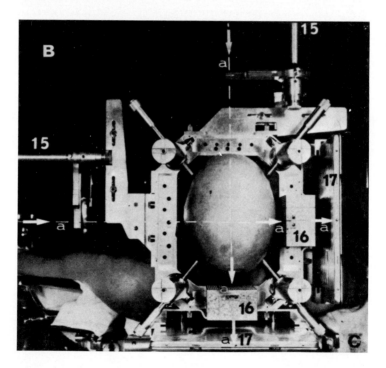

FIG. 2A and B. Contrast studies performed in stereotactic biplane orthogonal teleradiographic projections give undistorted natural size radiographs, allowing for precise localization of the different parts of the brain.

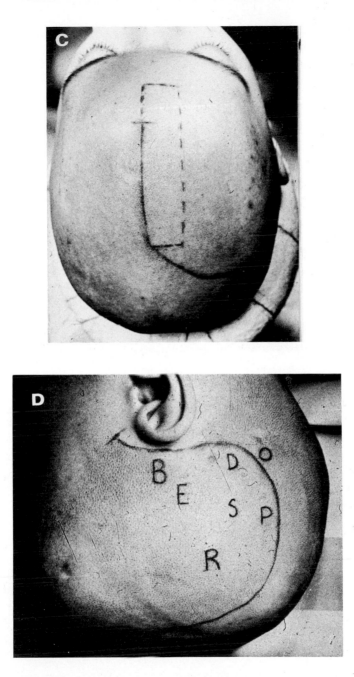

FIG. 2C and D. Direct transposition of three-dimensional radiographic data to the operating field is facilitated by adequate positioning of the head, according to radiographic planes. Note marks left on the skin by intracerebral electrode placement (capital letters in **D**), orienting scalp and bone flap.

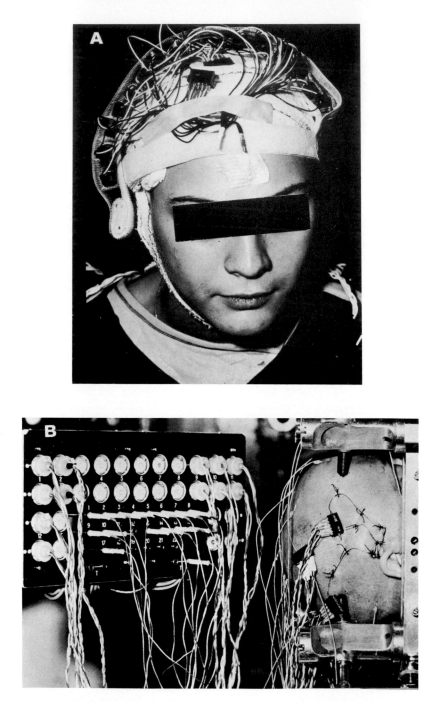

FIG. 3. Stereoelectroencephalographic localization of epileptogenic area. After stereotactic neuroradiological workup, electrode plan is established according to clinical and surface EEG findings, vascular pattern, and surgical considerations. Flexible multilead electrodes are inserted with stereotactic techniques. **(A):** Chronic telemetric recording. **(B):** Acute investigation in the operating theater; the patient's head is held by the stereotactic frame. Electrodes are fixed to the skin. **(C and D):** Left facial contraction, related to a discharge in the Rolandic operculum *(arrows).*

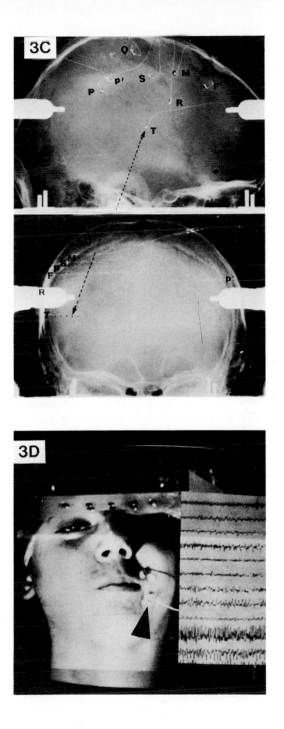

The precision of the stereotactic neuroradiological data allows for the correct and safe placement of intracerebral electrodes inserted with stereotactic techniques described elsewhere (5,6). The electrode plan is established according to: (a) clinical and EEG data; (b) neuroradiological information especially on the vascular pattern; and (c) surgical considerations.

A stereotactic diagram resumes significant neuroradiological features together with actual position of electrodes shown by control radiographs (Fig. 4). The extension of the epileptogenic area localized by the Stereo-EEG investigation is indicated on the same drawing. On this document, the limits of the surgical excision can be planned and mapped, taking into account, e.g., the relationship to the ventricle, the insula, and the topography of blood vessels to be respected or sacrificed depending upon their territory (Fig. 5A).

At craniotomy, this map provides an easy reference for delimiting the area to be excised. The penetration points of the electrodes, together with the superficial segments of arteries and veins, provide a satisfactory number of landmarks to eliminate all possible errors (Fig. 5B). Photographs taken at the end of the excision (Fig. 5C) allow for precise anatomical identification of the removed gyri.

Control angiography performed after surgery shows whether regional blood flow has been preserved (filling of arteries bridging the excised area; Fig. 6A and B). The surgical lesion can thus be rather precisely delimited. From the beginning to the end, the surgical procedure is guided by the stereoradiographic documents disclosing in fact the three-dimensional anatomy of the given brain, transferred to the operating field. In this way, surgery can acquire a higher degree of accuracy.

Beyond the immediate benefit to the individual patient, this type of neuroradiologically oriented and controlled surgical lesions may contribute more generally to our knowledge of functional localization in the brain cortex.

Detailed three-dimensional demonstration of the patient's brain before and after surgery may in fact add precise data on anatomical correlations of postoperative neurological deficits. Some examples could illustrate this point.

Figures 4–7 demonstrate a case where Stereo-EEG investigation indicated a large right temporoparietal epileptogenic area, including supramarginal and angular gyri (Fig. 4). At surgery, superficial vascular patterns shown by stereoangiography and electrode traces allow for the recognition of the exposed gyri and for a precise delimitation of the excision (Figs. 5 and 7). Regional blood flow has been preserved during subpial excision, as shown by control angiography (Fig. 6A and B). Postoperative neurological deficit 3 weeks after surgery is limited to partial left superior quadrantanopsia, without any apraxic or agnosic signs (Fig. 6C and D). In 17 similar cases, where the right temporoparietal junctional area has been removed without interfering with the arterial supply of neighboring gyri, detailed neurological examination done by Dr. H. Hécaën found only twice the neurological symptoms usually attributed to cortical lesions of this area (3). It might therefore be supposed that lesions producing the aprac-

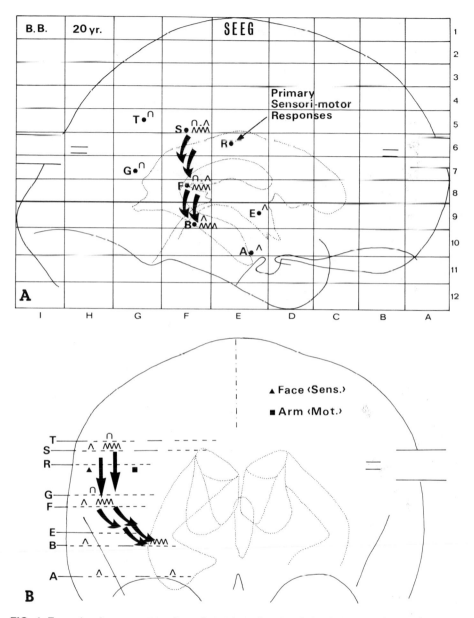

FIG. 4. Example of open surgery for epilepsy based on stereotactic investigations. Recorded information is summarized in stereotactic diagrams used for detailed planning of surgery. ∩, lesional; ∧, irritative; ∧∧, epileptogenic areas. Arrows indicate spread of seizure discharge.

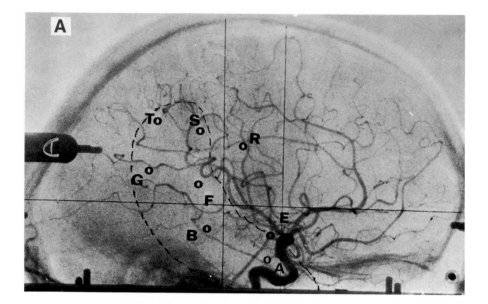

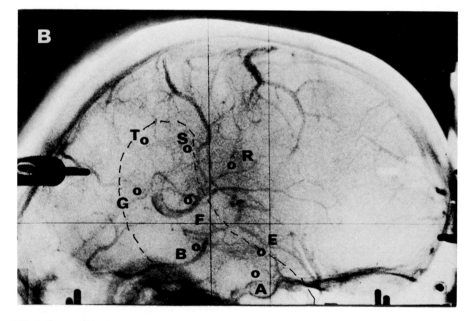

FIG. 5. Same patient.
(**A** and **B**): Arterial and venous angiograms. Electrode penetration points and planned excision are indicated.

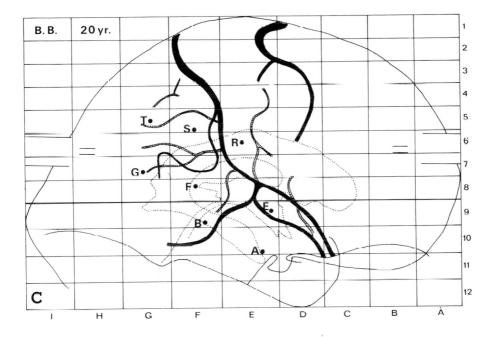

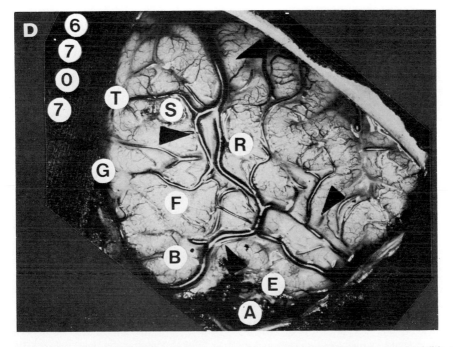

FIG. 5C-D. **(C):** Preoperative diagram of electrodes and principal blood vessels visible on the brain surface. Such landmarks allow for detailed localization of structures identified on stereotactic radiographs. **(D)** Photograph of the exposed cortex.

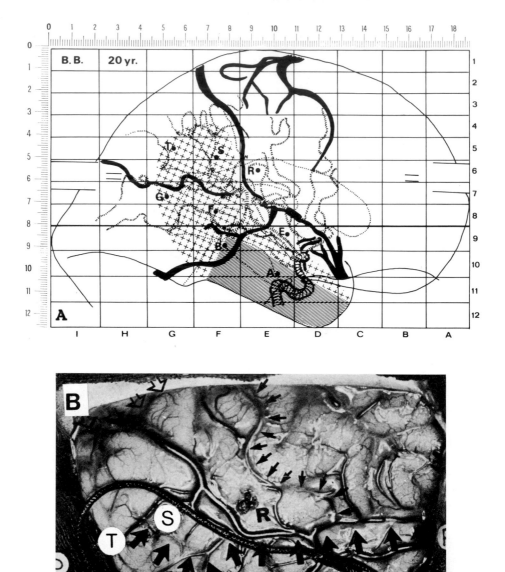

FIG. 6A and B. Same patient as Fig. 4 **(A):** Plan of surgery. Hatched area: temporal lobectomy including median structures. Crosses: cortical excision of temporoparietal junctional area. **(B):** Superficial vascular pattern and electrodes.

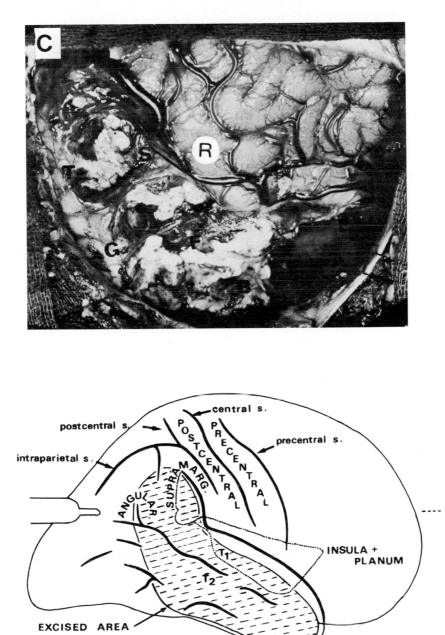

FIG. 6C and D. Same patient as Fig. 4. **(C):** Photograph of the brain after excision. **(D):** Excision related to gyri and sulci shown by three-dimensional angiography.

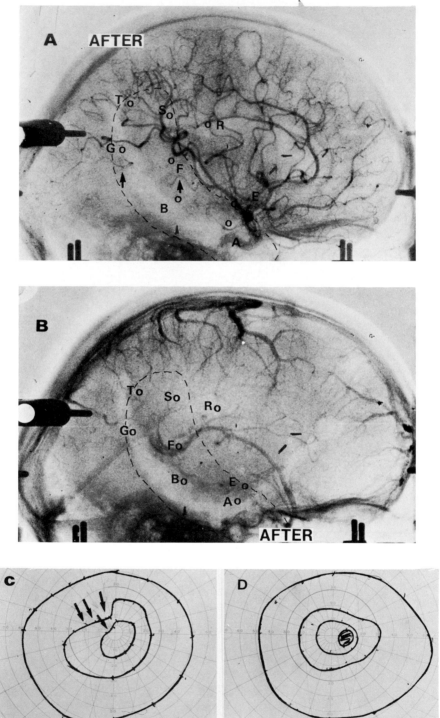

tognosic syndrome of the minor hemisphere include a more extensive territory and probably part of the underlying fiber tracts as well.

Some observations concerning impairment of contralateral motor functions after removal of the different parts of the Rolandic area could also be mentioned. In our cases, excision of the lower part of the central gyri up to 6 cm above the sylvian fissure was usually followed by mild transitory faciobrachial paresis only, provided that arteries supplying the superior part of the sensorimotor strip are respected. On the contrary, at the level of the paracentral mesial Rolandic cortex, even limited subpial removals that were less than 2 cm wide (Fig. 8C and D) left severe long-lasting motor sequelae in both lower and upper opposite limbs. The explanation of this difference might probably be found in the topography of the bundle of descending motor fibers and the vascular supply of the paracentral region (Figs. 8 and 9).

As illustrated in Fig. 9B, which shows an injected specimen, the Rolandic branches of the anterior cerebral artery coming from the interhemispheric surface may supply extensive parts of the superior part of the motor strip, up to 4 to 5 cm from the midline. Interruption of the blood flow in these branches might therefore damage a greater part of the motor cortex than would be expected. It might be added that in nonstereoscopic angiograms these vessels usually do not show up clearly because of the peripheral foreshortening and multiple superimpositions.

Another likely explanation can be the fact that descending motor fibers converge in the white matter near the ventricle. Even if the greater arteries running in the pia mater are preserved, interruption of the small branches penetrating the white matter can damage the bundle of motor fibers on their way toward the internal capsule.

Excision of the mesial frontal cortex anterior to the Rolandic area, as illustrated in Fig. 10, is usually followed by a contralateral motor inertia and aspontaneity, without Babinski's sign during a couple of weeks, provided that blood supply of the central gyri is spared.

CONCLUSION

In the light of several examples of surgical removal of cortical epileptogenic areas, we have tried to illustrate that stereotactic neuroradiological data may usefully contribute to open surgery.

Precise preoperative knowledge of the patient's brain allows for: (a) detailed "anatomical" planning of surgery; (b) identification of exposed cortex; (c) precise

---

FIG. 7. Same patient as Fig. 4. (**A** and **B**): Postoperative control angiography shows extent of excision. Major vessels bridging the removed area are preserved *(arrows)*. (**C** and **D**): Postoperative neurological deficit is limited to left superior quadrantanopsia.

delimitation of excision; (d) preservation of regional blood supply; and (e) preservation of underlying fiber tracts.

Moreover, since our knowledge of the anatomical localization and extent of surgical destruction is more accurate than was previously, postoperative deficits can be more precisely correlated to cortical lesions, thus contributing to a deeper knowledge of the functional anatomy of the human brain cortex. This in turn might be a factor of progress in neurosurgery, whether "general" or "functional."

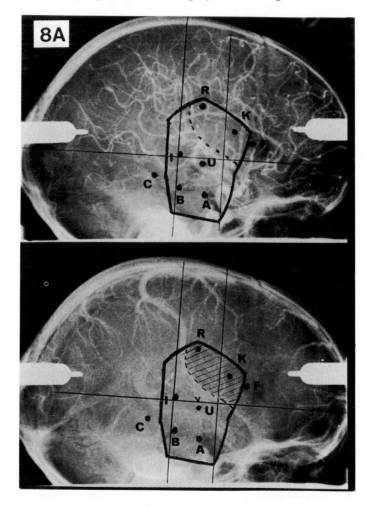

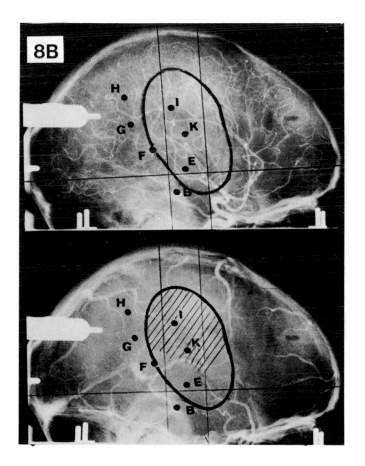

FIG. 8. (See pages 234–237.) Motor deficit after excisions in or next to the Rolandic area. (**A** and **B**): Subpial removal of the lower central area up to 6 cm above the sylvian fissure leaves only a transitory faciobrachial paresis, if the vascular supply of the upper part of the central gyri is preserved. (**C** and **D**): Less than 2-cm wide excision of the paracentral lobule is frequently followed by severe long-lasting paresis of contralateral lower and upper limbs.

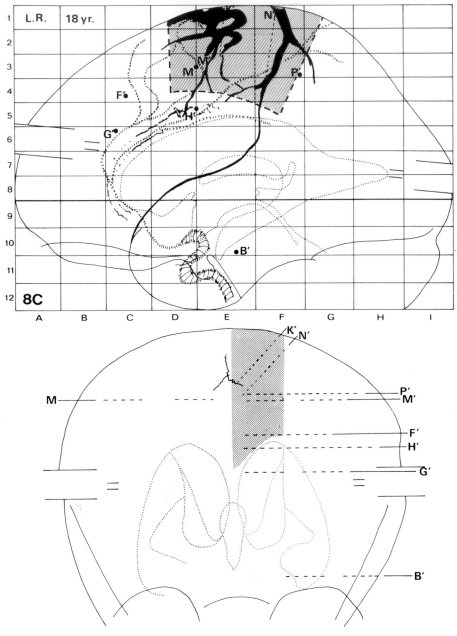

FIG. 8C.

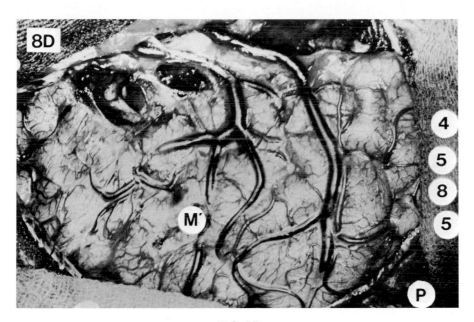

FIG. 8D

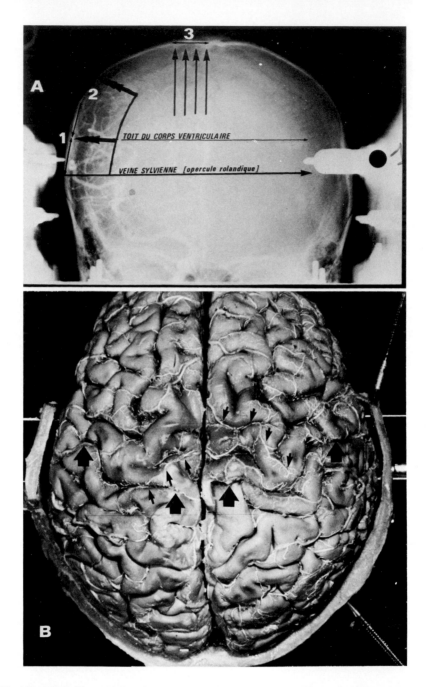

FIG. 9A and B. Topography of vascular supply and of descending motor fibers may explain the severe motor sequelae of paracentral excisions. **(A):** Extent of juxtasylvian (1, 2) and paracentral (3) excisions in cases of Fig. 8. **(B):** The territory supplied by the central branches of the anterior cerebral artery may extend up to 4 to 5 cm from the midline. Superior view of injected specimen. *Large arrows:* central sulcus. *Small arrows:* Rolandic branches of the anterior artery.

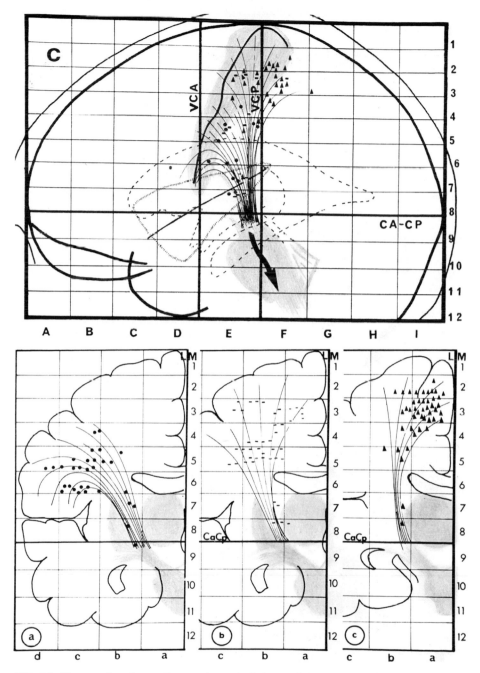

FIG. 9C. Topography of vascular supply and of descending motor fibers may explain the severe motor sequelae of paracentral excisions. **(C):** Motor fibers descending from the central gyri converge in the white matter. Proportional stereotactic diagrams of primary motor responses elicited by intracerebral low-frequency threshold bipolar stimulation in 30 epileptic patients. ●, face–tongue; −, upper limb; ▲, lower limb. Area of Rolandic sulcus shaded. Interruption of small arteries penetrating from the interhemispheric surface may interfere with the vascular supply of the fiber tract.

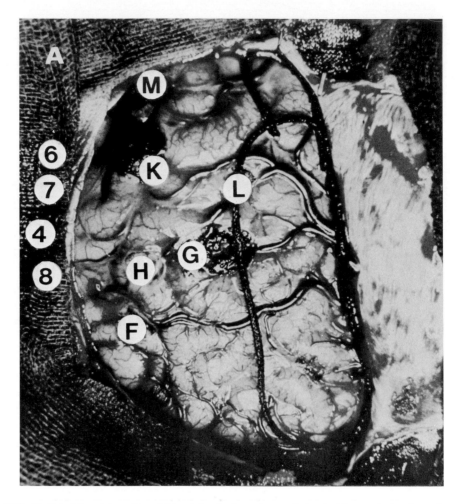

FIG. 10. Subpial excision of mesial frontal epileptogenic area in front of the central gyri, sparing, however, the regional blood supply, is followed by a contralateral motor inertia and aspontaneity (without Babinski's sign), regressing in 3 weeks.

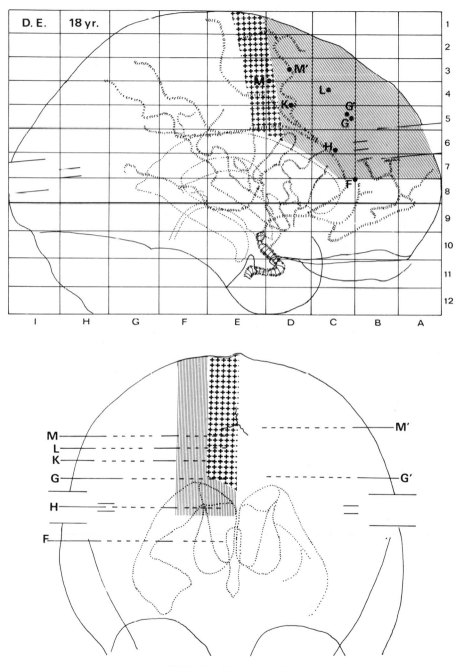

FIG. 10. (Continued)

REFERENCES

1. Bancaud, J., Talairach, J., et al. (1965): La Stéréoencephalographie dans l'épilepsie. Masson, Paris.
2. Bancaud, J., Talairach, J., et al. (1973): *E.E.G. et S.E.E.G. dans les tumeurs cérébrales et l'épilepsie.* Edifor, Paris.
3. Hécaën, H., Penfield, W., Bertrand, C., and Malmo, R. (1956): The syndrome of apractognosia due to lesions of the minor cerebral hemisphere. *A.M.A. Arch. Neurol. Psychiatr.,* 75:400–434.
4. Szikla, G., et al. (1977): *Angiography of the Human Brain Cortex.* Springer-Verlag, Berlin.
5. Talairach, J., Bancaud, J., Szikla, G., et al. (1974): Approche nouvelle de la neurochirurgie de l'épilepsie. *Neurochirurgie,* Vol. 20, Suppl. 1. Masson, Paris.
6. Talairach, J., Szikla, G., et al. (1967): *Atlas of Stereotaxic Anatomy of the Telencephalon.* Masson, Paris.

Functional Neurosurgery, edited by T. Rasmussen
and R. Marino. Raven Press, New York © 1979.

Long-Range Results of Medial Amygdalotomy on Epileptic Traits in Adult Patients*

H. Narabayashi

Juntendo Medical School 2–1 Hongo, Bunkyo-ku, Tokyo, Japan

In 1958 I performed my first amygdalotomy on an epileptic patient. This report concerns the long-range observations on some adult patients, i.e., those over 16 years of age at the time of operation, who have undergone this procedure, unilaterally or bilaterally, since that time.

CASE MATERIAL

A total of 29 adult patients who presented preoperatively both clinical seizures and epileptic abnormality in the EEG underwent this procedure. Eight of these, however, most of them early cases operated on more than 15 years ago, were lost to follow-up, and no long-range data are available. Of the 21 patients available for study (72.4% of total 29 cases), 3 patients died 8 to 10 years postoperatively of pneumonia or status epilepticus, as listed in Table 1. Postmortem studies were not available. Follow-up analyses of the remaining 18 patients are discussed here.

The essential data on each of these 18 patients are listed in Table 3. The

TABLE 1. *Results of amygdalotomy in 29 patients, 1960–1970*

Amygdalotomy in adult patients	No. of cases
Total operated on, 1960–1970	29
Lost to follow-up	8
Patients examined or responded by mail	21
Late postoperative deaths (from responses)	3
Case 24: died in 1969, 8 years postoperative, of status epilepticus	
Case 47: died in 1972, 10 years postoperative, of pneumonia	
Case 55: died in 1969, 7 years postoperative, of high fever followed by status epilepticus	
Patients studied and reported (see Table 3)	18

* A long-term follow-up study in epileptic child cases was reported at the First International Congress of Pediatric Neurology, October 1975, Toronto (8).

TABLE 2. *Postoperative classification of results*

Improvement in emotional and behavioral sphere
    A″: almost completely and dramatically normalized
    A : highly improved
    B : relatively better, doing housework or working part-time
    C : almost no change
    D : worsened
Improvement in EEG
    a : spikes or paroxysmal activity completely abolished
    b : moderate improvement
    c : slight improvement
    d : no change

---

postoperative follow-up period ranged from 5 to 17 years. As shown in Table 2, the results in the behavioral or emotional sphere were classified into five groups (A″, A, B, C, and D) and the effect on the EEG into four groups (a, b, c, and d).

RESULTS

Eleven, 61.1% of 18 patients, showed significant improvement (A″,5 patients; A,2 patients; and B,4 patients). The impressively improved status of these 11 continues, as almost all of them are living and working as normal, responsible, and independent members of society, depending on their intellectual capacity. Their jobs or social status are listed in the right-hand column of Table 3. The following patient is a typical example of this group.

Case Histories

Case 125, an 18-year-old boy: This patient's birth was normal as was his mental and physical development until the age of six. At the age of six he developed tonic seizures with loss of consciousness associated with an episode of high fever, which was presumed to be an encephalitic process of unknown etiology. Convulsive seizures occurred several times a week over the next 10 years, despite trials of various medications.

Around the age of 17 explosive, irritable, and aggressive behavior began, culminating in a near fatal attack with a baseball bat on his grandfather.

The patient's cooperation was very poor and the EEG had to be done under narcosis. This showed 2.6 cycles per second diffuse slow-wave abnormality with positive spikes (Fig. 1, top). Psychometric tests could not be carried out because of his poor cooperation, but his intellectual capacity did not seem to be low. Bilateral medial amygdalotomy was performed on February 2, 1972.

Postoperatively, this patient's improvement was dramatic, with almost complete calming and with a normalized emotional state. He was not abnormally hypoemotional, however, and could become angry and unhappy if other family members, shop mates, or customers treated him badly. To date, no violence has been observed and he is now working in his family's enterprise, management of hotels and shops. There is no spike activity in the EEG but the basic slowing is the same (Fig. 1, bottom). Medication was stopped about 2 years postoperatively, with no reappearance of seizures.

TABLE 3. *Results of amygdalotomy in 21 patients in a follow-up period of 5 to 17 years*

Number of the case	Age at the time of surgery (years)	Type of seizure (spikes on EEG)	I.Q.	Etiology	Side of surgery	Immediate postoperative result on behavior (on EEG)	Years after 1975	Social status
5	19 (M)	Focal and GM and r. hemiplegia (few sp. and w.)	60	Meningitis at 1 year	Left-sided	C	C (17 years)	Institutionalized
39	16 (F)	GM (bifrontal++)	Idiot	Seizures since 2 years	Bilateral	C (b)	B (16 years)	Some housework
40	18 (M)	PsM, (dreamy state and psychotic episode; few aT spikes)	Subnormal	(perinatal?)	Bilateral	A	C (psychotic episode recurred)	At home
42	26 (M)	GM and PsM, (dreamy state and psychotic episode; r. Fr. ++)	Normal	Encephalitis at 3 years and head injury	Bilateral	A (a)	C (a) (psychotic episode recurred)	Hospitalized or at home
53	18 (M)	GM and focal and r. hemiparesis (l. temp. slow-wave focus)	Subnormal	Encephalitis	Left-sided	B (d)	C (d)	—
57	35 (M)	GM and r. hemiparesis (CPO++)	Subnormal	Postvaccinal encephalitis at 8 months	Bilateral	C (b)	B (15 years)	Assisting in father's office
60	25 (F)	PsM (verbal automatism and hallucination) aT++ (l. > r.)	Normal	Injury?	Left-sided	A (a)	B (seizure recurred at 6 months but emotionally B)	Housework

TABLE 3. (Continued)

Number of the case	Age at the time of surgery (years)	Type of seizure (spikes on EEG)	I.Q.	Etiology	Side of surgery	Immediate postoperative result on behavior (on EEG)	Years after 1975	Social status
67	41 (M)	GM since 3 years (bilat. Fr and aT slow-wave burst)	Subnormal	Encephalitis at 3 years	Left-sided	B (d)	C (recurred at 8 months; hospitalized at present, 14 years later)	At home
73	33 (M)	GM since 6 years (diffuse sp.)	Subnormal	Encephalitis?	Left-sided	A″ (a″ no seizure no spikes)	A″ (13 years)	Working at office
109	18 (M)	GM + athetose (few diffuse +)	Idiot	Perinatal (kernicterus) encephalitis	Bilateral	B (a)	C (a) Idiot (8 years)	At home
110	38 (M)	GM (sp. and w. 2 c/s bifrontal)	Normal	Injury at soccer game at 13 years	Bilateral	A (b)	B (b) (7 years)	Gas station manager
112	34 (M)	GM since 12 years (diffuse paroxysm. slow)	Normal	Injury?	Left-sided	A (a)	A″(a) (9 years)	Worker at steel factory (died of heart attack just after this study was made)
114	39 (M)	GM with athetose (diffuse ++)	Subnormal	Perinatal asphyxia	Left-sided	A (a)	A (a) (6 years)	Mild housework because of athetosis

116	18 (M)	GM and atonic seizure since 5 years (Fr. and T. cortical spikes)	Normal	Encephalitis?	Bilateral	C	A (d) (6 years)	Office worker
121	21 (M)	GM since 7 years, with dreamy state and delusions (CPO++; r. > l.)	Normal	Encephalitis at 7 years	Bilateral	A"(a)	C (c) (recurred 2 years later)	At home
125	18 (M)	GM since 6 years (sp. and w.)	Normal	Encephalitis? at 6 years	Bilateral	A"(a)	A"(a) (5 years)	Manager of hotel and shops
126	24 (M)	GM since 4 years (r. aT+ and a few sp. and w.)	44	Encephalitis at 2 months	Bilateral	A"(b)	A"(a) (5 years)	Packing factory worker
127	24 (F)	GM (dreamy state severe self-aggression; aT+)	Normal	Perinatal (instrumental)	Bilateral	A"(a)	A"(a) (5 years)	Receptionist in doctor's office and flower arranger

aT, anterior temporal; C, central; F, female; Fr, frontal; GM, grand mal seizure; M, male; O, occipital; P, parietal; PsM, psychomotor seizure; sp and w, spike and wave.

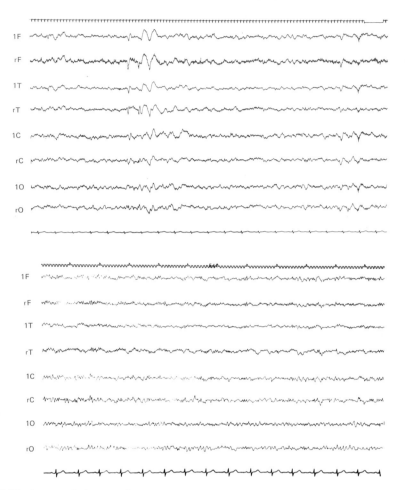

FIG. 1. Electroencephalogram of an 18-year-old male (case 125). **(Top):** preoperative; **(bottom):** 3 months postoperative. F, frontal; T, temporal; C, central; O, occipital; l, left-sided; and r, right-sided.

This patient provides a typical example of the indication for this type of surgery. His epilepsy was long-standing, of acquired etiology, and of grand mal rather than of the temporal lobe type. The psychological and behavioral problems became slowly and progressively more severe over the long course of his illness. Spike foci in the EEG became more prominent in the right temporal area.

The psychological tests were often difficult to apply in patients with poor concentration or who were too uncooperative. Satisfactory Rohrschach and psychological tests could be carried out in only five cases. The following patient illustrates the results of operation on the Rohrschach test results in a patient with posttraumatic epilepsy.

Case 110, a 38-year-old man: This man, 38 years of age at the time of surgery, had been quite normal until the age of 13, when he sustained a severe head contusion during a soccer game; this injury was followed by 30 minutes of coma. There were no neurological sequelae, but 3 months later generalized clonic convulsive seizures started. These recurred and persisted through the years at a rate of several times a week, despite heavy medication. The patient was married at 21 years of age but personality changes began to appear. He became more irritable and explosive, sometimes becoming violent and uncontrollable. These personality traits continued to worsen resulting in his wife divorcing him. The convulsive seizures persisted unchanged.

On June 21, 1970, bilateral stereotactic medial amygdalotomy was carried out. Following the procedure, the above-mentioned personality deviation gradually improved over the next few months, with no episodes of explosive violence following his discharge from the hospital a month after surgery. In attitude, he became very cooperative and pleasant, volunteering to help with his brother's job in a motorcar repair factory; he actually started to work in this job. Medication is still being continued, but at about half of the preoperative dosage. Rare clinical seizures persist but they are much slighter in severity. EEG spikes and paroxysms gradually improved and finally disappeared in the course of the first postoperative year.

In this case, the number of responses in the Rohrschach test increased postoperatively (Table 4). Reduction in aggressive attitude is shown by a decrease of FM and by slight increase of color response. The increase of M and of P indicates improvement in maturity and balance. Animal response (A) decreased from 94% preoperatively to 66% 6 months postoperative, suggesting a more balanced and mature status than before the procedure.

These results suggest the gradual but steady change of the patient from an aggressive, emotionally unsteady, and immature status to a better balanced, more social and mature personality after the surgery. Observations by Rohrschach test in the other four cases also indicated a similar tendency toward change or improvement.

Several factors could be identified as playing a role in those patients with unsatisfactory results, i.e., those in category C, Table 3. Three cases (40, 42,

TABLE 4. *Rohrschach test (Klopfer modification), Case 110*

		Preoperative (Jan. 18, 1970)	6-months postoperative (July 19, 1970)
	R	19	24
	Reject.	0	0
	M	1	3
	FM	9	6
	m	0	0
	cF	0	0
	Fc	0	0
	KF	0	0
	FC	0	1
Color	CF	0	0
	C	0	0
	P	4	7
	F%	47%	58%
	F-%	21%	25%
	W%	31%	25%
	D%	63%	71%
	Dd%	5%	4%
	A%	94%	66%
	At + Sex	0	0
	Organic signs (Piotrovski)	3	2

and 60) of psychomotor type epilepsy manifesting seizures of psychotic episode, i.e., prolonged dreamy state with hallucinations, delusions with feelings of fear, and verbal automatism, in addition to aggression and behavioral problems, were impressively improved immediately after unilateral or bilateral surgery, but in all three the psychic symptoms such as hallucinations or delusions similar to the preoperative symptoms recurred within about 6 to 12 months postoperatively, though the automatisms did not recur. Case 121 may also belong to the same category. These results suggest that psychotic seizures with hallucinations or delusions accompanied by fear or anger in epileptic patients are not influenced permanently by this surgery. Thus, the indication for this procedure on the medial amygdaloid nuclei may be different from that for temporal lobectomy.

Another important factor of practical importance in aiming to improve the patient's emotional status to the point that he can work, act, or study as an independent responsible member of society is the level of his intellectual capacity. Patients with marked mental deficiency usually become manageable and calm and develop better concentration, but naturally cannot be expected to function at levels beyond their intellectual capacity. Despite a subnormal intelligence, however, some patients can do simple jobs postoperatively, depending on the milieu around the patient. In children, difficulties in testing may lead to the intellectual level being misinterpreted as being lower than is actually the case. This aspect, reported previously (4), will not be discussed here in detail.

As has been discussed elsewhere (11), therapeutic lesions of the medial amygdaloid nucleus have resulted in more favorable results than when the lateral amygdaloid region has been the target.

No serious side effects were noted in this series of patients either in the immediate postoperative period or in the long-term follow-up period. The Klüver-Bucy syndrome was not produced, there was no loss or lowering of memory function and no persisting inertia, even after bilateral surgery. It was pointed out recently by Penfield (12) that memory function is not correlated to the amygdaloid nucleus.

SUMMARY

This long-term follow-up analysis of 18 patients with severe behavioral and epileptic problems who had undergone unilateral or bilateral stereotactic amygdalotomy in adult life suggests:

1. Severe behavioral problems in epileptic patients, such as uncontrollable violent explosion of temper, easy excitability or unsteadiness in mood, are well-benefited by this surgical procedure. Secondary to these improvements, many of the patients were able to return to productive work, earn salaries, support themselves and families, and pay taxes.

2. It is important to stress that these patients did not become hypoemotional or experience prolonged states of inertia. They do get angry, however, when

they are badly treated by the family, office mates, or schoolmates, but their outbursts of temper are not as destructive as before.

3. In about two-thirds of those cases who were greatly improved from the emotional standpoint, the clinical seizures, especially those of grand mal type, and the EEG paroxysms, especially in the frontotemporal area, were diminished. The effects on the epileptic seizures or paroxysms generally paralleled those on the behavioral problems (1,5,6,9). In the selection of cases for this procedure, the seizure pattern need not necessarily be of the temporal lobe type.

4. In the greatly improved cases, the threshold for barbiturate anesthesia usually fell, as a rule to about half of the preoperative dosage level. Chronic epileptic patients are known to be resistant to intravenous anesthesia by barbiturates.

5. No adverse psychological, intellectual, or autonomic side effects were noted in either adults or children, even after bilateral amygdaloid lesions. The results of Rohrschach test observations are presented. Neither the Klüver-Bucy syndrome nor disturbance of memory function was observed (5,8). The only noticeable side-effects were a transient inertia shortly after surgery, which lasted only for several days, and also a transient tendency for an increase of appetite or polyphagia for about 2 weeks in about one-third of the cases. This did not result in any serious increase of body weight, however. Changes in olfaction and taste were not experienced at all.

6. It is now generally agreed that the medial amygdaloid surgery is effective and useful for improving the seizure problems and behavioral problems of epileptic etiology, when all other pharmacological or conservative treatment has failed (7). But it cannot be the tool for solution of behavior problems of other unknown etiology, such as in major psychosis or psychoneurosis (2,3).

Finally, it should be emphasized, that the epilepsy in all the patients of this series was of acquired etiology, and no case was clearly of the primary, essential, or idiopathic type.

REFERENCES

1. Heimburger, R. F., Whitlock, C. C., and Kalsbeck, J. E. (1966): Stereotaxic amygdalotomy for epilepsy with aggressive behavior. *J.A.M.A.*, 198:741–745.
2. Hitchcock, E., and Cairns, V. (1973): Amygdalotomy. *Postgrad. Med. J.*, 49:894–904.
3. Kiloh, L. G., Gye, R. S., Rushworth, G. R., Bell, D. S., and White, R. T. (1974): Stereotactic amygdaloidotomy for agressive behaviour. *J. Neurol. Neurosurg. Psychiatry*, 37:437–444.
4. Nagahata, M. (1968): Behavior disorder and minor brain damage. *Shonika Shinryo*, 31:1193–1201. [in Japanese]
5. Narabayashi, H. (1971): Stereotaxic amygdalotomy for behavioral disorders of epileptic etiology. *Excerpta Med. Int. Congr. Ser.* No. 274, Psychiatry (Pt. 1): 175–184.
6. Narabayashi, H. (1972): Stereotaxic amygdalotomy. In: *The Neurobiology of the Amygdala*, edited by B. E. Eleftheriou, pp. 459–483. Plenum Press, New York.
7. Narabayashi, H. (1976): The place of amygdalotomy in the treatment of aggressive behavior with epilepsy. In: *Current Controversies in Neurosurgery*, edited by T. Morley, pp. 778–781. W. B. Saunders Co., Toronto, Canada.
8. Narabayashi, H. (1977): Stereotaxic amygdalotomy for epileptic heperactivity. (Long range

results in children.) In: *Topics in Child Neurology (Proceedings of the First International Congress of Pediatric Neurology),* edited by M. E. Blaw, I. Rapin, and M. Kinsbourne, pp. 319–331. Spectrum Publications, Jamaica, New York.

 9. Narabayashi, H., and Mizutani, T. (1970): Epileptic seizures and the stereotaxic amygdalotomy. *Confin. Neurol.,* 32:289–297.
10. Narabayashi, H., Nagao, T., Saito, Y., Yoshida, M., and Nagahata, M. (1963): Stereotaxic amygdalotomy for behavior disorders. *Arch. Neurol.,* 9:1–16.
11. Narabayashi, H., and Shima, F. (1973): Which is the better amygdala target, the medial or lateral nuclei? (For behaviour problems and paroxysm in epileptics.) In: *Surgical Approaches in Psychiatry,* edited by L. Laitinen and K. Livingston, pp. 129–134. Medical and Technical Publishing Co. Ltd., Lancaster.
12. Penfield, W., and Mathieson, G. (1974): Memory. *Arch. Neurol.,* 31:145–154.

Functional Neurosurgery, edited by T. Rasmussen
and R. Marino. Raven Press, New York © 1979.

Cortical Resection for Medically Refractory Focal Epilepsy: Results, Lessons, and Questions

Theodore Rasmussen

*Montreal Neurological Institute and Hospital, 3801 University Street,
Montreal, Quebec, Canada H3A 2B4*

The Montreal experience with the surgical treatment of medically refractory epilepsy by resection of epileptogenic areas of cerebral cortex had its genesis in Dr. Wilder Penfield's studies with Otfried Foerster (4,5). Since Dr. Penfield's first seizure operations were carried out in 1928, this experience has been developed and expanded through the years as a result of the combined efforts of both the clinical and the laboratory staffs of the Montreal Neurological Institute (3,24–30,32–37,39–41,43–53). The literature on the surgical treatment of epilepsy in other centers around the world has been summarized elsewhere (9,22,40,56).

In this chapter, I will first give a brief, updated summary of the results obtained through the years, at the Montreal Neurological Institute, in our attempts to reduce the clinical seizure tendency by cortical excision (24–27,32,36,39–41, 43,44,46,48,49,52,53), and will then outline a few of the interesting lessons we have learned as the years have gone by. Finally, I will comment on some questions arising from our experience with this series of patients that may be significant or relevant to considerations and theories of the basic nature of the neuronal seizure discharge and its recruitment proclivities that result in the production of clinical epileptic seizures in man.

RESULTS

A wide variety of lesions have been responsible for the seizures that have led to operation in this series of patients (Table 1). Slow-growing tumors and a few major vascular malformations constitute 20% of the total group. These patients often masqueraded for years as ordinary epileptic problems before the nature of the lesion responsible for the seizures was finally discovered by pneumograms, angiograms, or CT scans, or was discovered during an operation carried out for the seizures (16,47,51).

Brain scarring, gliosis, or atrophy as a result of birth trauma or anoxia was responsible for 27% of the nontumoral cases; postnatal head trauma accounted for 21%; and postinflammatory brain scarring was responsible for 15%. A wide variety of miscellaneous lesions accounted for 8%, and some of these will be referred to in a little more detail later. The etiology was considered to

TABLE 1
Total Surgical Seizure Series-Etiology
Patients operated upon from 1928 through 1976

Non-Tumoral Lesions				
Birth trauma or anoxia	415 pts. (27% of non-tumoral lesions)			
Postnatal trauma	321 pts. (21% "	"	"	)
Postinflammatory brain scarring	227 pts. (15% "	"	"	)
Miscellaneous	119 pts. (8% "	"	"	)
Unknown	433 pts. (29% "	"	"	)
	1515 pts. (100%)			
Tumors	364 pts.	20% of total group		
Vascular malformations	23 pts.			

Total 1902 pts.

be unknown in 29%, either because there was more than one potential cause or because there were no clues as to the etiology to be found in the history, the examination, or the findings at operation.

Total Nontumoral Series

From the beginning of the series in 1928, yearly follow-up reports or checkups were sought during the first 10 postoperative years, and subsequently reports were requested at 2- to 3-year intervals. Many of the patients have returned periodically over long periods of time for personal checkups including electroencephalographical (EEG) and neuropsychological reexaminations on either an outpatient or an inpatient basis.

In analyzing the effectiveness of the surgical procedure in reducing the patient's seizure tendency, we have endeavored to set up criteria that are as objective as possible. Thus, any episode that is visible to an observer, even a 2- to 3-sec twitching of the hand or side of the face, or any episode that disturbs the patient's contact with his environment, no matter how brief, is classified as an attack. A brief sensory episode that does not disturb the patient's contact with the environment, interfere with his ongoing activity, and is not noticeable to an observer is classified as an aura and not considered to be a clinical attack in the follow-up analyses.

By the end of 1974, 1,407 patients with medically refractory focal epilepsy caused by nontumoral epileptogenic lesions had been operated upon and cortical excision carried out (Table 2). There are satisfactory follow-up data of 2 years duration or more for 1,277 of these patients, with the median follow-up period being 12 years. Two hundred forty-seven patients, 19%, have had no seizures since discharge from the hospital. Another 14%, 178 patients, became and have

TABLE 2
Results of Cortical Excision for Focal Epilepsy
Patients with non-tumoral lesions operated upon 1928 through 1974

Seizure free since discharge	247 pts. (19%)	425 pts. (33%)		
Became seizure free after some early attacks	178 pts. (14%)			
			833 pts. (65%)	1277 pts. with follow-up data of 2-45 yrs.
Free 3 or more years then rare or occasional attacks	168 pts. (13%)	408 pts. (32%)		
Marked reduction of seizure tendency	240 pts. (19%)			
Moderate or less reduction of seizure tendency	444 pts. (34%)			median 12 yrs.

Inadequate follow-up data	87 pts.
Deaths in first 2 years	25 pts.
Postoperative deaths	18 pts.
Total	**1407 pts.**

remained seizure-free after having some attacks during the early postoperative months or a year or two. Thus, 33% of these 1,277 patients with medically refractory focal epilepsy became and have remained seizure-free after the cortical resection.

Another 168 patients, 13%, have had late recurrence of occasional attacks after having been seizure-free for periods ranging from 3 to 25 years. Two hundred and forty patients, 19%, have had less than 1 to 2% as many attacks compared to the preoperative rate, and not more than one to three attacks per year, but they have not been seizure-free for long enough periods to qualify for the previous group. These two groups, comprising 408 patients and making up 32% of the follow-up group, are considered to have experienced a marked, but not quite complete reduction in seizure tendency. Thus, in 65% of these 1,277 patients with medically refractory focal epilepsy, the cortical resection resulted in a complete or nearly complete reduction in seizure tendency.

The remaining one-third have had a lesser reduction of seizure tendency. Some of these have had only 5 to 10% as many attacks compared to the preoperative rate. Many have had about half as many, while the remainder have had a lesser reduction. A small minority have had little or no reduction.

Tumors

The reduction of seizure tendency was similar in the patients with tumors and vascular malformations (16,47,51). In these patients, the effectiveness of

TABLE 3

Astrocytomas and Miscellaneous Slowly-Growing Gliomas

Results of Operation on Seizure Tendency up to Evidence of Tumor Recurrence

(patients operated upon from 1931 through 1975

No attacks	56 pts. (26%)	88 pts. (41%)	157 pts. (73%)	218 pts (118 died 1-27 yrs postop.) (median FU 6 yrs)
Became seizure free	32 pts. (15%)			
Marked reduction in seizure tendency	69 pts. (32%)			(100 living 1-37 yrs postop) (median FU 8 yrs)
Moderate or less reduction in seizure tendency	61 pts. (28%)			
Inadequate follow-up data	17 pts.			
Died in 1st postoperative year	9 pts.			
Postoperative death (primary operation)	6 pts.			

Total 250 pts.

operation carried out with the seizure surgical techniques was tabulated up to the time of appearance of evidence of tumor recurrence, if that had occurred. In two-thirds of the patients in this group, the tumors were indolent gliomas, usually grade 1 or grade 2 astrocytomas (Table 3). There were satisfactory follow-up data of 1 year or more in 218 of the 250 patients in this group. The median follow-up period in the 118 patients who have died is 6 years. One hundred patients are still living 1 to 37 years after operation, with the median follow-up period being 8 years. Eighty-eight patients, 41% of the 218, became, and have remained seizure-free, as just defined. Another 32%, 69 patients, have had a marked reduction of seizure tendency, as previously defined. Thus 73% experienced a complete or nearly complete reduction of seizure tendency, similar to the results in the total series with nontumoral lesions (Table 2).

LESSONS

These patients have taught us a number of interesting lessons through the years. A few warrant discussion in this chapter.

Completeness of Excision

We soon learned that small cortical excisions limited to the area of lowest seizure threshold frequently produced only a minimal or moderate reduction of seizure tendency, whereas reoperation and more complete excision of the

TABLE 4
Cortical Excision for Non-tumoral Epileptogenic Lesions
Results of reoperation - 1928 through 1974

Seizure free since discharge	11 pts. (9%)	26 pts. (21%)	56 pts. (45%)	121 pts with follow-up data of 2-39 yrs. after last operation median 15 yrs.
Became seizure free after some early attacks	15 pts. (12%)			
Free 3 or more years then rare or occasional attacks	15 pts. (12%)	30 pts. (24%)		
Marked reduction of seizure tendency	15 pts. (12%)			
Moderate or less reduction of seizure tendency	65 pts. (55%)			
Inadequate data	6 pts.			
Postoperative deaths	4 pts.			

Total 131 pts.

epileptogenic area often produced enough further reduction of the patient's seizure tendency to convert an unsuccessful result into a successful one.

For example, by the end of 1974, 131 patients had undergone a second, occasionally a third, and rarely a fourth cortical resection (Table 4). There are satisfactory follow-up data of at least 2 years duration after the last operation in 121 of these patients. In 45% of these 121 patients, in whom the first cortical excision failed to produce a satisfactory reduction of seizure tendency, the further cortical excision resulted in a complete or nearly complete reduction of the seizure tendency.

Thus, we have learned that it is important to identify and map out the total epileptogenic area of the cortex as accurately as possible and to remove the involved cortex as completely as is feasible without running too great a risk of producing a significant neurological deficit.

Results in the Anatomical and Etiological Groups

Success in reducing the seizure tendency in this series is correlated with the completeness of the removal of the epileptogenic area rather than with the area of the principle epileptogenic area of the cortex or the cause of the original brain injury.

Cortical resections that were largely limited to the temporal lobe of one cerebral hemisphere were carried out in just over 50% of the patients in this series (Table 5). A complete or nearly complete reduction of seizure tendency resulted

TABLE 5
Temporal Lobe Epilepsy - Results of Cortical Excision
Patients with non-tumoral lesions operated upon from 1928 through 1972

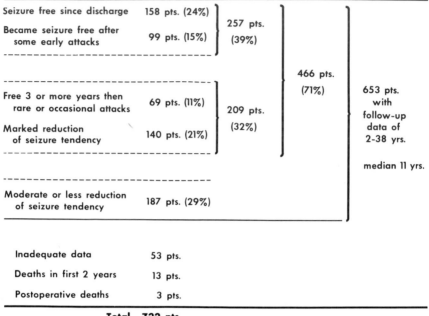

Seizure free since discharge	158 pts. (24%)	257 pts. (39%)		
Became seizure free after some early attacks	99 pts. (15%)		466 pts. (71%)	653 pts. with follow-up data of 2-38 yrs.
Free 3 or more years then rare or occasional attacks	69 pts. (11%)	209 pts. (32%)		median 11 yrs.
Marked reduction of seizure tendency	140 pts. (21%)			
Moderate or less reduction of seizure tendency	187 pts. (29%)			
Inadequate data	53 pts.			
Deaths in first 2 years	13 pts.			
Postoperative deaths	3 pts.			

Total   722 pts.

in 71% of these patients with medically refractory temporal lobe epilepsy. The statistics were similar in the smaller anatomical groups—frontal, central, parietal, and occipital—and in those with large destructive lesions involving more than one lobe of the brain, with the seizure-free percentage ranging from 25 to 44% and total percentage with a complete or nearly complete reduction in seizure tendency ranging from 55 to 74% (39,40,43,46,48,53).

Thus, the effectiveness of the cortical resection is about the same regardless of the anatomical area primarily involved in the epileptogenic process.

It is of interest also to look at the results in these same patients classified as to the *nature* of the original brain injury. By the end of 1970, there were 355 patients whose seizures clearly seemed to be caused by injury of the brain at birth (Table 6). Follow-up data on 337 of these patients showed that 47% became, and have remained, seizure-free, and a total of 72% have shown a complete or nearly complete reduction of seizure tendency.

The statistics again were similar in the other etiological categories, those with postnatal brain trauma, postinflammatory brain injury, those whose seizures were of unknown etiology, and those in the miscellaneous category (40,41,43, 45,49).

TABLE 6
Focal Epilepsy Due to Birth Trauma and Anoxia
Results of Cortical Excision - 1928 through 1970

Seizure free since discharge	90 pts. (27%)	156 pts. (47%)	240 pts. (72%)	337 pts. with follow-up data of 2-41 yrs. median 11 yrs.
Became seizure free after some early attacks	66 pts. (20%)			
Free 3 or more years then rare or occasional attacks	35 pts. (10%)	84 pts. (25%)		
Marked reduction of seizure tendency	49 pts. (15%)			
Moderate to no reduction of seizure tendency	97 pts. (29%)			

Inadequate follow-up data	14 pts.
Deaths in first 2 years	2 pts.
Postoperative deaths	2 pts.

Total   355 pts.

We interpret these experiences and statistics to indicate that the effectiveness of cortical resection in the treatment of medically refractory focal epilepsy is correlated primarily with the completeness with which the epileptogenic cortex can be removed, rather than with the anatomical location of the epileptogenic area of the brain or the nature of the underlying cause of the original brain damage.

Hemispherectomy and Superficial Hemosiderosis of the Brain

Hemispherectomy, more accurately termed *hemicorticectomy,* was introduced for the treatment of intractable seizures associated with infantile hemiplegia by Krynauw in 1950 (15). In properly selected patients, this procedure has proved to be highly successful in stopping the seizures (10,38,53,60). Many patients have also experienced marked behavioral improvement as well, after the damaged hemisphere has been removed.

Long-term observation of hemispherectomized patients, however, has shown that 20 to 30% develop, 4 or more years postoperatively, progressive brain dysfunction resulting from superficial hemosiderosis of the brain, first described by Noetzel (21), and produced experimentally by Iwanowski and Olszewski (12). This late complication is apparently a result of repeated small seepages of erythrocytes into the hemispherectomy cavity so that the cerebrospinal fluid (CSF) there becomes heavily laden with iron-containing pigment (2,11,23,42). This has not occurred in our patients who have had subtotal hemispherectomy.

The reduction of the seizure tendency in these patients has been nearly as good as in those who have had a complete hemispherectomy (42).

During the past 10 years, therefore, it has been our practice, in patients who were considered to be hemispherectomy candidates, to leave in situ a small portion of the least epileptogenic portion of the hemisphere, usually the frontal or occipital pole. Only in rare instances has it been necessary to reoperate and complete the hemispherectomy. None of these few patients who have had a two-stage complete hemispherectomy has developed this late complication of superficial cerebral hemosiderosis as yet.

Bilaterally Synchronous Spike-and-Wave Complexes in the EEG Produced by Unilateral Epileptogenic Lesions

It soon became apparent (13,28,57) that unilateral focal cortical epileptogenic lesions could produce, in some patients, bilaterally synchronous spike-and-wave bursts that resembled, more or less closely, the three per second generalized epileptiform discharges seen in patients with true absence or petit mal attacks and which were originally described by Gibbs and associates (6,7). We have learned that while these secondary bilaterally synchronous abnormalities are most commonly produced by mesial frontal epileptogenic lesions (57), they may also be produced in some patients by focal cortical lesions of the convexity of the frontal lobe, and by lesions of the temporal lobe and the parieto-occipital region. We have also learned that these bilaterally synchronous discharges may be produced by indolent gliomas in these regions, as well as by gliotic and cicatricial epileptogenic lesions. We have no answers as yet, however, to the neurophysiological question as to why these bilateral complexes are produced in one patient while the majority of patients with similar lesions exhibit the usual localized and lateralized random spike abnormality in the EEG.

The use of the intracarotid Amytal-Metrazol EEG test has aided in the identification of this interesting group of patients and has led to modification of the original concept of the mechanism of so-called secondary bilateral synchrony in the EEG (8).

Lateralization of Cerebral Speech Functions

Up until 20 years ago, when left-handed or ambidextrous patients were being operated on, cortical excisions carried out in either the right or left cerebral hemisphere often had to be more limited than was desired because of uncertainty as to the lateralization of the cerebral speech functions. The intracarotid Amytal speech test, introduced to us by Dr. Juhn Wada when he was at the Montreal Neurological Institute on a Rockefeller Fellowship, has enabled us to know in advance, with certainty, whether or not the cerebral hemisphere being operated on does or does not contain any speech functions (1,17,19,58,59). Thus, this test is done routinely preoperatively in all *non*-right-handed patients being consid-

TABLE 7

**Speech Lateralization in Patients
Without Early Left-Hemisphere Damage**
(262 Cases)

Handedness	No. of Cases	Speech Representation		
		Left	Bilateral	Right
Right	140	134 96%	0 0%	6 4%
Left or Mixed	122	86 70%	18 15%	18 15%

ered for operation, as well as in all those *right*-handed patients in whom some aspect of the clinical attack pattern, history, examination, or radiological findings have raised the possibility that the cerebral speech functions might not be in the left cerebral hemisphere, as normally would be the case.

We have learned (55) that 70% of non-right-handed seizure patients who have no historical or objective evidence of injury to the left cerebral hemisphere in the early years of life have speech functions in the left hemisphere (Table 7). Speech functions were in the right hemisphere in 15% of this group, while another 15% had some speech functions in both hemispheres (20,55). In 140 right-handed patients without early left hemisphere injury, in whom some question had been raised as to the lateralization of speech functions, 6 patients, or 4%, were found to have speech functions in the right hemisphere. None had any evidence of bilaterality of speech representation (Table 7).

The picture was quite different in those patients who did have some evidence of injury to the left cerebral hemisphere in the early years of life (Table 8). In the right-handed patients, speech functions were in the right hemisphere in 12%, in the left hemisphere in 81%, and three patients, 7%, had some speech representation in each hemisphere. Fifty-three percent of the non-right-handed

TABLE 8

**Speech Lateralization After Early Lesions
of the Left Cerebral Hemisphere**
(134 Cases)

Handedness	No. of Cases	Speech Representation		
		Left	Bilateral	Right
Right	42	34 81%	3 7%	5 12%
Left or Mixed	92	26 28%	17 19%	49 53%

patients in this group had speech in the right hemisphere, 28% had speech in the left hemisphere, and 19% had some speech representation in each hemisphere.

Thus, handedness is not a reliable guide to the lateralization of cerebral speech functions in ambidextrous or left-handed patients or in right-handed patients who have any evidence of injury to the left cerebral hemisphere in the early years of life.

An interesting aspect of the cerebral organization of speech functions has been demonstrated in the 38 patients whose carotid Amytal speech tests gave evidence of bilateral cerebral speech representation. Eighteen of these 38 patients were in the group *without* evidence of early injury to the left hemisphere (Table 7) and 20 were in the group *with* evidence of early left hemisphere injury (Table 8). Nearly half of these 38 patients, about equally divided between the two groups, showed a qualitative difference in the dysphasia induced by the injections of the two hemispheres (55). In those patients, the intracarotid Amytal injection of one hemisphere produced errors of naming but little or no disturbance in serial repetition tasks such as counting or reciting the days of the week forward and backward, or in oral spelling. Injection of the opposite hemisphere produced the reverse effect, that is, errors and hesitation in the verbal serial ordering tasks with little or no disturbance of naming. In two-thirds of these patients, the more marked deficit in serial repetition followed the right carotid injection and the principal deficit in naming followed the left-sided injection; in the remaining one-third, this pattern was reversed.

In those patients who subsequently underwent cortical excision bordering on the speech areas, the quality of the transient postoperative dysphasia matched that seen after the Amytal injection of the same hemisphere, thus validating the post-Amytal observation. The significance of this dissociation in regard to the organization of cerebral speech mechanisms in normal and in injured brains awaits further study.

Safeguarding Memory in Patients with Bitemporal EEG Abnormality

Another lesson, learned in a painful way and reported in detail by Penfield and Milner in 1958 (31), concerns the importance of the hippocampal regions in the consolidation of memory functions. Independent bitemporal spiking in the EEG may indicate the presence of sufficient damage to both hippocampal regions so that removal of this area on one side may reduce the amount of functioning hippocampal tissue to levels that may result in a permanent severe global memory impairment. Special memory testing devised by Milner and Taylor, and carried out during the intracarotid Amytal speech test, now gives us good evidence as to whether the hippocampal region on the side of the proposed temporal lobectomy is dispensable or carries a risk of producing a significant memory defect if it is removed (17,18). The intracarotid Amytal memory test is therefore carried out routinely in all patients being considered for temporal lobectomy in whom there is EEG, X-ray, or neuropsychological evidence of injury to both temporal lobes.

QUESTIONS

Of even greater interest than the lessons those patients have taught us, a few of which have just been discussed, are questions they have raised that must have some importance in regard to the fundamental nature of the neural mechanisms responsible for epileptic seizures.

Running-down Phenomenon

As already noted, nearly half of all patients who have become, and remained, seizure-free after cortical resection have had some attacks during the early postoperative months or a year or two before becoming seizure-free (Table 2). This postoperative running-down phenomenon of a residual seizure tendency occurs with about equal frequency in each of our anatomical and etiological subgroups (Tables 5 and 6).

The question we would ask is, what are the neurophysiological or neurochemical correlates of this common running-down phenomenon? When the answer is available, it should provide important clues to better understanding of the basic nature of seizure mechanisms.

Latent Period

The latent period that nearly always exists between an injury to the brain and the onset of seizures has been well known for many years, but the neurophysiological, neurochemical, or neuropathological reasons for it remain unexplained. Data from both military and civilian head injuries have amply documented the fact that about one-half to two-thirds of head-injured patients who are destined to develop posttraumatic epilepsy, experience the onset of the recurring seizures during the first 2 years after injury, with the onset in the remainder appearing over intervals extending up to 30 or more years (41,45). Thus, over half of the patients in this series with posttraumatic epilepsy (Fig. 1) experienced the onset of the recurring seizures during the first 2 years after injury, 43% during the first 12 months after injury, and another 13% during the next 12 months. In 8%, however, the latent period was over 10 years.

The picture is similar for those patients whose brain injury was the result of some inflammatory process or episode (Fig. 1). The onset of seizures occurred within the first 2 years in 51%, with 38% occurring in the first year and 13% in the second year.

What is the difference in the healing process or in the neuronal characteristics of the brain of the patient with posttraumatic epilepsy whose first seizure occurs 10 or more years after injury as compared to the more common situation in

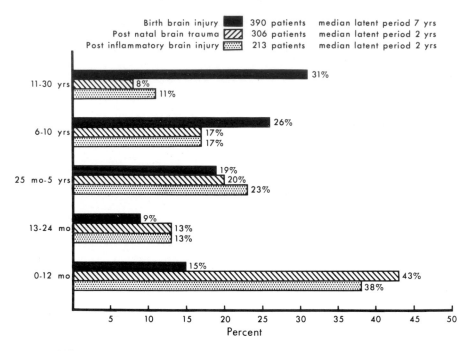

FIG. 1. Latent period between brain injury and onset of recurring seizures.

which the latent period is measured in months. This is another intriguing question the neurophysiological or neurochemical answers of which are, as yet, quite unknown.

The patient whose brain is injured at birth presents a different picture as far as the pattern of the latent period is concerned. Only 15% of such patients in this series experienced the onset of the recurring seizures during the first year of life, and only 9% during the second year (Fig. 1). In contrast, the latent period was more than 10 years in nearly a third, 31%, 3 times that of the posttraumatic and the postinflammatory group.

A series of related questions is posed by these data. Is this difference in pattern of the latent period related to the maturity of the brain at the time of injury? Is the difference related to the extensiveness or severity of the injury to the brain? Is the difference related to differing mechanisms of healing in the newborn and the more mature brain? Our data, at least as far as we have analyzed them to date, do not give any conclusive answers, but do suggest that immaturity of the brain plays some role. For example (Fig. 2), when the patients in the posttraumatic group are divided into those whose brain injury occurred *after* 5 years of age, 238 patients, and those whose injury occurred *during* the first 5 years of life, 68 patients, there is a significant difference in the latent periods of the two groups. The difference is much less marked, however, than that between the birth injury group and the two groups with postnatally injured brains (Fig. 1). It is a matter of speculation as to what aspect of the

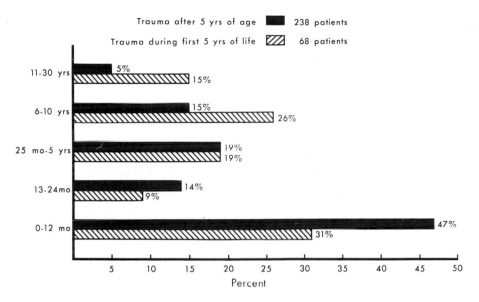

FIG. 2. Latent period between postnatal brain trauma and outset of recurring seizures, in 306 patients.

difference between the immature and the more mature brain plays a role in regard to these differing latent periods.

Late Recurrence

Another question of interest, and perhaps of potential importance, concerns those patients who have become seizure-free for periods of 3 years or longer, even up to 25 years, who then have had recurrences of one or more seizures (Tables 2, 4–6). These recurrent attacks have usually been isolated or rare occurrences, but in a small minority they have become a recurring and more significant seizure problem. The percentage of patients in this group is about the same whether, they are classified on an anatomical basis—11% of those with temporal lobe epilepsy (Table 5) and 12% of those with frontal lobe epilepsy (45), for example—or whether they are classified on an etiological basis—10% of those in the birth trauma group (Table 6) and 16% of those with posttraumatic epilepsy (43), for example.

This group of patients raises more intriguing questions the answers to which must ultimately be related to the basic neuronal mechanisms responsible for clinical epileptic seizures.

Variety of Lesions Producing Similar Seizures

Although the seizure tendency in many of the patients in our series could be satisfactorily classified as a result of injury to the brain at birth or a result of postnatal traumatic or inflammatory injury to the brain, or of indolent brain tumors, as noted in Table 1, an interesting group of miscellaneous lesions has been encountered in all the anatomical subgroups (Table 9).

These lesions include a variety of congenital lesions (Table 10) such as pial angiomatosis of the Sturge-Weber variety, with or without the typical nevus

TABLE 9
Non-Tumoral Epileptogenic Lesions
1928 through 1970 - 1230 pts.

Etiology	Temporal Lobe Epilepsy 667 pts.	Large Destructive Lesions 158 pts.	Frontal Lobe Epilepsy 229 pts.	Parietal Lobe Epilepsy 86 pts.	Central Lesions 67 pts.	Occipital Lobe Epilepsy 22 pts.
Birth compression, trauma or anoxia	32%	47%	12%	26%	21%	36%
Postnatal brain trauma	16%	12%	46%	41%	19%	5%
Postinflammatory brain scarring	16%	23%	12%	8%	9%	14%
Miscellaneous	5%	8%	9%	7%	12%	27%
Unknown	32%	11%	21%	19%	40%	18%

TABLE 10
Classification of Miscellaneous Non-Tumoral Epileptogenic Lesions - 1928 Through 1976 - 118 patients

Pial angiomatosis, full and forme fruste Sturge Weber cases ---------------------- 18

Small hamartoma --- 13

Tuberous sclerosis, full and forme fruste cases ------------------------------- 9

Old Intracerebral hemorrhage and/or operation for aneurysm -------------------- 9

Encephalopathy -- 9

Immunization complication --- 8

Anoxic episode due to anaesthesia complication, drowning, toxic fumes, etc. ------ 7

Previous operation for brain tumor -- 7

Arachnoid or intracerebral cyst --- 6

Complication of nephritis, diabetes or eclampsia ------------------------------ 6

Embolus to brain, heart operation, post-partum, septic ------------------------ 4

Parasitic cyst -- 3

Arteriolosclerosis - small vascular malformations - venous thrombosus - radiation gliosis, carotid artery ligation or traumatic occlusion - agenesis of corpus callosum - 2 each

Vasculitis, ricketts with cerebral bleeding - lead poisoning - electric shock, neurocutaneous melanosis - osteoma of skull - occult brain tumor -------- 1 each flammeus of the face (54), tuberous sclerosis, also with or without the typical skin lesions of this condition (37), small hamartomas, small vascular malformations, agenesis of the corpus callosum, and neurocutaneous melanosis. Injury to the brain is represented by an equally wide variety of types, previous intracerebral hemorrhage or craniotomy for aneurysm or tumor, various types of encephalopathy, complications of immunization procedures, anoxic episodes of various sorts, etc.

These patients point up another question of fundamental importance. What is the common denominator, the common neuronal abnormality, generated by such a wide variety of lesions which produces, in the end, a similar spectrum of EEG abnormalities and clinical seizures? And why does the latent period vary so greatly in different patients harboring the same type of lesions?

CONCLUSION

Epilepsy, this common, often disabling, yet intellectually fascinating, symptom of a wide variety of brain lesions, has for many years been one of the great teachers of neurology. Epilepsy is also an important generator of significant neurophysiological questions and a guide to further studies of fundamental aspects of nervous system function (14). In the future, as in the past, clinical and experimental studies of epilepsy will certainly continue to increase our understanding of the seizure discharge, its recruitment, and its spread through the nervous system, all of which result in clinical epileptic seizures. In the process, such studies will also aid in increasing our knowledge and understanding of both normal and abnormal nervous system function.

REFERENCES

1. Branch, C., Milner, B., and Rasmussen, T. (1964): Intracarotid sodium amytal for the lateralization of cerebral speech dominance. *J. Neurosurg.*, 21:399–405.
2. Falconer, M. A., and Wilson, P. J. E. (1969): Complications related to delayed hemorrhage after hemispherectomy. *J. Neurosurg.*, 30:413–426.
3. Feindel, W., and Penfield, W. (1954): Localization of discharge in temporal lobe automatism. *Arch. Neurol. Psychiatr.*, 72:605–630.
4. Foerster, O., and Penfield, W. (1930): Der Narbenzug am und im Gehirn bei traumatischer epilepsie in seiner Bedeutung für das Zustandkommen der Anfälle und für die Therapeutische Bekämpfung derselden. *Z. Gesamte. Neurol. Psychiatr.*, 125:475–572.
5. Foerster, O., and Penfield, W. (1930): The structural basis of traumatic epilepsy and results of radical operation. *Brain*, 53:99–120.
6. Gibbs, F. A., Davis, H., and Lennox, W. G. (1935): The electroencephalogram in epilepsy and in conditions of impaired consciousness. *Arch. Neurol. Psychiatr.*, 34:1133–1148.
7. Gibbs, F. A., Lennox, W. G., and Gibbs, E. L. (1936): The electroencephalogram in the diagnosis and localization of epileptic seizures. *Arch. Neurol. Psychiatr.*, 36:1225–1235.
8. Gloor, P., Rasmussen, T., Altuzarra, A., and Garretson, H. (1976): Role of the intracarotid Amobarbital-pentylenetetrazol EEG test in the diagnosis and surgical treatment of patients with complex seizure problems. *Epilepsia*, 17:15–31.
9. Green, J. R. (1977): Surgical treatment of epilepsy during childhood and adolescence. *Surg. Neurol.*, 8:71–80.
10. Gros, C., and Vlahovitch, B. (1955): *L'hémisphérectomie Cérébrale.* Imprimerie Causse, Graille, & Castelnau, Montpellier, France.

11. Hughes, J. T., and Oppenheimer, D. R. (1969): Superficial siderosis of the central nervous system: A report on nine cases with autopsy. *Acta Neuropathol., (Berl.)* 13:56–74.
12. Iwanowski, J., and Olszewski, J. (1960): The effects of subarachnoid injections of iron containing substances on the central nervous system. *J. Neuropathol. Exp. Neurol.,* 19:433–448.
13. Jasper, H. (1951): Etude anatomo-physiologique des epilepsies. Proceedings of the Second International Congress on Electroencephalography., Paris (1949). *Electroencephalogr. Clin. Neurophysiol.* 2 (Suppl.):99–111.
14. Jasper, H. H., Ward, A. A., Jr., and Pope, A., editors (1969): *Basic Mechanisms of the Epilepsies.* Little, Brown, Boston.
15. Krynauw, R. A. (1950): Infantile hemiplegia treated by removing one cerebral hemisphere. *J. Neurol. Neurosurg. Psychiatry,* 13:243–267.
16. Leblanc, F., and Rasmussen, T. (1973): Cerebral seizures and brain tumours. In: *Handbook of Clinical Neurology,* Vol. 15, edited by P. J. Vinken and G. W. Bruyn, pp. 295–301. North Holland Publishing Co., Amsterdam.
17. Milner, B. (1974): Psychological aspects of focal epilepsy and its neurosurgical management. In: *Neurosurgical Management of the Epilepsies,* edited by D. P. Purpura, J. K. Penry, and R. D. Walter, pp 299–321. Raven Press, New York.
18. Milner, B., Branch, C., and Rasmussen, T. (1962): Study of short term memory after intracarotid injection of sodium amytal. *Trans. Am. Neurol. Assoc.,* 87:224–226.
19. Milner, B., Branch, C., and Rasmussen, T. (1964): Observations on cerebral dominance. In: *Disorders of Language,* Ciba Foundation Symposium, edited by A. V. S. de Reuck and M. O'Connor, pp. 200–214. Churchill, London.
20. Milner, B., Branch, C., and Rasmussen, T. (1966): Evidence for bilateral speech representation in some non-right-handers. *Trans. Am. Neurol. Assoc.,* 91:306–308.
21. Noetzel, H. (1940): Diffusion von Blutfarbstoff in der innerne Randzone und äusseren Oberfläche des Zentralnervensystems bei subarachnoidaler Blutung. *Arch. Psychiatr.,* 111:129–138.
22. Ojemann, G. A., and Ward, A. A., Jr. (1974): Stereotactic and other procedures for epilepsy. In: *Neurosurgical Management of the Epilepsies,* edited by D. P. Purpura, J. K. Penry, and R. D. Walter, pp. 241–263. Raven Press, New York.
23. Oppenheimer, D. R., and Griffith, H. G. (1966): Persistent intracranial bleeding as a complication of hemispherectomy. *J. Neurol. Neurosurg. Psychiatry,* 29:229–240.
24. Penfield, W. (1930): The radical treatment of traumatic epilepsy and its rationale. *Can. Med. Assoc. J.,* 23:189–197.
25. Penfield, W. (1936): Epilepsy and surgical therapy. *Arch. Neurol. Psychiatr.,* 36:449–484.
26. Penfield, W., and Erickson, T. C. (1941): *Epilepsy and Cerebral Localization.* Charles C Thomas, Springfield, Illinois.
27. Penfield, W., and Flanigin, H. (1950): Surgical therapy of temporal lobe seizures. *Arch. Neurol. Psychiatr.,* 64:491–500.
28. Penfield, W., and Jasper, H. (1946): Highest level seizures. *Res. Publ. Assoc. Res. Nerv. Ment. Dis.,* 26:252–271.
29. Penfield, W., and Jasper, H. (1954): *Epilepsy and the Functional Anatomy of the Human Brain.* Little, Brown, and Co., Boston.
30. Penfield, W., and Kristiansen, K. (1950): *Epileptic Seizure Patterns.* Charles C Thomas, Springfield, Illinois.
31. Penfield, W., and Milner, B. (1958): Memory deficit produced by bilateral lesions in the hippocampal zone. *Arch. Neurol. Psychiatr.,* 79:475–497.
32. Penfield, W., and Paine, K. (1955): Results of surgical treatment of epileptic seizures. *Can. Med. Assoc. J.,* 73:515–531.
33. Penfield, W., and Perot, P. (1963): The brain's record of auditory and visual experience: A final summary and discussion. *Brain,* 86:595–696.
34. Penfield, W., and Rasmussen, T. (1951): *The Cerebral Cortex of Man.* Macmillan, New York.
35. Penfield, W., and Roberts, L. (1959): *Speech and Brain Mechanisms.* Princeton University Press, Princeton, New Jersey.
36. Penfield, W., and Steelman, H. (1947): The treatment of focal epilepsy with cortical excision. *Ann. Surg.,* 126:740–762.
37. Perot, P., Weir, B., and Rasmussen, T. (1966): Tuberous sclerosis: Surgical therapy for seizures. *Arch. Neurol.,* 15:498–506.
38. Ransohoff, J. C. (1955): Hemispherectomy in the treatment of convulsive seizures associated with infantile hemiplegia. *Res. Publ. Assoc. Res. Nerv. Ment. Dis.,* 34:176–195.

39. Rasmussen, T. (1963): Surgical therapy of frontal lobe epilepsy. *Epilepsia*, 4:181–198.
40. Rasmussen, T. (1969): The role of surgery in the treatment of focal epilepsy. In: *Clinical Neurosurgery*, Vol. 16, edited by R. G. Ojemann, pp. 288–311. Waverly Press, Baltimore, Maryland.
41. Rasmussen, T. (1969): Surgical therapy of post-traumatic epilepsy. In: *The Late Effects of Head Injury*, edited by A. E. Walker, W. F. Caveness, and M. Critchley, pp. 277–305. Charles C Thomas, Springfield, Illinois.
42. Rasmussen, T. (1973): Postoperative superficial hemosiderosis of the brain: Its diagnosis, treatment and prevention. *Trans. Am. Neurol. Assoc.*, 98:133–137.
43. Rasmussen, T. (1974): Cortical excision for medically refractory epilepsy. In: *The Natural History and Management of Epilepsy*, edited by P. Harris and C. Maudsley, pp. 227–239. Churchill Livingstone, Edinburgh.
44. Rasmussen, T. (1974): Cortical resection in the treatment of epilepsy. In: *Neurosurgical Management of the Epilepsies*, edited by D. P. Purpura, J. K. Penry, and R. D. Walter, pp. 139–154, Raven Press, New York.
45. Rasmussen, T. (1974): Post-traumatic epilepsy. In: *Brock's Injuries of the Brain and Spinal Cord*, 5th ed., edited by E. H. Feiring, pp. 544–569. Springer, New York.
46. Rasmussen, T. (1974): Surgery for epilepsy arising in other cortical regions. In: *Neurosurgical Management of the Epilepsies*, edited by D. P. Purpura, J. K. Penry, and R. D. Walter, pp. 206–226. Raven Press, New York.
47. Rasmussen, T. (1974): Surgery of epilepsy associated with brain tumors. In: *Neurosurgical Management of the Epilepsies*, edited by D. P. Purpura, J. K. Penry, and R. D. Walter, pp. 227–239. Raven Press, New York.
48. Rasmussen, T. (1974): Surgery of frontal lobe epilepsy. In: *Neurosurgical Management of the Epilepsies*, edited by D. P. Purpura, J. K. Penry, and R. D. Walter, pp. 197–205. Raven Press, New York.
49. Rasmussen, T. (1975): Surgical treatment of patients with complex partial seizures. In: *Complex Partial Seizures and Their Treatment*, edited by J. K. Penry and D. D. Daly, pp. 415–449. Raven Press, New York.
50. Rasmussen, T. (1976): The place of surgery in the treatment of epilepsy. In: *Current Controversies in Neurosurgery*, edited by T. P. Morley, pp. 465–477. Saunders, Philadelphia.
51. Rasmussen, T., and Blundell, J. (1961): Epilepsy and brain tumour. In: *Neurosurgery*, Vol. 7, edited by R. G. Fisher, pp. 138–156. Williams & Wilkins, Baltimore, Maryland.
52. Rasmussen, T., and Branch, C. (1962): Temporal lobe epilepsy: Indications for and results of surgical therapy. *Postgrad. Med. J.*, 31:9–14.
53. Rasmussen, T., and Gossman, H. (1963): Epilepsy due to gross destructive brain lesions. *Neurology (Minneap.)*, 13:659–669.
54. Rasmussen, T., Mathieson, G., and Leblanc, F. (1972): Surgical therapy of typical and a forme fruste variety of the Sturge-Weber syndrome. *Arch. Suisses Neurol. Neurochir. Psychiatr.*, 111:393–409.
55. Rasmussen, T., and Milner, B. (1977): The role of early brain injury in determining lateralization of cerebral speech functions. In: *Evolution and Lateralization of the Brain. Ann. N.Y. Acad. Sci.*, 299:355–369.
56. Talairach, J., et al. (1974): Approche nouvelle de la neurochirurgie de l'epilepsie: Methodologie stéréotaxique et results therapeutiques. *Neurochirurgie*, 20 (Suppl. 1):240.
57. Tükel, K., and Jasper, H. (1952): The electroencephalogram in parasagittal lesions. *Electroencephalogr. Clin. Neurophysiol.*, 4:481–494.
58. Wada, J. (1949): A new method for the determination of the side of cerebral speech dominance: A preliminary report on the intracarotid injection of sodium amytal in man. Igaku to Seibutsugaki. 14:221–222 *(in Japanese)*.
59. Wada, J., and Rasmussen, T. (1960): Intracarotid injection of sodium amytal for the lateralization of cerebral speech dominance: Experimental and clinical observations. *J. Neurosurg.*, 17:266–282.
60. Wilson, P. J. E. (1970): Cerebral hemispherectomy for infantile hemiplegia: A report of 50 cases. *Brain*, 93:147–180.

Subject Index